Psychiatric Nursing Diagnosis Care Plans for *DSM-IV*

The Jones and Bartlett Series in Nursing

Adult Emergency Nursing Procedures, Proehl

Basic Steps in Planning Nursing Research, Fourth Edition, Brink/Wood

Biotherapy: A Comprehensive Overview, Rieger

Bloodborne Pathogens, Second Edition, National Safety Council

Bone Marrow Transplantation, Second Edition, Whedon/Wujick

Bone Marrow Transplantation: Administrative Strategies and Clinical Concerns, Buchsel/Whedon

Breastfeeding and Human Lactation, Riordan/Auerbach

Study Guide for Breastfeeding and Human Lactation, Auerbach/Riordan

Building a Legacy: Voices of Oncology Nurses, Nevidjon

Cancer Chemotherapy: A Nursing Process Approach, Second Edition, Barton Burke et al.

Cancer Nursing: Principles and Practice, Fourth Edition, Groenwald et al.

A Challenge for Living, Corless at al.

Chemotherapy Care Plans, Barton Burke et al.

Chronic Illness: Impact and Interventions, Third Edition, Lubkin

A Clinical Guide to Cancer Nursing, Groenwald et al.

Comprehensive Cancer Nursing Review, Groenwald et al.

A Comprehensive Curriculum for Trauma Nursing, Bayley/Turcke

Comprehensive Perioperative Nursing Review, Fairchild et al.

Crisis Counseling, Second Edition, Janosik

Desk Reference for Critical Care Nursing, Wright/Shelton

Drugs and Protocols Common to Prehospital and Emergency Care, Cummings

Drugs and the Elderly, Swonger/Burbank

Essential Medical Terminology, Second Edition, Stanfield

Essentials of Oxygenation, Ahrens/Rutherford

Ethics Consultation, LaPuma/Shiedermayer

Family Life, Janosik/Green

Fundamentals of Nursing Research, Second Edition, Brockopp/Hastings-Tolsma

Handbook of Oncology Nursing, Second Edition, Gross/Johnson

Health Assessment in Nursing Practice, Third Edition, Grimes/Burns

Health Policy and Nursing: Crisis and Reform in the U.S. Health Care Delivery System, Second Edition, Harrington/Estes

Healthy People 2000, U.S. Department of Health and Human Services

Human Aging and Chronic Disease, Kart et al.

Human Development, Fourth Edition, Frieberg

Instruments for Clinical Nursing Research, Frank-Stromborg

Intravenous Therapy, Nentwich

Introduction to Human Disease, Fourth Edition, Crowley

Introductory Management and Leadership for Clinical Nurses, Swansburg

Management and Leadership for Nurse Managers, Swansburg

Management of Spinal Cord Injury, Zejdlik

Mastering the New Medical Terminology Through Self-Instructional Modules, Stanfield/Hui

Mathematics for Health Professionals, Third Edition, Whisler

Medical Ethics, Second Edition, Veatch

Medical Instruments for Nurses and Allied Health-Care Professionals, Aston/Brown

Medical Terminology with Vikki Wetle, R.N., M.A., Video Series, Wetle

Memory Bank for Chemotherapy, Third Edition, Preston/Wilfinger

Memory Bank for Critical Care, Third Edition, Ervin

Memory Bank for Hemodynamic Monitoring, Second Edition, Ervin/Long

Memory Bank for HIV Medications, Wilkes

Memory Bank for Intravenous Therapy, Second Edition, Weinstein

Memory Bank for Medications, Second Edition, Kostin/Sieloff

Mental Health and Psychiatric Nursing, Davies/Janosik

The Nation's Health, Fifth Edition, Lee/Estes

New Dimension's in Women's Health, Alexander/LaRosa

Nursing and the Disabled, Fraley

Nursing Assessment and Diagnosis, Second Edition, Bellack/Edlund

Nursing Research with Basic Statistical Applications, Dempsey/Dempsey

Nursing Staff Development, Swansburg

Nutrition and Diet Therapy, Second Edition, Stanfield

Oncogenes, Second Edition, Cooper

Oncology Nursing Drug Reference, Wilkes et al.

Oncology Nursing Homecare Handbook, Barton Burke

Oncology Nursing in the Ambulatory Setting, Buchsel/Yarbro

Oxygen Administration, National Safety Council

Pediatric Emergency Nursing Procedures, Bernardo/Bove

Perioperative Nursing: Principles and Practice, Fairchild

Perioperative Patient Care, Third Edition, Kneedler/Dodge

Perspectives on Death and Dying, Fulton/Metress

Primary Care of Women and Children with HIV Infection: A Multidisciplinary Approach, Kelly et al.

Ready Reference for Critical Care, Strawn/Stewart

Understanding/Responding: A Communication Manual for Nurses, Second Edition, Long

Varney's Midwifery, Third Edition, Varney

Women's Health and Development, McElmurray et al.

Working with Older Adults, Third Edition, Burnside/Schmidt

Writing a Successful Grant Application, Second Edition, Reif-Lehrer

Psychiatric Nursing Diagnosis Care Plans for *DSM-IV*

Mary Paquette, RN, PhD
Assistant Professor
Mount Saint Mary's College
Los Angeles, California

Christine Rodemich, RN, MN
Clinical Specialist
Associate Professor
Allied Health Department
Glendale Community College
Glendale, California

Jones and Bartlett Publishers
Sudbury, Massachusetts
Boston   London   Singapore

Editorial, Sales, and Customer Service Offices
Jones and Bartlett Publishers
40 Tall Pine Drive
Sudbury, Massachusetts 01776
(508) 443-5000
(800) 832-0034
info@jbpub.com
http://www.jbpub.com

Jones and Bartlett Publishers International
Barb House, Barb Mews
London W6 7PA
UK

Library of Congress Cataloging-in-Publication Data
Paquette, Mary.
    Psychiatric nursing diagnosis care plans for DSM-IV / Mary
Paquette, Christine Rodemich.
       p.   cm.
    Includes bibliographical references and index.
    ISBN 0-7637-0255-2 (pbk.)
    1. Psychiatric nursing. 2. Nursing care plans. 3. Nursing
diagnosis. I. Rodemich, Christine. II. Title.
    [DNLM: 1. Psychiatric Nursing—methods. 2. Nursing Diagnosis.
3. Patient Care Planning. WY 160 P219pa 1997]
RC440.P263 1997
610.73'68—dc21
DNLM/DLC
for Library of Congress
                                        96-45656
                                        CIP

Production Editor: Martha Stearns
Manufacturing Manager: Dana L. Cerrito
Editorial Production Service: Colophon
Typesetting: LeGwin Associates
Cover Design: Hannus Design Associates
Printing and Binding: D. B. Hess Co.
Cover Printing: Coral Graphic Services, Inc.

Printed in the United States of America
01 00 99 98 97   10 9 8 7 6 5 4 3 2 1

Contents

Preface

When patients with a psychiatric/mental health problem are admitted to a healthcare system, they are given one or more of the psychiatric diagnoses that appear in the *Diagnostic and Statistical Manual, IV (DSM-IV)*. Each of these diagnoses creates patient care problems that are treatable by nurses—the nursing diagnoses. These nursing diagnoses are the focus of all nursing care, and the subject of this book. The nursing diagnoses used here have been approved and defined by the North American Nursing Diagnosis Association (NANDA).

Psychiatric Nursing Care Plans for DSM-IV aims first to help nurses link nursing diagnoses with the psychiatric/mental health diagnoses contained in the *DSM-IV*, and second to provide generic nursing care plans for the nursing diagnoses. These nursing care plans will serve as the base of patient treatment plans.

Nurses care for people who are ill or incapacitated to help them recover their usual state of health. Moreover, nurses help patients maintain wellness and prevent illness. The American Nurses' Association defines this succinctly as "the diagnosis and treatment of human response to actual or potential health problems" (1980). This process more and more frequently is being defined by the use of nursing diagnosis.

Nursing diagnosis is being used not only as a tool for planning individualized patient care but also as a means to measure the contribution and productivity of nurses. In this cost-containment era, tools to measure nursing activity and productivity are in great demand. This book provides a foundation for doing just that, while providing an up-to-date re-source for the nurse to implement nursing diagnosis, to develop care plans easily, to document care given, and to specify in measurable terms what it is they do for patients.

How does *Psychiatric Nursing Diagnosis Care Plans for* DSM-IV accomplish this?

1. It clearly shows the relationship between psychiatric diagnoses (as they appear in *DSM-IV*) and nursing diagnoses.
2. It identifies more than 75 psychiatric diagnoses, so most common patient situations are accounted for.
3. It provides a list of the most commonly occurring nursing diagnoses (with rationales) for each of these psychiatric diagnoses.
4. It provides generic nursing diagnosis care plans and expects the nurse to do more than simply copy a standard care plan. It asks the nurse to make the necessary changes and to *adapt* the generic plan to a particular patient and circumstances.

Psychiatric Nursing Diagnosis Care Plans for DSM-IV facilitates the planning of nursing diagnosis-based care for most patients and does it better than any other currently available resource. At the same time, nurses and administrators alike can facilitate the process of documenting the time and cost expenditures involved in providing that care. In today's cost-conscious healthcare environment, such a resource is invaluable.

Mary Paquette
Christine Rodemich

Introduction

Psychiatric Nursing Diagnosis Care Plans for DSM-IV is divided into three interlinked units; each unit builds on the previous one. To use this book most effectively, scan the table of contents, and note the three separate units.

➤ **Unit I** gives an overview of nursing assessment, the step that must be done before a nursing diagnosis can be made. Nursing assessment directs the formulation of nursing diagnoses; patient outcomes and interventions emanate from the assessment. *DSM-IV* offers five axes to assess various aspects and characteristics of a psychiatric/mental health patient. Data from axes V (Severity of Psychosocial Stressors) and VI (Global Assessment of Functioning) are especially relevant to nursing, and the nursing assessment may confirm or question a *DSM-IV* diagnosis.

➤ **Unit II** lists the *DSM-IV* psychiatric diagnoses and associated nursing diagnoses for the adult patient—more than 75 diagnoses. We have selected those diagnoses that are most commonly seen in psychiatric settings and that are the focus of treatment. While other mental disorders may be equally important in accurately diagnosing an individual, it would have been cumbersome to include the less commonly used diagnoses in this book.

➤ Psychiatric diagnoses are listed within the framework used by *DSM-IV*.

➤ Each psychiatric diagnosis is followed by a list of the nursing diagnoses that are most likely to be associated with it.

➤ Each nursing diagnosis statement contains a "related to" component—that is, the most probable cause in the context of the particular psychiatric diagnosis.

➤ Each nursing diagnosis has a rationale that explains its link with a given *DSM-IV* diagnosis. When you are ready to do care planning for a patient, look up the appropriate psychiatric diagnosis in Unit II. Note the nursing diagnoses that are listed there, choose those that are appropriate for your patient at any given time, and refer to Unit III for the generic care plans for these nursing diagnoses.

➤ **Unit III** contains generic care plans for each of the NANDA-approved nursing diagnoses that are used in this book—45 in all. Each care plan contains these components.
  ▷ Definition of the nursing diagnosis
  ▷ Etiologies ("related to")
  ▷ Characteristics/assessment findings
  ▷ Expected outcomes/goals of care (including measurable criteria)
  ▷ Nursing orders with rationale
  ▷ Charting components (evaluation criteria)

These components form the steps of the nursing process and are presented in a logical format that proceeds from assessment to planning to intervention to evaluation. The first three components (Definition, Related to, Characteristics/Assessment Findings) are defined by NANDA; additional information not included by NANDA appears in a distinguishing typeface.

Review the characteristics of the nursing diagnoses you select to be sure they are consistent with the assessment data on your particular patient. Next, read the entire care plan and select the parts that are appropriate for the patient. Add any additional outcomes, interventions, and pertinent time frames as necessary and appropriate, based on your own clinical judgment.

The charting components are a guide to what needs to be documented in the patient's chart and can serve as evaluation criteria.

The generic care plans provide a convenient, easy-to-use and up-to-date nursing care plan base. Use any or all of the care plans as appropriate for any given patient.

A formal, individualized plan of care is imperative for professional nursing care. The resources found in *Psychiatric Nursing Care Plans for* DSM-IV streamline the process used to develop a written plan. We welcome your feedback and suggestions as you use this resource.

Contributors

Jeannette Allen, RN, MSN, CS
Clinical Nurse Manager
UCLA Neuropsychiatric Institute
Los Angeles, California

Regina Asaro, RN, C
Executive Director
Victims for Justice
Anchorage, Alaska

Danelda Bond, RN, BSN
Assistant Director of Nursing
Los Angeles County/University of Southern
California Medical Center
Los Angeles, California

Eleanor Brazal-Villanueva, RN, C, MA, MEd
Nursing Education Coordinator
Kaiser Permanente Medical Center
Woodland Hills, California

Tess L. Briones, RN, MS, CCRN, CEN
Clinical Nurse Specialist, Surgical ICU
University of Michigan Medical Center
Adjunct Professor, School of Nursing
University of Michigan
Ann Arbor, Michigan

Cheryl Burlingame, RN, MN
Director of Resource Centers/Crisis Team
Pine Grove Hospital & Mental Health Center
Canoga Park, California
Psychotherapist, private practice
Woodland Hills, California

Rose Mary Carroll-Johnson, RN, MN
Editor, Oncology Nursing Forum
Valencia, California

Mary R. de Meneses, RN, EdD
Professor and Coordinator, Graduate Program in
Medical-Surgical Nursing
Southern Illinois University
Edwardsville, Illinois

Donna Gray, RN, MN, CS
Administrative Nurse 1
UCLA Neuropsychiatric Institute
Los Angeles, California

Mark Greenfeld, RN, MN
Psychotherapist, private practice
Los Angeles, California

Lyda Hill, RN, CS, PhD
Associate Professor
Department of Nursing
California State University, Long Beach
Long Beach, California
Private practice, clinical psychology
South Laguna, California

Elizabeth F. Hiltunen, RN, MS
Clinical Nurse Specialist
Medical-Surgical Nursing
Waltham-Weston Hospital Medical Center
Waltham, Massachusetts

Norine J. Kerr, RN, MN
Clinical Nurse Specialist, Partial
Hospitalization Services
The Menninger Clinic
Topeka, Kansas
Doctoral candidate, University of Kansas
Kansas City, Kansas

Mary E. A. Laskin, RN, MN
Los Angeles County–University of Southern
California Medical Center
Los Angeles, California

Mary E. Mirch, RN, EdD
Associate Dean, Health Services
Glendale Community College
Glendale, California

Margo Neal, RN, MN
Publisher
NurseCom, Inc.
Malibu, California

Jean Nix, RN, MS, MFCC
Nursing Instructor
Pacific Union College
Angwin, California
Psychotherapist, private practice
Ontario, California

Mary Paquette, RN, PhD
Assistant Professor
Mount Saint Mary's College
Los Angeles, California

Martina Ramirez, RN, MN
Faculty Coordinator
California State University
Dominguez Hills, California

Christine Rodemich, RN, MN
Clinical Specialist, Associate Professor
Allied Health Department
Glendale Community College
Glendale, California

Faith I. Rossman, RN, MN
Clinical Educator, Patient Education
Kaiser Foundation Hospital
Woodland Hills, California

Lorraine Sharp, RN, MN
Assistant Professor
Mount Saint Mary's College
Los Angeles, California

Ginny Taylor, RN, PhD
Psychotherapist, private practice
Laguna Hills, California
Instructor, California State University
Long Beach, California

Sheryl Tyson, RN, MN
Clinical Nurse Manager
UCLA Neuropsychiatric Institute
Los Angeles, California

Jane C. Walton, MS, RN
Assistant Unit Leader, Geriatric Rehabilitation
Johnson R. Bowman Health Care Center for
the Elderly
Faculty member, Rush University College of Nursing
Rush-Presbyterian–St. Luke's Medical Center
Chicago, Illinois

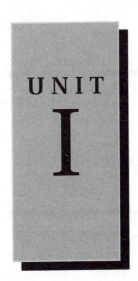

Nursing Assessment

Contents

Introduction to the Nursing Assessment Guide

The in-depth assessment guide that follows is based on NANDA's definitions and classification of nursing diagnoses. Like any other assessment guide, it must be individualized in the order and depth of assessment to serve the needs of the nurse, the facility, and, ultimately, the patient who depends on an accurate diagnosis of his or her health-related needs. Individual situations will dictate how this assessment guide—and what sections of it—will be used.

Many assessment models have been developed. Examples include review of body systems, evaluation of human needs, and reliance on nursing theorists' conceptual frameworks (i.e., Gordon's Functional Health Patterns, Roy's Adaptation Model, Johnson's Behavioral Systems, and Orem's Self-Care). In the clinical setting, assessment tools are developed that are time effective and efficient to meet agency needs. Nurses working collaboratively with the mental health team need to adjust their assessment to complement the multidisciplinary approach of care planning. Assessment is an essential skill that must be systematic and holistic regardless of the tool used. The complexity of the data collected will depend on the role and education of the nurses and services provided by the facility.

Busy acute care facilities may want to devise checklists, develop a two-tiered assessment strategy, or arrange for preadmission assessment. The standard assessment tool used by most mental health professionals in acute hospital settings and outpatient psychiatric clinics is the mental status examination and suicide assessment of lethality. Specialty units (e.g., chemical dependency) may want to reorganize the assessment to facilitate identification of commonly encountered problems. Many creative strategies for accurate, complete, yet practical data gathering are available.

The assessment guide contains three distinct types of information:

1. Subjective assessment data
2. Objective assessment data
3. Nursing diagnoses

Subjective and objective assessment data are suggested for each of the NANDA diagnoses. Subjective and objective data are further defined as *essential* (baseline information to be gathered) and *expanded* (data to be gathered if problems are identified in the baseline assessment). The expanded data also apply to community, intermediate, and long-term-care settings.

With the advent of managed care, more mentally ill patients are being served by community programs. Acute care stays are significantly shorter, with the focus on biochemical stabilization rather than on traditional psychotherapy. This presents a challenge to nursing, the focus of which has been on the nurse-patient relationship and on managing the therapeutic milieu.

Complete assessment of the psychiatric client leads to a greater possibility of accurate nursing diagnoses. When the etiology of the behaviors is understood and recognized, standard nursing care plans can be individualized to meet the unique needs of each patient. As the assessment process continues, diagnoses may change and the healthcare manager will be responsible for developing cost-effective strategies. The correlation between *DSM-IV* and NANDA nursing diagnoses is an efficient and practical means to treatment and care planning.

Guide to Nursing Assessment of the Psychiatric/Mental Health Patient

I. Exchanging

Exchanging means to give, relinquish, or lose something while receiving something in return; the substitution of one element for another; the reciprocal act of giving and receiving. It is therefore used to classify many of the physiologic processes within the body, e.g., nutrition, oxygenation, regulation. It is the single largest taxonomic category. Level Two categories within this pattern are interdependent and intertwined so that alterations in one usually indicate at least the potential for alterations in another.

A. Nutrition

1. *Subjective*

   Essential
   a. Effect of disease/treatment/medication (e.g., MAO inhibitors) on intake of food and drink
   b. Alcohol intake (frequency, amount)
   c. Recent change in eating patterns; appetite generally, recently

   Expanded
   a. Typical daily meal plan before diagnosis or illness (24-hour dietary history); socioeconomic influences, cultural influences, balance, amounts, schedule
   b. Foods particularly liked or avoided; situations/feelings resulting in increased/ decreased intake
   c. History of weight problems, family weight problems
   d. Recent weight changes
   e. Preferred weight-loss regimen

2. *Objective*

   Essential
   a. General appearance
   b. Weight/height compared to age-appropriate norms
   c. Condition of hair, nails, skin
   d. Dentition

   Expanded
   a. Ability to plan meals using basic food groups
   b. Amount of empty calories consumed
   c. Number of meals eaten per day
   d. Types of snacks

3. *Nursing Diagnoses*
   Altered Nutrition: More than Body Requirements
   Altered Nutrition: Less than Body Requirements
   Altered Nutrition: Potential for More than Body Requirements*

   Related Nursing Diagnoses
   Constipation
   Self-Care Deficit
   Chronic Low Self-Esteem
   Situational Low Self-Esteem
   Ineffective Individual Coping

B. Elimination

1. *Subjective*

   Essential
   a. Complaints of constipation or diarrhea
   b. Discomfort in elimination

   Expanded
   a. Degree of concern about bowel movement

This assessment guide is adapted from Carroll-Johnson, R.M. (1990). Guide to nursing assessment. In M. Neal, M. Paquette, & M. Mirch, *Nursing care plans for DRG's.* Venice, CA: General Medical Publishers.

*Care plans for this diagnosis are not included in this volume.

2. *Objective*

Essential
a. Usual bowel elimination patterns: frequency, timing, amount, color, consistency, discomfort
b. Contour, distention of abdomen
c. Medications contributing to constipation
d. Amount of exercise
e. Fluid intake, diet, fiber intake
f. Use of aids to elimination: laxatives, drugs (prescribed or over-the-counter), enemas
g. Perspiration patterns

Expanded
a. Scars, artificial orifices (location, appearance)
b. Bowel sounds

3. *Nursing Diagnoses*
   Constipation
   Perceived Constipation*
   Diarrhea*
   Bowel Incontinence*
   Altered Patterns of Urinary Elimination*
   Stress Incontinence*
   Total Incontinence*

   Related Nursing Diagnoses
   Altered Nutrition: More than Body
      Requirements
   Altered Nutrition: Less than Body
      Requirements
   Fluid Volume Deficit
   Self-Care Deficit

C. Circulation

1. *Subjective*

Essential
a. Chest pain, palpitations
b. Confusion

Expanded
a. Cold/tingling extremities, pain
b. Leg cramps, numbness
c. Abdominal tenderness, nausea
d. Nocturnal dyspnea, orthopnea
e. Weakness, malaise, fatigue

2. *Objective*

Essential
a. Vital signs: pulse, blood pressure, breath sounds and rate
b. Level of consciousness, orientation
c. Heart rate, rhythm, sounds
d. Peripheral pulses (strength, quality)
e. Fainting spells, blackouts
f. Fluid balance, low urine output
g. Skin temperature, color, capillary refill
h. Edema of extremities

Expanded
a. Mottling, clubbing of fingers/toes
b. Thrombophlebitis

3. *Nursing Diagnoses*
   Fluid Volume Excess*
   Potential Fluid Volume Deficit*
   Fluid Volume Deficit
   Decreased Cardiac Output*

   Related Nursing Diagnoses
   Altered Nutrition: Less than Body Requirements
   Impaired Communication*
   Altered Thought Processes
   Altered Cerebral Tissue Perfusion*

D. Physical Integrity

1. *Subjective*

Essential
a. Vision, hearing, proprioception
b. Photosensitivity
c. Altered thought processes
d. Panic
e. Delirium, confusion
f. Judgment, cognition

Expanded
a. Memory impairment
b. Carelessness, lack of attention to detail

2. *Objective*

Essential
a. Skin condition: intactness, bruising, petechiae, rashes, sunburn
b. Poor healing
c. Incidence of accidental injury (e.g., falls, trauma)

*Care plans for this diagnosis are not included in this volume.

d. Balance and coordination
e. Level of consciousness

Expanded
a. Observed memory impairment
b. History of reckless behavior (e.g., driving too fast)
c. Living situation (e.g., environmental hazards, home, board and care, homeless)

3. *Nursing Diagnoses*
Potential for Injury/Trauma
Potential for Impaired Skin Integrity*
Impaired Skin Integrity*

Related Nursing Diagnoses
Altered Nutrition: Less than Body Requirements
Altered Nutrition: More than Body Requirements
Sensory/Perceptual Alterations
Altered Thought Processes

II. Communicating

Communicating means to converse; to impart, confer, or transmit thoughts, feelings, or information, internally or externally, verbally or nonverbally. Communication with others is accomplished verbally and nonverbally. A variety of disease conditions, physical or psychologic, can impair an individual's ability to relay information accurately or to express needs. In its present state of development, nursing diagnosis has addressed itself only to verbal communication impairments. In this text, impaired communication is used related to psychiatric disorders (e.g., schizophrenia, mania, depression, mental retardation).

A. Communication

1. *Subjective*

Essential
a. Anxiety
b. Auditory hallucinations
c. Hearing ability
d. Language(s) spoken/understood
e. Affect/mood (elation, depression)
f. Ability to answer questions appropriately

Expanded
a. Double-bind messages in family system

b. Degree of volition/motivation to communicate
c. Ability to read

2. *Objective*

Essential
a. Quality and tone of voice (e.g., hoarse, whispered)
b. Clarity of speech, articulation
c. Ability to be assertive
d. Speech peculiarities (e.g., neologisms, echolalia)
e. Manifestations of altered thought processes (e.g., loose associations, flight of ideas)

Expanded
a. Writing ability
b. Educational level

3. *Nursing Diagnoses*
Impaired Verbal Communication

Related Nursing Diagnosis
Sensory/Perceptual Alterations

III. Relating

Relating means to connect, to establish a link between, to stand in some association to another thing, person, or place; to be borne or thrust in between things. For taxonomic purposes this category encompasses an individual's abilities to perform various roles (e.g., job, family) and to associate with others.

A. Socialization

1. *Subjective*

Essential
a. Most important people in patient's life, their reaction to what has happened to patient
b. Patient's concerns about these people
c. Ability/inability to tolerate aloneness
d. Desire to participate in group activities
e. Perception of personality (e.g., shy, introverted)
f. Feelings of vulnerability
g. Willingness to trust self/others

Expanded
a. Needs when feeling bad physically or mentally (e.g., wants to be left alone)
b. Needs when bothered by something (e.g., talk it out with someone, work it out for self)

---

*Care plans for this diagnosis are not included in this volume.

c. Reaction to perceived stigma of diagnosis
d. Effect of illness on participation in groups
e. Excessive participation in social activities
f. Levels of emotional intimacy

2. *Objective*

Essential

a. Demeanor and general appearance (e.g., poor hygiene, inappropriate dress)
b. Communication patterns (e.g., direct, circular, vague)
c. Degree of openness, willingness to discuss relationships, feelings
d. Ability to express empathy/sympathy
e. Withdrawn behavior
f. Ability to establish eye contact (Note: this can be culturally influenced)
g. Interpersonal behavior (e.g., overcompliant, passive, avoidant, rebellious, hostile, aggressive)
h. Excessive defensiveness (e.g., overuse of defense mechanisms)

Expanded

a. Stability and length of relationships
b. Strength of support system (e.g., family friends, professionals)
c. Membership in social groups

3. *Nursing Diagnoses*

Impaired Social Interaction
Social Isolation

Related Nursing Diagnoses

Diversional Activity Deficit
Chronic Low Self-Esteem
Situational Low Self-Esteem
Altered Thought Processes
Ineffective Individual Coping

B. Role

1. *Subjective*

Essential

a. Expressed number of roles (e.g., student, parent, employee)
b. Reasons for working
c. Perceived effect of disease/treatment on ability to work
d. Changes disease/treatments/medications have made on life
e. Patient's feelings about these changes
f. Activities that give satisfaction in daily life

g. Sources of financial/emotional support
h. Ability to relinquish control
i. Perceived division of family responsibilities

Expanded

a. Ability to identify and meet own needs
b. Ease in asking for help from others
c. Responsibility for financial/emotional support of others
d. Degree of comfort with dependency
e. Who provides help in decision making
f. Comfort/willingness to explore expanded and new roles

2. *Objective*

Essential

a. Marital status, children
b. Actual roles being assumed
c. Type of work, length of time in job
d. Number of hours worked per day, number of jobs
e. Plans to return to work

Expanded

a. Appropriateness of role expectations
b. Stated expectation of ability to resume/continue usual roles
c. Alternatives to remaining in same roles
d. Resources available to facilitate role change/adjustment
e. Ability to establish priorities and manage time effectively

3. *Nursing Diagnoses*

Altered Role Performance*
Altered Parenting*
Potential Altered Parenting*
Altered Family Processes
Altered Family Processes: Alcoholism
Parental Role Conflict*

Related Nursing Diagnoses

Ineffective Individual Coping
Ineffective Family Coping
Chronic Low Self-Esteem
Situational Low Self-Esteem

---

*Care plans for this diagnosis are not included in this volume.

C. Sexuality Patterns

1. *Subjective*

Essential
a. Degree of satisfaction with sexual relation-ships
b. Effect of illness on sexual relationships
c. Sexual difficulties/functioning caused by illness/medications
d. Anxiety associated with sexual functioning

Expanded
a. Adaptation to altered sexual pattern
b. Effect of illness on potential for relationships
c. Effects of relationship problems on sexuality
d. Values, religious beliefs about sex
e. Knowledge of sexually transmitted disease, safe sex practices
f. Fear of pregnancy

2. *Objective*

Essential
a. Hypersexual behavior/inappropriate display of sexuality (e.g., masturbation, abuse of self/others)
b. Availability of partner
c. Sexual preference (e.g., heterosexual, homosexual)
d. Presence of sexually transmitted diseases
e. Use of drugs/alcohol
f. Last menstrual period
g. Onset of menopause
h. Altered body image
i. Exacerbation of psychiatric symptoms
j. Age of client

Expanded
a. Patterns of sexual activity (e.g., monoga-mous, multiple partners)
b. Loss of functional or psychosocial role(s)
c. Partner's perception of altered sexuality
d. Associated diagnostic tests
   1) hormonal levels
   2) culture of discharge
   3) pregnancy

3. *Nursing Diagnoses*
Altered Sexuality Patterns
Sexual Dysfunction

Related Nursing Diagnoses
Chronic Low Self-Esteem
Situational Low Self-Esteem
Altered Role Performance*

Ineffective Individual Coping
Anticipatory Grieving
Anxiety
Fear
Social Isolation

IV. Valuing

Valuing means to be concerned about, to care; the worth or worthiness; the relative status of a thing, or the esteem in which it is held, according to its real or supposed worth, usefulness, or importance; one's opinion or liking for a person or thing; to equate in importance. Assessment attempts to determine spiritual, religious, or perhaps cultural influences on an individual's approach to healthcare or reaction to illness. While alterations in this pattern are rarely primary or priority diagnoses, they can often have a profound effect on one's ability to impact other, more physiologically oriented problems.

A. Spiritual State

1. *Subjective*

Essential
a. Religious preference
b. Cultural background
c. Philosophical and spiritual beliefs
d. What gives meaning to life
e. Sources of strength and hope
f. Loss of meaning in life, loss of faith
g. Lack of will to live
h. Feelings of despair, emptiness, hopeless-ness, isolation

Expanded
a. Effects of beliefs on reaction to illness
b. Thoughts/feelings about cause of illness
c. Interest in self-discovery
d. Beliefs in potential conflict with medical treatment
e. Verbalization of inner conflict about beliefs
f. Anger toward God

2. *Objective*

Essential
a. Delusions/religiosity
b. Display/wearing of religious items, cloth-ing, books

---

*Care plans for this diagnosis are not included in this volume.

c. Practice of religious/spiritual rituals
d. Religious/spiritual-related visitors

Expanded
a. Degree of focus on external world versus inner awareness
b. Ability to listen for/belief in inner guidance
c. Membership in a religious or spiritually based group (e.g., church, 12-step program)

3. *Nursing Diagnoses*
Spiritual Distress

Related Nursing Diagnoses
Ineffective Individual Coping
Decisional Conflict
Chronic Low Self-Esteem
Situational Low Self-Esteem
Knowledge Deficit
Dysfunctional Grieving

V. Choosing

Choosing means to select between alternatives; the action of selecting or exercising preference in regard to a matter in which one is a free agent; to determine in favor of a course; to decide in accordance with inclinations. It therefore depends to a great extent on the individual's problem-solving/coping skills. Humans, after all, are able to make choices about complying with medical care and establishing healthy life habits. Coping styles of both the individual and the family system, however, do affect decisions.

A. Coping

1. *Subjective*

Essential
a. Presence of self-destructive thoughts and suicidal feelings
b. Degree of anxiety, depression
c. Precipitating event of crisis
d. Understanding of current stressors and problem
e. Distorted perceptions
f. Effectiveness of coping mechanisms
g. Factors that interfere with effective use of coping mechanisms
h. Behaviors when upset (e.g., self-destructive)
i. Usual methods of stress reduction
j. Previous experience with hospitalization, illness

Expanded
a. Effect of crisis on functional roles
b. Exacerbation of chronic problems
c. Perception of available resources
d. Ability to use community resources
e. Family style of coping with crisis

2. *Objective*

Essential
a. Personal/family history of ineffective coping (e.g., suicide, alcoholism, drug abuse, violence)
b. Affect, mannerisms
c. Ability to attend to interview, comprehend information, ask pertinent questions
d. Past need for professional intervention (e.g., psychiatrist, counselor, hospitalization)
e. Behavioral signs of anxiety
f. Suicide plan

Expanded
a. Effectiveness of family unit, support systems
b. Availability of appropriate community support
c. Available resources

3. *Nursing Diagnoses*
Ineffective Individual Coping
Impaired Adjustment
Defensive Coping*
Ineffective Denial
Ineffective Family Coping: Disabling
Ineffective Family Coping: Compromised

Related Nursing Diagnoses
Sleep-Pattern Disturbance
Chronic Low Self-Esteem
Situational Low Self-Esteem
Anxiety
Dysfunctional Grieving
Spiritual Distress

B. Participation

1. *Subjective*

Essential
a. Expressions of willingness to comply with treatment
b. Reasons given for lack of compliance

---

*Care plans for this diagnosis are not included in this volume.

c. Perceived compatibility of treatment plan with current life-style

d. Level of commitment to treatment plan

Expanded

a. Identification of priorities

b. Effect of priority setting on ability/willingness to comply

c. Perceived consequences of noncompliance

2. *Objective*

Essential

a. Knowledge of risks and benefits of treatment (e.g., informed consent)

b. Past record of compliance with medical care, appointments

c. Factors interfering with compliance (e.g., transportation, finances, scheduling)

Expanded

a. Resources available to increase likelihood of compliance

b. Ability to alter factors interfering with compliance

c. Ability to create supportive environment and social support

3. *Nursing Diagnoses*

Noncompliance

Related Nursing Diagnoses

Spiritual Distress

Anxiety

Knowledge Deficit

Altered Thought Processes

Ineffective Individual Coping

Impaired Adjustment

C. Judgment

1. *Subjective*

Essential

a. Emotional states (e.g., anxiety, denial, fear, unwillingness to take responsibility for decision) interfering with judgment

b. Conflict and feelings of ambivalence

c. Distorted perception/beliefs that interfere with decision making

d. Reliance on others for decision making

e. Perceived ability to follow through on a decision

f. Expressions of not knowing what to do

Expanded

a. Expressions of doubt regarding judgment of healthcare providers

b. Healthcare decisions with more than one alternative

c. Expressions of anger toward physician, care providers

d. Perception of family reaction to decisions

e. Family's willingness to participate in decision making

f. Ability to tolerate ambiguity

g. Level of maturity

h. Denial

2. *Objective*

Essential

a. Degree of reality orientation

b. Altered thought processes (e.g., delusions, loose associations)

c. Conceptual ability, abstract

d. Actual decisions made

e. History of decisions being made by others

f. Ability to state alternatives/consequences

g. History of decision-making patterns

Expanded

a. Opinions, desires of family members/support persons

b. Intellectual capacity

c. Ability to plan long-term goals

3. *Nursing Diagnoses*

Decisional Conflict

Related Nursing Diagnoses

Knowledge Deficit

Spiritual Distress

Anxiety

Fear

Altered Thought Processes

Chronic Low Self-Esteem

Situational Low Self-Esteem

D. Health-Seeking Behaviors

1. *Subjective*

Essential

a. Personal activities perceived to be directly beneficial/detrimental to health

b. Expressions of desire to improve health status

c. Knowledge of strategies to implement change

Expanded
a. Prior attempts at improving health status
b. Success, appropriateness of attempts

2. *Objective*

Essential
a. General appearance
b. State of health

Expanded
a. Congruence of appearance with stated age, assessment of health status
b. Diagnosis amenable to cure/improvement by adoption of healthier life-style habits

3. *Nursing Diagnoses*
Health-Seeking Behaviors*

Related Nursing Diagnoses
Altered Nutrition: Less than Body
Requirements
Altered Nutrition: More than Body
Requirements
Diversional Activity Deficit
Knowledge Deficit

VI. Moving

Moving means to change the place or position of a body or any member of the body; to put or keep in motion; to provoke an excretion or discharge; the urge to action or to do something; to take action. It is therefore affected by a variety of etiologic agents that interfere with the ability to move purposefully in the environment, to care for self, and to recreate. As in the Exchanging pattern, the Level Two concepts are very interdependent: Alterations in one level often mean difficulties in another.

A. Activity

1. *Subjective*

Essential
a. Description of typical day
b. Ability to perform activities of daily living (ADL)
c. Fatigue, weakness, pain

Expanded
a. Presence of major depression, psychosis

2. *Objective*

Essential
a. General appearance, posture, coordination
b. Physical illness and trauma
c. Psychomotor retardation
d. Medications/treatments affecting activity (e.g., ECT, sedatives)
e. Use of mobility aids

Expanded
a. Sleep disturbance
b. Factors contributing to poor nutritional status
c. Type and extent of physical disability
d. Usual exercise level/energy level

3. *Nursing Diagnoses*
Impaired Physical Mobility*
Activity Intolerance*
Fatigue*
Potential Activity Intolerance*

Related Nursing Diagnoses
Chronic Pain
Altered Nutrition: Less than Body Requirements
Altered Nutrition: More than Body Requirements

B. Rest

1. *Subjective*

Essential
a. Amount of sleep needed/usual amount of sleep
b. Usual sleep routines
c. Sleeping problems, trouble falling/staying asleep
d. Dependency on sleeping aids
e. Fatigue
f. Anxiety, grief, depression

Expanded
a. Onset of sleeping problems
b. Preoccupation with sleep disturbance
c. Dreams, nightmares
d. Perception of alertness

2. *Objective*

Essential
a. Use of sleeping aids: which ones? for how long?

---

*Care plans for this diagnosis are not included in this volume.

b. Clarity of thought content
c. Presence of snoring, restlessness, excessive diaphoresis, sleep apnea periods
d. Use of stimulants, other medications
e. Alcohol consumption daily and at bedtime
f. Exercise, amount and type

Expanded
a. Physical signs of sleep deprivation (e.g., yawning, ptosis of eyelids, dark circles under eyes)
b. Psychologic signs of sleep deprivation (e.g., irritability, inattention)
c. Disruptive environmental factors (e.g., noise, temperature, light)
d. Inappropriate daytime behaviors indicating sleep deprivation (e.g., nodding off, cataplexy)

3. *Nursing Diagnoses*
Sleep-Pattern Disturbance

Related Nursing Diagnoses
  Ineffective Individual Coping
  Chronic Low Self-Esteem
  Situational Low Self-Esteem
  Anxiety
  Altered Thought Processes

C. Recreation

1. *Subjective*

Essential
a. Usual enjoyable diversions, skills, activities
b. How often enjoyed
c. Complaints of boredom, fatigue
d. Perception of helpfulness and meaning of activity
e. Willingness to participate in new therapeutic activities

Expanded
a. Patient's concept of play and relaxation
b. Ability to play and relax
c. Preference for solitary or group activity
d. Motivation to develop or initiate plans for recreation

2. *Objective*

Essential
a. Extent to which diagnosis interferes with recreational activities
b. Attendance at group activities
c. Actual participation in scheduled activities

Expanded
a. Transportation and finances available for recreation
b. Amount of time spent in passive activity (e.g., watching TV)
c. Scheduled recreational time
d. Balance between work and play each week
e. Memberships in clubs, organizations
f. Accessibility of recreational pursuits

3. *Nursing Diagnoses*
Diversional Activity Deficit

Related Nursing Diagnoses
  Spiritual Distress
  Altered Thought Processes
  Fatigue*
  Social Isolation

D. Activities of Daily Living

1. *Subjective*

Essential
a. Desire to care for self
b. Home-care needs
c. Home/family situation

Expanded
a. Division of labor (e.g., how/who does shopping, cooking, cleaning, transporting?)
b. Impression of home situation

2. *Objective*

Essential
a. Relationship of condition to home situation
b. Number and type of available home help
c. Monetary needs/means
d. Financial resources (e.g., insurance)
e. Compliance history, visit history

Expanded
a. Specific needs at home
b. Survey of home situation: cleanliness, safety, adequacy

3. *Nursing Diagnoses*
Impaired Home Maintenance Management*
Altered Health Maintenance*

Related Nursing Diagnosis
  Altered Role Performance*

---

*Care plans for this diagnosis are not included in this volume.

E. Self-Care

1. *Subjective*

Essential

a. Attitude toward attending to self-care activities
b. Distorted body image
c. Ability to follow expected daily routines of eating, bathing, dressing/grooming, toileting
d. Level of self-esteem
e. Anxiety, depression, fatigue

Expanded

a. Degree of dependency on other
b. Description of assistance needed
c. Complaints of ADL difficulties
d. Motivation to perform ADL

2. *Objective*

Essential

a. General appearance, hygiene
b. Use of aids for ADL
c. Ability to move about, care for self
d. Appropriateness of dress to situation
e. Degree of reality orientation
f. Frequency and amount of medication
g. Hyperactivity, loss of impulse control
h. Ritualistic behavior
i. Suspiciousness, delusions
j. Regressive behavior
k. Defiance/negativism
l. Purging and vomiting
m. Psychomotor retardation/agitation

Expanded

a. Condition and appropriateness of ADL aids
b. Ability to set up and maintain ADL routine
c. Presence of supportive, significant others
d. Abilities of caregiver/assistant
e. Available resources for basic needs/care
f. Adherence to medication regime
g. Exacerbation of symptoms

3. *Nursing Diagnoses*
Self-Care Deficit
Impaired Swallowing*

*Care plans for this diagnosis are not included in this volume.

Related Nursing Diagnoses
Altered Nutrition: Less than Body Requirements
Fatigue*
Activity Intolerance*

VII. Perceiving

Perceiving means to apprehend with the mind; to become aware of by the senses; to apprehend what is not open or present to observation; to take in fully or adequately. Information relayed from early life to the brain via the five senses shapes one's view of the world and of oneself as a person.

A. Self-Concept

1. *Subjective*

Essential

a. Perceptions of effects of illness/hospitalizations
b. Mood shifts
c. Awareness of presence of multiple personalities
d. Questioning "Who am I?"
e. Description of ideal self
f. Evaluation of roles and role performance
g. Perception of self as valuable/worthless
h. Gender identity, sense of maleness, femaleness
i. Comfort with sexual orientation/role
j. Perception of body appearance

Expanded

a. Perception of ability to overcome problems
b. Perception of ability to cope with life situations
c. Feelings of emptiness, boredom, abandonment
d. Outlook about future
e. Capacity to tolerate stress

2. *Objective*

Essential

a. Age, developmental status
b. Accurate/distorted perceptions
c. Severity of self-esteem and object-relations disturbance
d. Interpersonal skills, level of socialization
e. Acknowledgment of self-concept difficulties
f. Quality of relationships (e.g., unstable)
g. Grandiosity, negative labeling of self

Expanded
a. Use of community resources
b. Ability to function in roles
c. Presence of chronic psychiatric/medical condition
d. Visibility of stigma

3. ***Nursing Diagnoses***
Body-Image Disturbance
Situational Low Self-Esteem
Chronic Low Self-Esteem
Personal Identity Disturbance

Related Nursing Diagnoses
Ineffective Individual Coping
Impaired Social Interaction
Social Isolation

B. Sensory/Perceptual

1. *Subjective*

Essential
a. Hallucinations
b. Illusions
c. Level of anxiety

Expanded
a. Description of effects of medication
b. Stated ability to cope with chronic halluci-nations
c. Feelings of depersonalization

2. *Objective*

Essential
a. Chronic or acute anxiety
b. Awareness of position of body parts
c. Ability to move all body parts
d. Lab tests for metabolic imbalances (e.g., lithium toxicity)
e. Sensory overload
f. Sleep deprivation
g. Prolonged immobilization
h. Elevated vital signs
i. Chronicity of hallucinations

Expanded
a. Ability to control hallucinations
b. Methods used to control hallucinations

3. ***Nursing Diagnoses***
Sensory/Perceptual Alterations
Unilateral Neglect*

Related Nursing Diagnoses
Self-Care Deficit
Altered Though Processes

C. Meaningfulness

1. *Subjective*

Essential
a. Feelings about seriousness of diagnosis
b. Characteristics of approach to life
c. Outlook on the future
d. Verbal expressions of having no control or influence over the situation or outcome
e. Feelings of emptiness, meaninglessness
f. Philosophical beliefs
g. How illness alters life goals, present situation
h. Losses because of illness/hospitalization

Expanded
a. Locus of control, internal or external
b. Feelings regarding ability to affect course of disease
c. Expressions of milestones to achieve, reasons for living

2. *Objective*

Essential
a. Demeanor
b. Affect
c. Extent of participation in decision making or care when opportunities are present
d. Ability to set future-oriented goals

Expanded
a. Present illness in the context of life occur-rences
b. Available resources for support, assistance
c. Ability to seek information regarding care

3. ***Nursing Diagnoses***
Hopelessness
Powerlessness

Related Nursing Diagnoses
Spiritual Distress
Ineffective Individual Coping
Noncompliance
Anxiety
Fear

---

*Care plans for this diagnosis are not included in this volume.

VIII. Knowing

Knowing means to recognize or acknowledge a thing or a person; to be familiar with by experience or through information or report; to be cognizant of something through observation, inquiry, or information; to be conversant with a body of facts, principles, or methods of action; to understand. Delivery of information through teaching and counseling patients is integral to almost all nursing functions. Patients' ability to learn, to internalize, and to understand the information provided varies widely. It can be difficult to differentiate real knowledge deficits from other nursing diagnoses—particularly anxiety, noncompliance, and decisional conflict. Careful assessment can distinguish whether delivery of information really can solve a given problem or whether the problem is interfering with the reception of information.

A. Knowing

1. *Subjective*

Essential
a. Requests for information
b. Expressions of anxiety
c. Awareness of memory impairment
d. Reports of disturbed thinking (e.g., racing thoughts, inability to concentrate)
e. Verbalization of sensory/perceptual alterations
f. Use of fantasy, nonreality-based thought, concrete thinking

Expanded
a. Preferred learning style
b. Level of current knowledge
c. Accuracy of follow through of instructions
d. Verbalization of incorrect healthcare knowledge

2. *Objective*

Essential
a. Identified learning needs based on psychologic diagnosis
b. Inability to trust caregivers
c. Hyperactivity
d. Psychomotor retardation

e. Confabulation
f. Distractibility
g. Impaired memory
h. Ability to retain to recall information

Expanded
a. Degree of compliance with medical regimen
b. Impediments to learning (e.g., retardation, psychosis, anxiety, regressive thought processes)
c. Learning needs of family, community caretakers
d. Culture and values
e. Educational background

3. *Nursing Diagnoses*
Knowledge Deficit

Related Nursing Diagnoses
Anxiety
Noncompliance
Ineffective Coping
Impaired Adjustment
Altered Thought Processes
Sensory/Perceptual Alterations

B. Thought Processes

1. *Subjective*

Essential
a. Self-appraisal of mood (e.g., elation, anxiety, depression)
b. Self-appraisal of ability to think clearly, reason logically (e.g., racing thoughts, loose associations)

Expanded
a. Level of trust, self-esteem
b. Verbalization of confusion
c. Inability to focus, concentrate
d. Inability to state consequences of actions

2. *Objective*

Essential
a. Oriented to person, place, time
b. Attention span
c. Intact memory, short- and long-term
d. History of psychiatric problems
e. Affect
f. Speech patterns
g. Problem-solving ability

h. Thought content (e.g., delusions)
i. Abstract reasoning ability
j. Serum alcohol, drug levels
k. Flight of ideas

Expanded
a. Age
b. IQ and educational level
c. Learning disability
d. Racing thoughts
e. Calculation ability
f. Decision-making ability
g. Context when delusions occur (e.g., in a crowd)
h. Cultural perspectives

3. *Nursing Diagnoses*
   Acute Confusion
   Chronic Confusion
   Altered Thought Processes

   Related Nursing Diagnoses
   Chronic Low Self-Esteem
   Situational Low Self-Esteem
   Impaired Social Interaction
   Social Isolation
   Ineffective Individual Coping
   Dysfunctional Grieving

IX. Feeling

Feeling means to experience, a consciousness, sensation, apprehension, or sense; to be consciously or emotionally affected by a fact, event, or state. As interpreted within the context of Taxonomy I, this information can be in the form of physical or emotional cues that can be interpreted by the individual in a variety of ways.

A. Comfort

1. *Subjective*

Essential
a. Complaints of pain/discomfort on a scale of 0 to 10 (intensity)
b. Location of pain
c. Length of occurrence
d. Manifestations of anxiety
e. Quality of pain
f. Relieving measures
g. Degree of interference in ADL

Expanded
a. Exacerbating factors
b. Emotional reaction to pain
c. Level of preoccupation with symptoms
d. Meaning of the pain
e. Presence of la belle indifférence
f. Degree of interference in usual roles

2. *Objective*

Essential
a. Behavioral manifestations (e.g., grimacing, guarding, moaning)
b. Degree of discomfort reported associated with type of condition
c. Amount of acute psychosocial stress
d. Degree of exaggeration of symptoms, pain
e. Vital signs
f. Diaphoresis, nausea, vomiting

Expanded
a. Long-term coping strategies (e.g., guided imagery, medications)
b. Social impairment
c. Number of healthcare providers consulted
d. Secondary gains
e. Amount of enduring psychosocial stress

3. *Nursing Diagnoses*
   Pain*
   Chronic Pain

   Related Nursing Diagnoses
   Ineffective Individual Coping
   Impaired Physical Mobility*
   Activity Intolerance*
   Fatigue*

B. Emotional Integrity

1. *Subjective*

Essential
a. Verbal expression of feelings (e.g., of depression, anger, guilt)
b. Report of loss
c. Significance of lost object/person
d. Fear of repetition of event
e. Flashbacks, nightmares
f. Excessive verbalization of the traumatic event
g. Survivor's guilt
h. Suicidal ideation

---

*Care plans for this diagnosis are not included in this volume.

Expanded
a. Somatic symptoms (e.g., tension head-aches, irritable colon)
b. Psychic/emotional numbness
c. Previous unresolved losses
d. Excessive ambivalence regarding lost object/person
e. Socially unacceptable losses (e.g., murder, suicide)
f. Sudden loss, multiple losses
g. Degree of social/occupational impairment

2. *Objective*

Essential
a. Age, sex, marital status
b. Length of time since loss
c. Course of grief process
d. Affect/mood
e. Overt emotions being expressed (e.g., anger, crying)
f. Details of suicide plan
g. Addictive disorders (e.g., gambling, chemical abuse)
h. Obsessive-compulsive behavior

Expanded
a. How previous losses were resolved
b. History of maladaptive coping
c. Antisocial activity
d. Support system available
e. Source of hope

3. *Nursing Diagnoses*
    Anticipatory Grieving
    Dysfunctional Grieving
    Potential for Violence
    Self-Mutilation
    Post-Trauma Response

    Related Nursing Diagnoses
    Ineffective Individual Coping
    Spiritual Distress

C. Emotional State

1. *Subjective*

Essential
a. Verbalization of concerns, fears
b. Somatic complaints (e.g., chest pain, dyspnea)
c. Feelings of powerlessness
d. Reports of phobias
e. Fears of dying, feelings of impending doom

Expanded
a. Identification of specific threats
b. Intensity of concerns on a scale of 0 to 10
c. Reality base of fears
d. Nightmares

2. *Objective*

Essential
a. Reason for admission
b. History of ineffective coping
c. Exaggerated behavior, angry expressions
d. Specificity of concerns
e. Avoidant behavior
f. Use of tranquilizers
g. Hyperventilation, palpitations
h. Chemical dependency/abuse
i. Ritualistic behavior
j. Altered states of consciousness (e.g., depersonalization)
k. Flashbacks
l. Vigilant, tense demeanor

Expanded
a. Vital signs
b. Stability of emotions
c. Support system

3. *Nursing Diagnoses*
    Anxiety
    Fear

    Related Nursing Diagnoses
    Ineffective Individual Coping
    Knowledge Deficit

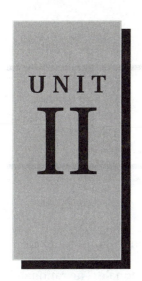

UNIT

II

Organic Mental Syndromes and Disorders

Contents

Introduction

Unit II provides a guideline to help nurses select NANDA nursing diagnoses that correlate with the *Diagnostic and Statistical Manual-IV (DSM-IV)* disorders.

DSM-IV, compiled by the American Psychiatric Association (1994), provides a common language for practitioners and researchers who deal with mental health issues and psychiatric disorders. *DSM-IV* is a classification manual; it describes characteristic features of specific mental disorders. Each patient admitted to a psychiatric/mental heath facility will be given one or more diagnoses from this manual. For this reason, nurses who care for patients in these settings need to be familiar with *DSM-IV* nomenclature and terminology.

Each psychiatric diagnosis in this unit is linked with several nursing diagnoses. Each nursing diagnosis has an accompanying rationale. The rationales reflect the possibilities of altered health patterns often seen with the specific mental disorder. Linking diagnosis with rationale is designed to promote the development of independent thinking while collaborating with the psychiatric diagnosis and treatment. Nurses do not make psychiatric diagnoses; rather, they identify the altered health pattern (nursing diagnosis) that they can address independently.

Unit II is a guide to help nurses validate and augment their own judgment in selecting nursing diagnoses for any patient with a psychiatric/mental health disorder.

Delirium and Dementia

DSM-IV **Delirium**

293.00   Due to general medical conditions
291.00   Substance intoxication delirium
291.00   Substance withdrawal delirium

Nursing Diagnoses for **DSM-IV 293.00, 291.00**

➤ **Knowledge deficit** regarding associated general medical conditions

RATIONALE: Delirium can be associated with many different general medical conditions, each of which has characteristic physical examination and laboratory findings. These findings show that the cognitive disturbance is the direct physiological consequence of a general medical condition.

➤ **Acute confusion** related to substance intoxication

RATIONALE: Drug and alcohol abuse, a medication side effect, or toxin exposure can cause a disturbance in consciousness and a change in cognition that develop over a short period. Delirium that occurs during substance intoxication may arise within minutes to hours after taking relatively high doses of certain drugs (e.g., cannabis, cocaine, and hallucinogens).

➤ **Acute confusion** related to substance withdrawal

RATIONALE: Delirium that is associated with substance withdrawal develops as tissue and fluid concentrations of the substance decrease after reduction or termination of sustained, high-dose use of certain substances. The delirium may continue for only a few hours or may persist for as long as two to four weeks.

➤ **Fluid volume deficit** related to withdrawal symptoms (e.g., dehydration, nausea, and vomiting)

RATIONALE: Fluid and electrolyte imbalance, increased metabolic state, and dehydration are common problems. Decreased magnesium level in the blood and increased level of acetaldehyde cause withdrawal symptoms. The regulation of the antidiuretic hormone is disrupted. The effect of stress causes retention of sodium and depletion of potassium.

➤ **Sensory/perceptual alterations** related to delirium (metabolic dysfunction, social isolation, reduced environmental input, cerebral pathology, etc.)

RATIONALE: With delirium, there is reduced ability to maintain attention to external stimuli; disorganized thinking, sensory misperceptions, and disorientation to time and place may occur. Perceptual disturbances resulting in illusions and hallucinations are common.

➤ **Sleep-pattern disturbance** related to altered levels of consciousness

RATIONALE: In delirium, there is a disturbance in the sleep-wake cycle that can range from drowsiness to semicoma. Some individuals may be hypervigilant, have difficulty falling asleep, and experience vivid dreams and nightmares. The decreased environmental stimulation that occurs during the evening hours contributes to increased confusion at night for the client with dementia who frequently experiences hypnogogic states.

➤ **Fear** related to threatening hallucinations or delusions

RATIONALE: With high levels of fear, the individual may attack those who are seen as threatening and may attempt to escape from the present surroundings. The patient will often cry and call for help, particularly during the night.

Additional Nursing Diagnoses

Ineffective family coping: compromised
Potential for violence: directed at others

DSM-IV Dementia

290.xx   Alzheimer's type, with late onset
290.20   Alzheimer's type, with delusions
290.21   Alzheimer's type, with depressed mood
290.30   Alzheimer's type, with delirium
290.40   Vascular dementia
294.90   Dementia due to HIV disease
294.10   Dementia due to Parkinson's disease, Huntington's disease, substance-induced persisting dementia, multiple etiologies

Nursing Diagnoses for DSM-IV *290.xx, 290.20, 290.21, 290.30, 290.40, 294.90, 294.10*

➤ **Chronic confusion** related to cerebral pathology

RATIONALE: With dementia, there is an impairment in short- and long-term memory associated with impairment in abstract thinking and impaired judgment.

➤ **Self-care deficit** related to memory impairment and regression

RATIONALE: The patient has a decreased ability to perform ADLs adequately as mental and physical deterioration increase. Poor impulse control and bad judgment result in neglect of personal appearance and hygiene. In advanced dementia, the individual becomes oblivious to his or her surroundings and requires total care.

➤ **Dysfunctional grieving** related to multiple losses of function and role

RATIONALE: Patients with Alzheimer's experience gradual loss of memory, perceptional ability, and physical functioning as they deteriorate emotionally and mentally. The family and patient experience multiple losses (e.g., loss of independence, role, function, living arrangements) that need to be mourned simultaneously. When dementia is accompanied by depression, the nurse and the mental health team need to assess whether the depression that exists is secondary to the dementia or whether a pseudodementia exists that is a symptom of a major depressive episode in the geriatric client.

➤ **Potential for injury/trauma** related to cerebral pathology, memory impairment, agitation

RATIONALE: Disorientation, confusion, and forgetfulness result in environmental hazards (e.g., fires, falls); patients become unable to care for themselves safely. Severe brain dysfunction results in dimin-ished psychomotor activity, lethargy, and apathy. People with dementia may wander and become lost. They are susceptible to accidents and infectious diseases. Delirium represents a medical emergency and health team members must respond rapidly with assessment to determine the underlying cause. During a state of delirium, the person may be experiencing psychomotor agitation and may injure him or herself during a hyperactive state.

➤ **Impaired verbal communication** related to cerebral pathology

RATIONALE: With dementia, there is language impairment that interferes with the ability to interact with others. There is a loss in use, understanding, and comprehension of language. The inability to express oneself (aphasia) may extend to all areas of communication. The individual may not comprehend questions and may demonstrate a pathologic, repetitious use of spoken words and phrases (palilalia) or misuse words or word combinations (paraphasia). In delirium, speech often is rambling, irrelevant, or incoherent.

➤ **Ineffective individual coping** related to confusion, lability of affect (loss of emotional control)

RATIONALE: Fear, anxiety, sadness, anger, and frustration increase as mental and physical function decrease. Labile emotional states make is difficult to cope with everyday stresses. Multiple losses may overwhelm the patient with uncontrollable feelings of grief and loss. Feelings of frustration may arise when the individual attempts to perform simple tasks that were once under his or her control. This frustration further diminishes the ability to cope effectively and to perform tasks that could previously be performed functionally.

➤ **Anxiety/fear** related to loss control, threat to self-concept

RATIONALE: Decreased control over sexual and aggressive impulses may accompany cognitive deficits. Social judgments may be impaired. Anxiety, depression, and feelings of shame may be present and be a serious threat to self-esteem.

➤ **Diversional activity deficit** related to cognitive impairment

RATIONALE: Patients with dementia are unable to perform tasks that require the incorporation of new information and may repeatedly ask questions about what to do. They have difficulty recalling both personal and nonpersonal recent events, which makes it difficult to keep them occupied with interesting pastimes.

➤ **Altered family process** related to prognosis, treatment plan, resources

RATIONALE: The family of the patient with dementia needs information regarding safe and adequate care for the patient. Community resources can provide support and guidance to enable the family to care for their loved one at home for as long as possible during the gradual decline of abilities.

➤ **Impaired adjustment** related to progressive cognitive and physical impairment

RATIONALE: When symptoms of dementia are mild, the person is aware of deteriorating faculties. She or he may react with marked anxiety or depression; attempts to conceal or compensate for intellectual deficits are very common. Even mild psychosocial stressors may make adjustment to the cognitive deficits extremely difficult. When deterioration increases, the person may become withdrawn and apathetic, which interferes with adequate adjustment.

➤ **Hopelessness** related to chronic progressive deterioration of mental and physical well-being

RATIONALE: Although the onset and subsequent course of dementia depend on the underlying etiology, most common are the cases in which subsequent cognitive and physical deterioration is inevitable. The person and family face a process that is progressive and can ultimately result in death. Death without dignity, where the person fears loss of control, is a common fear. A depressed mood is a common feature of dementia and further adds to the sense of hopelessness the person is experiencing.

Additional Nursing Diagnoses

Knowledge deficit
Powerlessness
Noncompliance

Substance-Related Disorders

DSM-IV Alcohol-Induced Disorders

303.00   Alcohol intoxication
291.80   Alcohol withdrawal
291.30   Alcohol-induced psychotic disorder with
          hallucinations

DSM-IV Amphetamine-Induced Disorders

292.89   Intoxication
292.00   Withdrawal

DSM-IV Cocaine-Induced Disorders

292.00   Withdrawal
292.81   Intoxication

DSM-IV Opioid-Induced Disorders

292.00   Withdrawal
292.89   Intoxication

DSM-IV Sedative, Hypnotic-, or Anxiolytic-Induced Disorders

292.89   Intoxication
292.00   Withdrawal

Nursing Diagnoses for DSM-IV 303.00, 291.00, 291.30, 292.89, 292.00, 291.80, 292.81, 292.89

➤ **Potential for violence: directed at others** related to "disinhibitory" phenomena

RATIONALE: Alcohol intoxication is frequently associated with criminal acts, homicide, and physical abuse of spouse and children. Maladaptive behavioral changes (e.g., aggressiveness, impaired judgment, emotional lability) result in violence against others. Aggressiveness and hyperactivity are features of intoxication associated with all the psychoactive substances with the exception of opioid intoxication. However, even during intoxication with opioids, patients have impaired judgment and may exhibit euphoria and grandiosity, which puts them at risk for committing aggressive acts. Often the behavioral manifestations of intoxication are difficult to predict when an individual combines psychoactive substances.

➤ **Potential for violence: self-directed** related to central nervous system (CNS) depressant effects of the psychoactive substance or "disinhibitory" phenomena

RATIONALE: Suicide and self-destructive behaviors are extremely common when depressed individuals become intoxicated. One study indicates that about one-fourth of all suicides occur while the person is drinking alcohol (American Psychiatric Association, 1987). The combination of grandiosity, impaired judgment, and agitation that result from intoxication with psychoactive substances often leads to self-destructive acts that have the high potential for being lethal. Combining substances further adds to the danger of overdose.

➤ **Potential for injury/trauma** related to substance intoxication

RATIONALE: Falls and accidents result in fractures, hematomas, and other head injuries, as well as automobile injuries and fatalities.

➤ **Altered thought processes** related to intoxication

RATIONALE: Maladaptive cognitive changes may include hypervigilance, impaired judgment, confusion, incoherent speech, transient ideas of reference, and paranoid and grandiose ideation. Delirium may develop shortly after the ingestion of many psychoactive substances. Permanent changes in cognition can result from continuous ingestion of psychoactive substances that predispose individuals to episodes of psychosis while intoxicated.

➤ **Sensory/perceptual alterations** related to withdrawal symptoms

RATIONALE: Vivid visual, auditory, or tactile hallucinations are present in alcohol hallucinosis and withdrawal delirium. Hallucinations and illusions are common features of withdrawal from any psychoactive substance, especially when delirium is present.

➤ **Altered through processes** related to withdrawal symptoms

RATIONALE: Delusions, paranoid ideation, confusion, impaired judgment, disorientation, and memory impairment are common features of psychoactive substance withdrawal.

➤ **Potential for injury** related to complications of withdrawal

RATIONALE: Complications of overdose and withdrawal are fluid and electrolyte imbalance, respiratory failure, shock, toxic psychosis, and nutritional imbalance. Seizures precede the development of delirium tremens, which can be life-threatening. Delirium tremens begins 2 to 3 days after drinking stops and subsides 1 to 5 days thereafter.

➤ **Sleep-pattern disturbance** related to psychomotor agitation or psychomotor retardation

RATIONALE: The rebound effect is present during withdrawal. If the ingested substance was a CNS depressant, then psychomotor agitation will be present and make sleep difficult. If the ingested substance was a stimulant, then the person may experience a "crashing" syndrome in which hypersomnia is present. Psychoactive substances disturb the normal sleep cycle and thus persons may experience REM rebound or the increased need for deep, stage IV sleep.

➤ **Anxiety/fear** related to the rebound effects of withdrawal

RATIONALE: Anxiety, tremulousness, and irritability often appear when the immediate psychoactive effects of the drug have subsided. The fear of not obtaining relief from the withdrawal symptoms further intensifies anxiety, which complicates the withdrawal symptoms.

Additional Nursing Diagnoses

Hopelessness
Ineffective family coping: compromised
Knowledge deficit
Powerlessness

Psychoactive Substance Use Disorders

DSM-IV Alcohol Use Disorders

303.90 Dependence
305.00 Abuse

DSM-IV Amphetamine Use Disorders

304.40 Dependence
305.70 Abuse

DSM-IV Cocaine Use Disorders

304.20 Dependence
305.60 Abuse

DSM-IV Opioid Use Disorder

304.00 Dependence
305.50 Abuse

DSM-IV Phencyclidine Use Disorders

304.90 Dependence
305.90 Abuse

DSM-IV Sedative, Hypnotic, or Anxiolytic Use Disorders

304.10 Dependence
305.40 Abuse

DSM-IV Polysubstance-Related Disorder

304.80 Dependence

Nursing Diagnoses for DSM-IV *303.90, 305.00, 304.40, 305.70, 304.20, 305.60, 304.00, 305.50, 304.90, 305.90, 304.10, 305.40, 304.80*

➤ **Ineffective individual coping** related to continued abuse of substance despite adverse consequences

RATIONALE: With abuse, the individual may recognize that his or her substance abuse is excessive, but is either unable or unwilling to make an effort to reduce or control it. The person continues to use even though social, physical, and psychologic problems are present. The substance abuser uses alcohol and drugs to cope with everyday stressors and to relieve tension and anxiety.

➤ **Impaired adjustment** related to chronic dependence on chemical substances

RATIONALE: The substance-dependent individual does not know how to cope with everyday stressors without resorting to alcohol or drug use. The person has difficulty tolerating anxiety or frustration and uses drugs to escape tension. There often are problems with relationships and underlying conflicts with feelings of dependency and low self-worth.

➤ **Ineffective family coping: disabling** related to ongoing substance dependency

RATIONALE: Alcoholics and drug users have a high rate of marital separation and divorce. Major family obligations may be neglected or inadequately fulfilled due to intoxication, withdrawal symptoms, and amount of time spent in getting, taking, and recovering from the substance's effects.

➤ **Chronic low self-esteem** related to feelings of powerlessness, disturbance of mood and personality

RATIONALE: In chronic use and dependence, mood lability and suspiciousness are common. Long-term dependence on alcohol and drugs is often associated with the "amotivational syndrome," whereby the individual loses interest in work, school, hobbies, and family affairs. Chronic low self-esteem and feelings of sadness can result from loss of meaningful activity and relationships. As attempts to control the use of the substance fail, the person reaches a state of powerlessness in which she or he no longer tries and the disease progresses.

➤ **Ineffective denial** related to substance dependency

RATIONALE: Denial is the defense mechanism most frequently used by the dependent person. Chemically dependent individuals use denial and manipulation to minimize the seriousness of their habit. They will blame society, make excuses, intellectualize, and pick fights to avoid facing the truth about their problem.

➤ **Sexual dysfunction** related to excessive alcohol/drug intake

RATIONALE: Alcoholism causes peripheral neuropathy, which is nonreversible. Alcohol and marijuana lead to low testosterone, which could lead to low desire. Cocaine first affects ejaculation, then leads to low desire and erectile dysfunction. Moderate amounts of alcohol decrease inhibition; too much interferes with functioning.

➤ **Altered nutrition: less than body requirements** related to improper diet, physiologic effects of alcohol

RATIONALE: Physical complications of chronic alcohol dependence includes gastritis and cirrhosis. A large intake of alcohol can produce a malabsorption syndrome whereby food nutrients are not fully absorbed. This can result in vitamin deficiency disease such as Wernicke-Korsakoff (thiamine) and peripheral neuropathy (B vitamins).

➤ **Potential for violence: self-directed** related to polysubstance use and depression

RATIONALE: There is an increasing tendency for drug users to mix multiple drugs and to mix drugs with alcohol, resulting in dangerous potentiation of drug action and side effects. Lack of coordination, unsteady gait, and impaired attention when intoxicated can lead to falls, accidents, and highway fatalities. Prolonged drinking often produces anxiety and depression. Underlying depression may be intensified by the depressant effects of alcohol. Use of psychoactive substances lowers impulse control as higher cortical centers are depressed.

➤ **Powerlessness** related to inability to abstain from alcohol/drugs

RATIONALE: Repeated experiences of failure to stop drinking easily lead to feelings of despair and hopelessness. By the time the individual is ready to ac-

knowledge the alcoholism or drug use, she or he feels powerless to stop it.

➤ **Noncompliance** related to denial of psychologic dependency, lack of situational supports

RATIONALE: Feelings of helplessness to establish a life of work, family, friends, and pastimes without drugs often lead to noncompliance in following a recovery program successfully. Lack of adherence can be due to denial of the seriousness of the problem, lack of environmental support to stop using, and psychologic dependency on the chemical.

➤ **Dysfunctional grieving** related to loss of lifestyle/friends, substance-abuse habits

RATIONALE: Substance abusers usually have a difficult time recognizing and expressing their feelings. They defend against pain and sadness by becoming intoxicated. When the chemically dependent decide to stop using, there is a tremendous adjustment in how time is spent, who one spends time with, and learning how to deal with feelings. Often the number of losses incurred when using and the change in lifestyle when stopping become overwhelming and the individual is unable to grieve spontaneously.

➤ **Spiritual distress** related to lack of faith, hope, and meaning

RATIONALE: The success of Alcoholics Anonymous is attributed to the 12-step program that includes developing a relationship with a higher power. Often substance abusers are not connected to a deeper sense of themselves or to a spiritual being that provides comfort and hope. The lack of spiritual guidance and meaningful values contributes to a state of spiritual distress.

➤ **Altered family processes: alcoholism** related to addictive personality and resistance to treatment

RATIONALE: When one or more family members is addicted to chemical substances, the entire family functioning is affected. The family unit becomes disorganized, leading to conflict, denial of problems, and ineffective coping. It is not uncommon for the family to experience a series of self-perpetuating crises.

Additional Nursing Diagnoses

Anxiety
Hopelessness
Knowledge deficit
Potential for violence: directed at others

Schizophrenia and Other Psychotic Disorders

DSM-IV Schizophrenia

295.30	Paranoid
295.20	Catatonic
295.10	Disorganized
295.90	Undifferentiated
295.60	Residual

DSM-IV Other Psychotic disorders

295.40	Schizophreniform disorder
295.70	Schizoaffective disorder
293.xx	Psychotic disorder caused by a general medical condition

Nursing Diagnoses for DSM-IV 295.10, 295.20, 295.30, 295.90, 295.60, 295.40, 295.70, 293.xx

➤ **Altered thought processes** related to biochemical imbalances, unmet needs (i.e., power, control, and sexual and aggressive drives)

RATIONALE: Delusions (i.e., simple persecutory, ideas of reference, thought broadcasting, thought insertion, thought withdrawal) are the major disturbances in content of thought. Loosening of associations, poverty of content of speech, neologisms, perseveration, clanging, and blocking are disturbances in the form of thought.

➤ **Self-care deficit** related to poor judgment, impaired cognition, apathy

RATIONALE: Impairment in several areas of ADL is due to problems with self-initiation and goal-directed behavior as a result of cognitive impairment and poor reality orientation. Patients in a catatonic stupor maintain a rigid posture and resist efforts to be moved. Malnutrition, exhaustion, and self-inflicted injury are common problems. Schizophrenics may be regressed to an earlier age, and be disorganized and dependent on others for basic care. Supervision may be required to ensure nutrition and hygiene needs are met.

➤ **Chronic low self-esteem** related to reduced occupational and social functioning level

RATIONALE: Functioning in areas of work, social relationships, and self-care is reduced markedly during the course of the illness, and a return to full premorbid functioning is not common. There is also a failure to achieve the expected level of social development.

➤ **Sensory perceptual alterations** related to biochemical imbalances and anxiety

RATIONALE: Hallucinations (e.g., auditory and visual) are a primary symptom of schizophrenia and other psychotic disorders.

➤ **Impaired social interaction** related to lack of perceived positive social reinforcement, disturbances in communication

RATIONALE: Difficulties in interpersonal relationships are a result of withdrawal into fantasy, flat or inappropriate affect, poverty of speech content, and loose associations. Communication with others is impaired by the individual's inability to relate effectively to others in a meaningful manner.

➤ **Social isolation** related to social withdrawal, lack of trust

RATIONALE: Mistrust of others is a core problem in schizophrenia. The individual feels vulnerable in the presence of others, fearing the other person will control, threaten, or abandon him or her. The schizophrenic will choose to be isolated rather than risk the pain of being hurt. Feelings of isolation and lack of meaningful relationships lead to feelings of loneliness, emptiness, and desperation. The degree of withdrawal can range from intense shyness to complete reclusiveness.

➤ **Impaired verbal communication** related to psychotic process

RATIONALE: Linguistic changes reflect a disruption in abstract thought patterns. The private and symbolic meaning of the person's verbalizations reflects an abandonment of conceptually based language patterns. Linguistic changes are echolalia (purposeless repetition of a word), clang associations (repetition of words that have similar sound), neologism (privately coined word with meaning known only to the speaker), and the word salad (words are linked illogically).

➤ **Noncompliance** related to inability to follow through with self-care

RATIONALE: Schizophrenics are sometimes noncompliant about following the prescribed treatment regime. They will refuse to take medications or go to day care. This behavior may be due to not comprehending or believing in the importance of the treatment for facilitating their optimal level of functioning.

➤ **Ineffective family coping: disabling** related to dysfunctional patterns

RATIONALE: All family members participate in the dysfunctional patterns that contribute to the development of a schizophrenic child. Overt symptoms of the family's dysfunction can be expressed in one member who becomes the identified patient. There may be distorted communication patterns among family members, and an investment in keeping one child helpless and dependent to maintain stability within the family structure.

➤ **Constipation** related to side effects of antipsychotic medication

RATIONALE: Most schizophrenics are prescribed medication to control disturbed thinking. Constipation is a common side effect, as are dry mouth, drowsiness, photosensitization, and extrapyramidal symptoms.

➤ **Knowledge deficit** regarding treatment, medications, prognosis

RATIONALE: The schizophrenic patient often stops taking medications once stabilized, not understanding what happens when medications are omitted (e.g., reappearance of symptoms). The individual needs to be aware of side effects of psychotropic drugs and the importance of reporting any signs of toxicity. Knowledge of the dangers of mixing alcohol and certain drugs, protecting self from the sun when taking thorazine, and follow-up appointments are all part of patient education.

➤ **Knowledge deficit** regarding associated medical conditions

RATIONALE: A variety of medical conditions may cause psychotic symptoms, including neurological, endocrine, and metabolic conditions; fluid or electrolyte imbalances; hepatic or renal diseases; and autoimmune disorders with CNS involvement.

Additional Nursing Diagnoses

Body-image disturbance
Decisional conflict
Impaired adjustment
Personal identity disturbance

Delusional Disorder

DSM-IV 297.10 Delusional Disorder

Nursing Diagnoses for DSM-IV 297.10

➤ **Altered thought processes** related to excessive use of defenses

RATIONALE: Delusions (a false, fixed belief that cannot be corrected by logic) are persistent and nonbizarre. There is an insidious development of a permanent and unshakable delusional system, with preservation of clear and orderly thinking. The delusional system interferes with only one aspect of the patient's life.

➤ **Potential for violence: directed at others** related to suspiciousness, anger, ideas of reference

RATIONALE: Paranoid people are overconcerned with hidden motives and special meanings of others. They have a tendency to be easily slighted and quick to take offense. There is a readiness to counterattack when any threat is perceived. They are most upset by interpersonal issues involving dependency and intimacy.

➤ **Impaired social interaction** related to chronic low self-esteem

RATIONALE: Paranoids suffer a feeling of deep inadequacy in all areas of interpersonal relationship. They are aloof, haughty, rigid, and suspicious. These individuals harbor a secret desire for revenge against society.

➤ **Chronic low self-esteem** related to problems with trust

RATIONALE: Basic trust fails to develop in paranoid individuals. Many have been physically beaten or treated with cruelty, and had very unreliable or moralistic, demanding, and perfectionistic parents. The grandiosity of the paranoid serves to mask the underlying feelings of humiliation, shame, and low self-esteem.

➤ **Fear** related to delusions of persecution

RATIONALE: The paranoid personality will attribute malicious intent to trivial actions by real people in the community. Next, they see these people as organized into a community of plotters (e.g., FBI, Mafia, communist) who are after them. They experience a great deal of fear at being the object of persecution.

Additional Nursing Diagnoses

Anxiety
Ineffective family coping: compromised
Knowledge deficit
Powerlessness
Social isolation

Brief Reactive Psychosis

DSM-IV 298.80 Brief Reactive Psychosis

Nursing Diagnoses for DSM-IV *298.80*

➤ **Anxiety/fear** related to sudden onset of psychotic symptoms

RATIONALE: Brief reactive psychosis is characterized by great emotional turmoil, grossly disorganized behavior, and a lack of contact with reality. The person is usually incapacitated and dependent on others for help. It can be a frightening experience to lose the sense of who you are and of your surroundings so suddenly.

➤ **Ineffective individual coping** related to severe anxiety and situational crisis

RATIONALE: The precipitating event for the psychosis is usually a major stress that leads to emotional turmoil, feelings of being overwhelmed, and confusion. Unstable personalities seem to be more susceptible to this kind of psychotic break.

➤ **Ineffective family coping: compromised** related to temporary family disorganization and role changes

RATIONALE: Even though the brief psychotic reaction may only last a few hours to days, hospitalization may be required. The person is often self-destructive and dangerous to others in the environment. The family must deal with the patient's intense change in personality and behavior that occurs without much warning.

Additional Nursing Diagnoses

Altered thought processes
Impaired adjustment
Knowledge deficit
Powerlessness
Self-care deficit
Situational low self-esteem

Mood Disorders

DSM-IV Bipolar Disorders

296.4x   Manic
296.6x   Mixed

Nursing Diagnoses for DSM-IV *296.4x, 296.6x*

➤ **Potential for injury** related to hyperactivity, poor judgment

RATIONALE: During a manic episode there is a considerable impairment in social and occupational functioning. Often there is a need for protection from the consequences of poor judgment (e.g., car accidents, gambling, spending sprees, hypersexual activity). Involuntary hospitalization may be necessary to protect the individual and to contain the hyperactivity during a manic phase.

➤ **Altered nutrition: less than body requirements** related to increased activity, decreased sleep, lack of food intake

RATIONALE: The manic person engages in continuous activity that is rapid and excessive. She or he does not take time to sit down to eat, often going for days without adequate food or fluids. High expenditure of energy coupled with lack of sleep and decreased food intake results in burning a greater amount of calories than usual, with subsequent weight loss.

➤ **Sleep-pattern disturbance** related to hyperactivity

RATIONALE: There is a decreased need to sleep during the manic episode. The person awakens after only two or three hours of sleep, full of energy. She or he may go days without any sleep and not feel tired.

➤ **Impaired social interaction** related to expansive mood

RATIONALE: Enthusiasm and increased sociability are seen in the manic phase, but the person soon become intrusive, domineering, and demanding in interactions with others. Overactive manic patients can be loud and constantly irritating to those around them. Activities are often disorganized, flamboyant, and reckless, with a high potential for painful consequences.

➤ **Altered thought processes** related to excessive use of defenses, low self-esteem

RATIONALE: The manic episode is one of a predominantly elevated and euphoria mood. However, there is inflated self-esteem that leads to grandiosity that may be delusional. The person will exhibit flight of ideas, distractibility (responds to irrelevant stimuli), and pressured speech. Grandiose delusions usually involve a special relationship to God or some well-known figure. Hallucinations may also be present.

➤ **Ineffective family coping: disabling** related to chronically unexpressed feelings of guilt, anxiety, and despair

RATIONALE: The manic phase is usually a defense against severe depression. The behavior of a manic person disables his or her own capacities and that of the family to deal effectively with the underlying feelings of despair.

➤ **Ineffective denial** related to lack of insight

RATIONALE: As a rule, manic people do not realize that they are not well. They will become irritated and threaten to sue anyone who tries to get them into the hospital for treatment. They will overestimate their abilities in all areas and take extraordinary risks. They will deny that they have problems by presenting a facade of wellness.

➤ **Altered sexuality patterns** related to hypersexual activity

RATIONALE: Normal inhibitions are lowered, and a usually modest person may engage in frequent and inappropriate sexual encounters and use profane language. Manic people may dress in an outlandish and provocative manner, and act very seductively toward the opposite sex.

➤ **Impaired adjustment** related to refusal to follow recommended treatment

RATIONALE: Often, the manic-depressive individual will refuse to take prescribed lithium, or will stop taking it without the physician's knowledge.

➤ **Potential for violence: directed at others** related to expansiveness, anger

RATIONALE: When someone tries to control the manic's expansive behavior, the manic person becomes angry. She or he will react with rage and may scream, curse, or strike out violently at others in the environment.

Additional Nursing Diagnoses

Chronic pain
Knowledge deficit
Noncompliance

DSM-IV Depressive Disorders

296.2x	Major depression, single episode
296.5x	Bipolar disorder, depressed
298.3x	Major depression, recurrent
300.40	Dysthymia (depressive neurosis)

Nursing Diagnoses for DSM-IV 296.2x, 296.5x, 298.3x, 300.40

➤ **Potential for violence: self-directed** related to hopelessness

RATIONALE: Suicidal thoughts are present in mot moderately and severely depressed people. Suicide risk is greatest when the patient expresses hopelessness, when the patient exhibits sudden cheerfulness or unusual calmness, and up to three months after hospitalization. When delusions/hallucinations are present they may be nihilistic delusions of the world or personal destruction. Substance abuse during depressive episodes increases the likelihood of acting on suicidal thoughts.

➤ **Chronic low self-esteem** related to feelings of worthlessness

RATIONALE: Low self-esteem is characteristic of most depressed patients. Loss of self-respect and self-confidence leads the person's self-concept and perspective of the world to a very negative view. Negative self-evaluations, feelings of inadequacy, and excessive guilt are common features of depression. The sense of worthlessness may be of delusional proportions. The chronically depressed person becomes less capable of enjoying life and forming attachments to other people.

➤ **Dysfunctional grieving** related to multiple losses, socially unacceptable losses

RATIONALE: Dysfunctional grief is a failure to complete the grieving process and cope successfully with the loss. Factors that contribute to unresolved grief are socially unacceptable loss (e.g., suicide), uncertainty over loss (e.g., person missing in action), and being overwhelmed by multiple losses. When there is ambivalence over the lost object or person, or a need to be strong and in control, grieving is more difficult. When a current loss reawakens an old, unresolved loss, grieving is compounded and depression often results.

➤ **Sleep-pattern disturbance** related to internal stressors

RATIONALE: Sleep is commonly disturbed in depressed people. Insomnia is usually the first symptom reported and occurs in 90% of cases. Initial insomnia is having difficulty falling asleep. Middle insomnia is waking up during sleep and falling asleep again with difficulty. Terminal insomnia is early morning awakening. Hypersomnia may be present and is manifested by prolonged sleep (14 to 15 hours) and frequent daytime naps and sleepiness.

➤ **Hopelessness** related to feelings of despair

RATIONALE: Feelings of hopelessness, guilt, and worthlessness are commonly seen during depressive episodes. There is a sustained mood of feeling sad, gloomy, despairing, and pessimistic. A loss of interest and pleasure in life events leads to a feeling that life is not worth living. Hopelessness is manifested by a belief that recovery and a better future are not possible. Excessive guild feelings about past events, and a belief that there is no way to undo or compensate for their actions, add to the hopelessness. The degree of despair determines the immediate risk for suicide.

➤ **Altered sexuality patterns** related to decreased sexual libido, antidepressant medication

RATIONALE: Loss of sexual drive is universally seen in depressed persons. Most men lose interest and stop all sexual activity. Women may continue having sexual relations but without desire or interest. Decreased sexual drive is a common side effect for antidepressant medications.

➤ **Altered nutrition: less than/more than body requirements** related to disturbed appetite

RATIONALE: Loss of appetite occurs most commonly but sometimes increased appetite is seen. There can be significant weight loss or gain. Many depressed persons are incapable of enjoying formerly favorite foods, which now seem tasteless.

➤ **Constipation** related to antidepressant medication, psychomotor retardation

RATIONALE: Constipation is very common among depressed persons. Antidepressants often aggravate the problem and much attention is paid to the difficulty in having a regular bowel movement. Vegetative functioning decreases with depression.

➤ **Diversional activity deficit** related to loss of interest or pleasure in activities

RATIONALE: The depressed person has decreased energy, difficulty thinking or concentrating, and a loss of interest in usual activities. Apathy leads to withdrawal from friends and family and neglect of pleasurable pastimes.

➤ **Decisional conflict** related to powerlessness, negative self-evaluation

RATIONALE: One of the most painful symptoms suffered by depressed persons is the incapacity to make decisions. Even minor decisions, such as what clothing to wear, become difficult; major decisions about work and family become almost impossible.

➤ **Self-care deficit** related to apathy, loss of interest in self

RATIONALE: If impairment is severe, the depressed person may be totally unable to function socially, to feed or dress self, or to maintain minimal personal hygiene. There may be regressive dependence on others.

➤ **Anxiety** related to low self-worth

RATIONALE: Most depressed persons suffer from anxiety—the two states exist together. In agitated depression, anxiety is manifested by pacing, hand-wringing, and rumination.

➤ **Chronic pain** related to depression

RATIONALE: Complaints of chronic pain in the head, chest, abdomen, shoulder, or neck are common in depression.

➤ **Spiritual distress** related to despair

RATIONALE: Depressed people have generally lost their faith in whatever previously gave meaning to their lives. They may feel that God has deserted them or is punishing them for some past sin. Sometimes the guilt and self-condemnation come from certain ingrained religious beliefs.

➤ **Powerlessness** related to learned helplessness

RATIONALE: Seligman (1975) defines helplessness as a belief that no one will do anything to aid you. The individual's perceived lack of control over environmental reinforcement leads to withdrawal, loss of motivation for any activity, and feelings of hopelessness. The behavioral manifestations of helplessness and depression parallel each other.

Additional Nursing Diagnoses

Altered thought processes
Impaired social interaction
Ineffective family coping: compromised
Knowledge deficit

DSM-IV 293.83 Mood Disorders Caused by a General Medical Condition

Nursing Diagnosis for DSM-IV 293.83

➤ **Knowledge deficit** regarding associated general medical conditions

RATIONALE: Depression can be associated with a variety of physical illnesses. However, to receive this diagnosis, the disturbance in mood must be caused by the direct physiological effects of a general medical condition. Evidence from the history, physical examination, or laboratory findings must support the conclusion that the mood disturbance is not better accounted for by another mental disorder.

Anxiety Disorders

DSM-IV Panic Disorder

300.01   Without agoraphobia
300.21   With agoraphobia
300.22   Agoraphobia without history of panic
          attacks

DSM-IV Phobias

300.23   Social phobia
300.29   Specific phobia

Nursing Diagnoses for DSM-IV *300.01, 300.21, 300.22, 300.23, 300.29*

➤ **Anxiety/fear** related to unexpected and intense panic attacks

RATIONALE: Recurrent panic attacks with periods of intense fear and discomfort are an essential feature of panic disorder. Symptoms such as dyspnea, chest pain, dizziness, palpitations, sweating, choking, and numbness result in the individual believing she or he is going crazy or will die. The person fears having a panic attack, but is uncertain when and if it will occur at all.

➤ **Powerlessness** related to inability to control anxiety and panic, chronic low self-esteem

RATIONALE: Panic attacks usually begin with the sudden onset of intense apprehension and fear. The person feels an impending sense of doom before the anxiety escalates to a full-blown attack. Agoraphobia is the fear of being in situations where help will be unavailable. As a result of feelings of powerlessness and fear, the person restricts activities and travel outside the home. Low self-esteem results from being unable to function normally or continue with one's regular routine.

➤ **Ineffective individual coping** related to severe anxiety

RATIONALE: The feeling of impending doom paralyzes the person, preventing him or her from successfully coping with the situation. As the level of anxiety rises, perceptions are narrowed and attention becomes selective. Physical symptoms are overwhelming and all attention is focused on the body rather than on the total situation.

➤ **Sleep-pattern disturbance** related to physiologic disturbances caused by anxiety

RATIONALE: Anxious persons frequently suffer from insomnia and difficulty with sleeping through the night. Dependency on hypnotics, anxiolytics, and sedatives interferes with the normal wake-sleep cycle.

➤ **Social isolation** related to avoidance behavior

RATIONALE: Panic disorder with agoraphobia is associated with varying degrees of constriction in life-style. The fear of having an attack in public (e.g., standing in line, being in a crowd, driving a car) forces the person to become almost completely homebound or unable to leave the house without a companion.

➤ **Impaired social interaction** related to fear of humiliation, shame, social stigma

RATIONALE: In social phobias, the individual has a persistent fear that she or he will be exposed to embarrassing scrutiny by others. The person may fear talking in public, choking on food when eating in front of others, or trembling when with others. There is some interference with social and occupational functioning due to the considerable inconvenience caused by avoiding certain situations.

Additional Nursing Diagnoses

Chronic low self-esteem
Hopelessness
Knowledge deficit

DSM-IV Anxiety Disorders

300.30   Obsessive-compulsive disorder

Nursing Diagnoses for DSM-IV *300.30*

➤ **Anxiety** related to unmet psychologic safety and security needs

RATIONALE: Obsessive-compulsive behaviors are an unconscious attempt to reduce an intolerable level of anxiety. Extreme anxiety and discomfort are experienced when a ritualistic routine is disrupted. Several defense mechanisms are used to control anxiety (e.g., isolation, reaction formation, undoing, and regression) and when stressful events occur, defenses and ritualistic behaviors become intensified.

➤ **Altered thought processes** related to anxiety

RATIONALE: The individual experiences persistent ideas, thoughts, and impulses that are intrusive and senseless. The most common are repetitive thoughts of violence, contamination, and doubts about something. The repetitive, purposeful behaviors that are done in response to the obsessions are called compulsions. This behavior helps to relieve anxiety and binds it by displacement and undoing.

➤ **Self-care deficit** related to ritualistic behavior

RATIONALE: The most common behaviors involve hand washing, counting, checking, and touching. The repetitive nature of these acts becomes all absorbing and the individual neglects self-care activities. Frequent hand washing can cause impairment of skin integrity.

➤ **Ineffective individual coping** related to inability to express feelings directly

RATIONALE: Even though people may recognize that their thoughts are unreasonable, they cannot stop the excessive, ritualistic behavior. The inability to express their feelings more directly results in this maladaptive coping behavior.

➤ **Decisional conflict** related to fear of making a mistake, ambivalence, low self-worth

RATIONALE: People with obsessive-compulsive disorder tend to procrastinate and avoid making decisions due to an inordinate fear of making a wrong choice. Ambivalence is common and the conflict of opposing emotions contributes to the tremendous doubt in the face of choices.

➤ **Ineffective family coping: disabling** related to obsessive-compulsive behavior

RATIONALE: Obsessive-compulsive behavior is often so disruptive and time consuming that the family cannot focus on other matters of concern. People with this disorder tend to have overcontrolling families, where parents established rigid standards of behavior that must be followed.

Additional Nursing Diagnoses

Chronic low self-esteem
Knowledge deficit
Potential for injury
Powerlessness

DSM-IV Anxiety Disorders

300.02   Generalized anxiety disorder
309.81   Posttraumatic stress disorder

Nursing Diagnoses for DSM-IV *300.02, 309.81*

➤ **Anxiety/fear** related to reexperiencing of traumatic event

RATIONALE: The person may have recurrent and intrusive recollections of the event. As the original event is being remembered, it is being relived as if the individual were there. There is often intense psychologic stress when the person is exposed to similar events, and a phobic avoidance of situations resembling the trauma.

➤ **Powerlessness** related to serious threat to life or physical integrity

RATIONALE: The stressor producing post-traumatic syndrome is experienced with intense fear, terror, and helplessness. Common traumas are sudden destruction of one's home, military combat, concentration camps, rape, or seeing someone seriously injured or killed. The individual is subjected to a situation where she or he is unable to experience and assimilate all feelings due to the overwhelming threat to life. The person feels vulnerable and helpless. There is a fear of death and loss of bodily control.

➤ **Post-trauma response** related to chronic severe anxiety

RATIONALE: The individual reexperiences the traumatic event with flashbacks, intrusive thoughts, and repetitive nightmares and dreams. Excessive verbalization about the traumatic event is common as a way to release anxiety. The person experiences self-blame, shame, and sadness. An exaggerated startle reaction and hyperalertness are common symptoms.

➤ **Rape-trauma syndrome** related to unresolved rape trauma

RATIONALE: The trauma syndrome that develops after a forced, violent sexual attack or attempted rape includes an acute phase of disorganization of the victim's life-style and a long-term process of reorganization of life-style. The victim may experience repetitive nightmares, sudden onset of phobias, increased anxiety and fear, pronounced changes in sexual behavior, or no verbalization of the occurrence of rape.

➤ **Situational low self-esteem** related to altered life-style, chronic anxiety, depression

RATIONALE: There is a numbness of response to the external world that is manifested by decreased interest, feelings of detachment and estrangement form others, and constructed emotional responses. The person may suffer from depressive symptoms, restlessness, impulsive behavior, insomnia, and survivor's guilt. The individual no longer feels safe in his or her world and frequently will alter previous life-style by becoming passive, submissive, and dependent.

➤ **Potential for violence: self-directed** related to self-destructive behavior

RATIONALE: Social isolation, a negative self-concept, impulsive behavior, and chronic anxiety result in increased alcohol/drug abuse, suicide attempts, illegal activities, and reckless driving.

➤ **Potential for violence: directed at others** related to explosive outbursts, substance abuse

RATIONALE: Emotional lability, impulsive acting out, and an impaired interpretation of reality combined with intoxication often lead to violent episodes.

➤ **Sleep-pattern disturbance** related to high levels of anxiety

RATIONALE: Trouble falling or staying asleep is a common problem with anxious individuals. People suffering from post-traumatic stress are often awakened with nightmares and anxiety.

Additional Nursing Diagnoses

Hopelessness
Ineffective family coping: compromised
Knowledge deficit

DSM-IV 293.89 Anxiety Disorder Due to a General Medical Condition Substance-Induced Anxiety Disorder

Nursing Diagnosis for DSM-IV *293.89*

➤ **Knowledge deficit** regarding associated general medical conditions

RATIONALE: A variety of medical conditions, including endocrine, cardiovascular, respiratory, metabolic, and neurological conditions, may cause anxiety symptoms. The associated physical examination and laboratory findings must reflect the etiological medical condition. There might be features that are atypical of primary anxiety disorder, such as atypical age at onset or absence of family history.

Somatoform Disorders

DSM-IV Somatoform Disorders

300.11 Conversion disorder
300.18 Somatization disorder
307.xx Pain disorder

Nursing Diagnoses for DSM-IV 300.11, 300.18, 307.xx

➤ **Ineffective individual coping** related to unmet dependency needs, inability to deal effectively with conflicts, chronic anxiety

RATIONALE: Two mechanisms have been suggested to explain what a person gains from having a conversion symptom. The "primary gain" is keeping an internal conflict or need out of awareness (e.g., after an argument, the person develops paralysis of the arm rather than acknowledge the rage). The "secondary gain" is to avoid a particular activity, or to get attention that would not otherwise be available.

➤ **Fear** related to unrealistic interpretation of physical symptoms

RATIONALE: In somatoform disorder, there is a preoccupation with the fear of having, or the belief that one has, a serious disease. The unrealistic fear persists despite medical tests and reassurance that there is no pathology.

➤ **Anxiety** related to inability to control pain, unresolved conflicts

RATIONALE: The lack of control and the dread associated with pain increase the perception of pain and diminish the effect of pain-reduction methods. The occurrence of symptoms in a somatization disorder is related to the amount of anxiety the person is experiencing. The anxiety is unconsciously channeled through the visceral organs and indirectly expressed as symptoms.

➤ **Chronic pain** related to recurrent and multiple somatic complaints, depression, unexpressed anger

RATIONALE: Patients with somatization disorder have a history of several years' duration of symptoms that can include some or all of the following: GI symptoms (e.g., nausea and vomiting, abdominal pain, diarrhea), female reproductive-system symptoms (e.g., menstrual irregularity, dysmenorrhea), pain (e.g., backache, joint pain, headaches), and cardiopulmonary symptoms (e.g., shortness of breath, chest pain, palpitations).

➤ **Altered sexuality patterns** related to pain, indifference

RATIONALE: With somatization, people may experience a lack of pleasure or pain during intercourse. Preoccupation with somatic symptoms contributes to sexual indifference.

➤ **Impaired adjustment** related to adapting to sick role, exaggeration of physical symptoms

RATIONALE: Clients who exhibit conversion and somatization disorders are usually well known within the healthcare system. Physical illness is a semi-legitimate way of getting needs for attention and nurturing met.

➤ **Ineffective family coping: compromised** related to recurrent somatic complaints

RATIONALE: It is difficult to distinguish between conversion, somatization, and malingering. The family may believe that the patient uses symptoms to manipulate them and to receive secondary gain. Frequent visits to the physician can become almost a way of life that interferes with meeting other family obligations. Dependency needs are often unrecognized and get gratified through physical illness. An individual's symptom may become an ongoing focus in the family. The overfunctioning family member may in subtle ways reinforce and perpetuate the somatic symptoms until an entrenched pattern exists.

➤ **Impaired social interaction** related to withdrawal and chronic pain

RATIONALE: A massive withdrawal from the environment occurs as the individual focuses on self and body sensations. This further escalates the pain and physical symptoms.

Additional Nursing Diagnoses

Chronic low self-esteem
Ineffective denial
Knowledge deficit
Powerlessness

Dissociative Disorders

DSM-IV Dissociative Disorders

300.14   Dissociative identity disorder
300.15   Dissociative disorder
300.60   Depersonalization disorder

Nursing Diagnoses for DSM-IV *300.14, 300.15, 300.60*

➤ **Anxiety/fear** related to acute situational stressors

RATIONALE: The transition from feeling normal to an altered state is usually sudden and is often triggered by psychosocial stress. Anxiety is experienced as the person feels no longer in control of behavior or feelings.

➤ **Personal identity disturbance** related to alteration in the normally integrative functions of identity

RATIONALE: In dissociative disorders, the normal integrative functions of identity, memory, or consciousness are disturbed. With multiple-personality disorder, the person's identity is forgotten and a new one assumed. With depersonalization disorder, the feeling of one's own reality is lost. With a disturbance in memory, important personal events cannot be recalled.

➤ **Ineffective individual coping** related to alterations in consciousness, severe anxiety

RATIONALE: The disruption of feeling unreal, losing one's memory, or dealing with multiple personalities often leads to substance abuse, self-mutilation (in an effort to feel real), suicide attempts, and violence toward others.

Additional Nursing Diagnoses

Body-image disturbance
Chronic low self-esteem
Decisional conflict
Hopelessness
Ineffective family coping: disabling
Knowledge deficit

Adjustment Disorder

DSM-IV Adjustment Disorder

309.00   With depressed mood
309.24   With anxiety

Nursing Diagnoses for DSM-IV 309.00, 309.24

➤ **Impaired adjustment** related to identifiable, acute, or enduring psychosocial stressor(s)

RATIONALE: An adjustment disorder occurs when a person has an unusually intense reaction to a stressor(s) that impairs functioning in occupational and social activities. The maladaptive reaction occurs within three months of the onset of the stressor.

➤ **Anxiety** related to ineffective coping strategy

RATIONALE: Anxiety, manifested by worry, nervousness, and jitteriness, is a common symptom that develops in response to a psychosocial stressor. The degree of anxiety is usually out of proportion to the intensity of the stressor.

➤ **Situational low self-esteem** related to impaired occupational/social role functioning

RATIONALE: Depression, feelings of hopelessness, and crying are common manifestations of an adjustment disorder. Difficulties at work and in relationships contribute to feelings to low self-esteem.

Additional Nursing Diagnoses

Decisional conflict
Ineffective family coping: compromised
Ineffective individual coping
Knowledge deficit
Powerlessness
Spiritual distress

Personality Disorders

DSM-IV Personality Disorders

301.83   Borderline
301.70   Antisocial

Nursing Diagnoses for DSM-IV *301.83*

➤ **Personal identity disturbance** related to overused defenses: splitting and projective identification

RATIONALE: There is an inability to integrate aspects of the self into a relatively coherent and acceptable sense of self in the borderline personality. This instability of self-image leads to chronic feelings of emptiness and boredom.

➤ **Chronic low self-esteem** related to low achievement

RATIONALE: Borderline behavior is highly unpredictable. These people rarely achieve up to their level of ability. They are often employed in low-level positions and use their leisure time poorly. Repetitive self-destructive acts contribute to feelings of low self-esteem and worthlessness.

➤ **Ineffective individual coping** related to impulsive behavior, self-destructive behavior, acting out

RATIONALE: Impulsiveness is usually in areas that are potentially dangerous to the self (e.g., sex, spending, reckless driving, substance abuse, binge eating). The person is unable to control the impulsive behavior whatever the consequences.

➤ **Impaired social interaction** related to intense anger, uncertainty, unstable affect

RATIONALE: Because both dependency and hostility are intensely felt, the interpersonal relationships of borderlines are tumultuous. Marked mood swings, inappropriately intense anger, and uncertainty about choice of friends or lovers result in chaotic relationships. The borderline uses the mechanism of splitting to react to people as "all good" and idealize them, or as "all bad" and devalue them.

➤ **Spiritual distress** related to feelings of emptiness, meaninglessness, lack of long-term goals and values

RATIONALE: Chronic feelings of emptiness and boredom can stimulate a crisis in meaninglessness. An inability to decide which values to adopt and concerns about religious identification and moral issues can lead to spiritual distress.

➤ **Decisional conflict** related to self-doubt, low self-worth, depression

RATIONALE: The uncertainty regarding long-term goals may be expressed as inability to choose a career, to decide what friends to have, or which religion to follow.

➤ **Fear** related to perceived abandonment issues

RATIONALE: People with disturbed identity have difficulty tolerating being alone, and will avoid abandonment at all costs. The fear of abandonment keeps borderlines in destructive relationships long after these would normally have ended. Often they will demonstrate clinging behavior when they sense rejection is forthcoming.

➤ **Potential for violence: self-directed** related to impulsiveness, self-mutilating behavior

RATIONALE: In more severe cases of borderline personality disorder, recurrent suicidal gestures and self-mutilating behavior are common. This may serve to manipulate others, to express intense anger, or to counteract feelings of numbness that are experienced during stress.

➤ **Potential for violence: directed at others** related to intense/inappropriate expression of anger

RATIONALE: Borderlines frequently display a terrible temper and constant anger and engage in recurrent physical fights. Impulsive behavior such as reckless driving can result in injury to others.

➤ **Impaired adjustment** related to unmet childhood dependency needs

RATIONALE: These clients long for an intimate relationship but have approach-avoidance conflicts. While longing for intimacy, they also fear being engulfed so will do something to alienate the other person. Their life becomes chaotic and crisis prone. Fearing dependency, but also needing to be dependent, they will set up a crisis in which the caregiver must take control and set limits on behavior.

➤ **Risk for self-mutilation** related to impulsiveness, intense anger, and self-destructive behavior

RATIONALE: Deliberate destruction of body tissue without conscious intent of suicide is a symptom associated with borderline personality disorder as well as with other diagnoses. The behavior is generally impulsive and the onset is linked to a stressful situation. It serves many purposes, such as releasing tension or anger, punishing oneself, feeling powerful, and in controlling and manipulating others.

Nursing Diagnoses for DSM-IV 301.70

➤ **Impaired adjustment** related to repeated failure in age-appropriate roles

RATIONALE: Antisocial individuals demonstrate a pattern of irresponsibility, characterized by failure to honor financial obligations and inability to sustain consistent work.

➤ **Ineffective individual coping** related to substance abuse, repeated violation of social norms

RATIONALE: There is a high rate of substance abuse among sociopaths, as well as a failure to conform to social norms. Persons with this disorder are frequently in trouble with the law and more often end up in prison than in a hospital for treatment.

➤ **Impaired social interaction** related to inability to sustain long-term relationships, lack of empathy

RATIONALE: Antisocial individuals have a greatly impaired capacity to sustain lasting, close, responsible relationships. Even though they are often superficially quite charming, they are known for conning and manipulating others for personal profit and pleasure.

➤ **Potential for violence: directed at others** related to aggressiveness

RATIONALE: Repeated physical fights, including spouse and child abuse, are often seen with antisocial personalities. There is a reckless disregard for others' safety as indicated by reckless driving and driving while intoxicated.

Additional Nursing Diagnoses

Ineffective family coping: compromised
Knowledge deficit

DSM-IV Personality Disorders

301.60   Dependent
301.82   Avoidant

Nursing Diagnoses for DSM-IV 301.60

➤ **Decisional conflict** related to excessive dependency

RATIONALE: Excessive dependence on others results in the dependent personality allowing others to make all or most significant decisions. Without a great deal of support and advice from others, these people are unable to make everyday decisions.

➤ **Powerlessness** related to inability to communicate effectively, lack of assertive skills

RATIONALE: Dependent people rely so heavily on others that they feel helpless when alone. They feel powerless to succeed in the world on their own and do not have the initiative to begin new projects or make plans.

➤ **Chronic low self-esteem** related to inability to express feelings

RATIONALE: The dependent personality has a low self-concept and sees him- or herself as incapable, less than, and in need of protection. The inability to be alone and to initiate activity lead to limited opportunities to develop abilities and talents that would build healthy self-esteem.

➤ **Fear** related to perceived threat of abandonment

RATIONALE: Dependent people are frequently preoccupied with fears of being abandoned and feel devastated and helpless when close personal relationships end.

Nursing Diagnoses for DSM-IV 301.82

➤ **Social isolation** related to fear of criticism, rejection

RATIONALE: The avoidant personality fears negative evaluation from others and is easily hurt by any hint of disapproval. She or he avoids relationships to protect self from criticism, thus has no close friendships.

➤ **Anxiety/fear** related to social discomfort

RATIONALE: Avoidant personalities yearn for social contact and acceptance but fear being unacceptable. They feel too intimidated to initiate and maintain relationships. They worry about embarrassing themselves, saying the wrong thing, or having unsurmountable difficulties in new situations. Specific phobias may be present.

➤ **Chronic low self-esteem** related to negative labeling of self

RATIONALE: Depression is often present because the person desires social contact but is unable to achieve it. The person is angry at him- or herself for being fearful.

Additional Nursing Diagnoses

Altered sexuality patterns
Impaired adjustment
Impaired social interaction
Ineffective family coping: compromised
Ineffective individual coping
Knowledge deficit

Eating Disorders

DSM-IV Eating Disorders

307.10 Anorexia nervosa
307.51 Bulimia nervosa

Nursing Diagnoses for DSM-IV *307.10, 307.51*

➤ **Body-image disturbance** related to distorted perceptions of body sensations

RATIONALE: Patients with an eating disorder are preoccupied with their body size and shape, and are dissatisfied with their appearance. They say that they "feel fat" even when very thin and emaciated looking. Excessive exercising, not eating, vomiting, and use of laxatives are all attempts at reducing body size.

➤ **Altered nutrition: less than body requirements** related to self-induced vomiting, low calorie intake

RATIONALE: Severe weight loss and life-threatening metabolic changes result from a reduction in total food intake. Binge eating and vomiting can lead to electrolyte imbalances, dental problems, hypokalemic alkalosis, esophageal tears, and cardiac arrhythmias.

➤ **Ineffective individual coping** related to compulsive behavior concerning food intake

RATIONALE: The individual feels a lack of control over eating behavior during binges. Disordered eating is a method of coping with anxiety, stress, and underlying conflicts of dependency, separation, identity, and sexuality.

➤ **Ineffective denial** related to distorted body perceptions

RATIONALE: People with eating disorders will deny or minimize the severity of their illness. They tend to be very resistive to therapy and quite manipulative once they are hospitalized for treatment. They will adamantly refuse to maintain a normal body weight.

➤ **Anxiety/fear** related to loss of control

RATIONALE: The person with anorexia has an intense fear of gaining weight and becoming obese. This fear contributes to a distorted body perception. A lack of self-esteem and ineffectiveness lead to the need to control at least one aspect of life. A focus on mastery of weight and eating can lead to feelings of extraordinary accomplishment.

➤ **Altered thought processes** related to distorted body image

RATIONALE: With anorexia, there is often a lack of recognition of fatigue, weakness, and hunger that allows the individual to continue with excessive exercising and low food intake. The person also has a distorted perception of own body size.

➤ **Social isolation** related to chronic low self-esteem

RATIONALE: Alienation and isolation from family and peers happens as others fail to understand the meaning of the self-destructive behavior. Guilt at not being able to control the problem leads to self-dislike and more sporadic self-denial or indulgence, which further contributes to a negative self-concept.

➤ **Noncompliance** related to chronic nature of eating disorder, lack of situational/financial resources, need to minimize seriousness of condition.

RATIONALE: People who are noncompliant with recommended healthcare activities are generally aware that they have chosen not to care for themselves. Being asymptomatic or unable to afford treatment are often used as rationalizations to alleviate underlying anxiety.

➤ **Risk for self-mutilation** related to compulsive behaviors

RATIONALE: Feelings of depression, rejection, self-hatred, separation anxiety, and fluctuating emotions contribute to the patient deliberately injuring self to release tension.

Additional Nursing Diagnoses

Ineffective family coping: compromised
Knowledge deficit

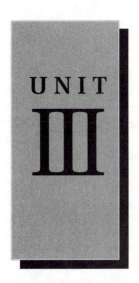

UNIT III

Nursing Care Plans for NANDA Nursing Diagnoses

(Categorized According to Human Response Patterns)

Contents

I. Exchanging

A. NUTRITION

1. Altered Nutrition: More than Body Requirements

Definition

The state in which an individual experiences an intake of nutrients that exceeds metabolic needs

Related to

- Excessive intake in relation to metabolic need
- Altered satiety patterns
- Anxiety
- Boredom
- Decreased activity patterns
- Decreased metabolic needs
- Decreased self-esteem
- Decreased sense of taste and smell
- Depression
- Guilt
- Lack of basic nutritional knowledge
- Lack of motivation
- Lack of self-confidence
- Loneliness
- Stress

Characteristics/Assessment Findings

- Weight 10% over ideal for height and frame
- *Weight 20% over ideal for height and frame
- Triceps skin fold greater than 15 mm in males, 25 mm in females
- Sedentary activity level
- Reported or observed dysfunctional eating patterns (e.g., pairing food with other activities)
- Concentrating food intake at end of day
- Eating in response to external cues (e.g., time of day, social situation)
- History of obesity in one or both parents
- Verbalization that food is used as a reward/comfort measure
- Verbalization of inability to cope with internal and external stressors
- Weight fluctuation over past 10 years

Expected Outcomes/Goals

The patient will
- regain and maintain ideal body weight as evidenced by keeping a weekly weight graph.
- change both attitude and behavior toward weight control as evidenced by maintenance of a weekly food and behavior diary.
- demonstrate a sense of self-control and personal satisfaction as evidenced by
  - consistent weight-loss pattern
  - verbalization of positive feelings about self.
- develop a systematic approach to maintain weight loss and to prevent weight gain as evidenced by adherence to a weight-control program.

Content appearing in this typeface is additional information not included in the NANDA nursing diagnoses.

*Critical.

Nursing Orders with Rationale

➤ Assess and monitor for presence/absence/ changes in assessment findings outlined above *in order to detect any change in status.*

➤ Perform a nutritional assessment (i.e., triceps skin fold measurement, height, weight, diet history) *to establish a baseline for future weight-loss pattern (Krause & Mahan, 1984).*

➤ Provide frequent non–food-related, positive reinforcement (e.g., praise) *to reinforce behavior changes, weight loss, motivation, self-confidence (Brownell, 1984).*

➤ Encourage participation in weight-control classes, exercise programs, established dietary regimens *to foster adherence to a weight-loss program by development feelings of belonging (Bjorntorp, 1983).*

➤ Discuss myths about food and eating, especially those that prevent weight loss *to change beliefs, attitudes, and thoughts by interpreting reality in new and different ways (Griffiths, 1981).*

➤ Help to identify internal and external cues that increase desire to eat, response to these cues *to develop strategies for behavioral change (i.e., methods for controlling environment, physiological or psychological responses to food) (Ames & Kneisl, 1986).*

➤ Help patient to set realistic goals for self *to give patient an opportunity for success (Sanger & Cassino, 1984).*

➤ Encourage family/significant other(s) to praise weight-loss achievements, to avoid tempting patient with foods, to provide nonfood rewards, and to support patient during situational crises. *This support will help patient's effort to adhere to the weight-control program (Caine & Bufalino, 1987).*

➤ Help patient to express feelings about eating behaviors and factors that cause overeating *to develop an objective, in-control attitude that is conducive to building self-esteem (Wineman, 1980).*

➤ Weigh weekly *to document and reinforce a pattern of weight loss (Christian & Greger, 1985).*

➤ Instruct regarding
  ▷ keeping a weekly weight graph, food and behavior diary
    to help analyze accurately biopsychosocial events associated with food-intake behavior (Christian & Greger, 1985).

  ▷ ways to take control of eating behaviors (e.g., appetite management techniques such as distraction, activities)
    to promote successful accomplishment of weight loss (Christian & Greger, 1985).

  ▷ healthy eating behaviors (e.g., location of eating, activities while eating, speed of eating, attractiveness of setting, amount of food, preplanning meals)
    to assist incorporating healthy eating behaviors into life-style (Harris, 1983).

Charting Components

➤ Detailed record of food and fluids ingested, feelings and behaviors while eating
➤ Eating patterns
➤ Expressed feelings about eating behaviors, body image, weight
➤ Goals formulated by patient
➤ Observed or reported behaviors that promote/ hinder weight loss
➤ Verbalization of intent to maintain weight-control program after discharge
➤ Weekly weight
➤ Patient/family teaching, response

2. Altered Nutrition: Less than Body Requirements

Definition

The state in which an individual experiences an intake of nutrients insufficient to meet metabolic needs

Related to

➤ Inability to ingest or digest food or to absorb nutrients due to biological, psychological, or economic factors (e.g., limited financial resources, low socioeconomic background)

➤ Purging and vomiting
➤ Increased anxiety, loneliness
➤ Impulsive behavior
➤ Ambivalent feelings regarding food
➤ Inappropriate food choices
➤ Partial consumption of meals

Characteristics/Assessment Findings

➤ Loss of weight with adequate food intake
➤ Body weight 20% or more under ideal
➤ Reported inadequate food intake less than recommended daily allowance (RDA)
➤ Reported or evidence of lack of food
➤ Aversion to eating
➤ Satiety immediately after ingesting food
➤ Abdominal pain with or without pathology
➤ Capillary fragility
➤ Abdominal cramping
➤ Diarrhea/steatorrhea
➤ Hyperactive bowel sounds
➤ Lack of interest in food
➤ Perceived inability to ingest food
➤ Pale conjunctival and mucous membranes
➤ Poor muscle tone
➤ Excessive loss of hair
➤ Lack of information, misinformation
➤ Decreased lymphocyte count, serum albumin, serum transferrin, or iron-binding capacity
➤ Inability to prepare meals
➤ Pattern of decreased dietary intake
➤ Weight fluctuation over past 10 years
➤ Misconceptions
➤ Excessive laxative use
➤ Problems with teeth and gums
➤ Amenorrhea
➤ Hirsutism (e.g., lanugo, hair)
➤ Excessive exercise

Expected Outcomes/Goals

The patient will
➤ accept and adjust to a comprehensive program of weight management as evidenced by
  ▷ decreasing or being free from binging and purging episodes
  ▷ absence of electrolyte imbalance, cardiac dysrhythmia, and other complications of altered nutrition.
➤ regain/maintain ideal body weight for height and age as evidenced by weekly weight graph.

➤ identify sources of problem and means of coping with factors that hinder ingestion of an adequate dietary intake as evidenced by verbalization of problems and coping mechanisms.
➤ develop a nutritional program adequate to maintain designated weight when discharged as evidenced by a written plan.

Nursing Orders with Rationale

➤ Assess and monitor for presence/absence/ changes in assessment findings outlined above *in order to detect any change in status.*

➤ Observe all food intake *to determine adequacy of amount and type (Ames & Kneisl, 1986).*

➤ Provide opportunities for discussion of factors that prevent ingestion of adequate intake *to develop strategies that may be developed to alter events that adversely affect nutritional status (Wineman, 1980).*

➤ Remove all noxious stimuli from immediate environment during mealtime; offer structured support *to provide a pleasant setting (Harris, 1983).*

➤ Avoid discussing food or somatic complaints during meals; focus on pleasant topics and praise patient's ability to consume meals within prescribed time period. *Eating/not eating is a symptom of a problem of control, anxiety, loneliness, and need for nurturance (Davies & Janosik, 1991).*

➤ Determine food preferences *so these can be included in diet if allowed (Harris, 1983).*

➤ Weigh daily at the same time, with same type of clothing, after emptying bladder *to determine pattern of weight fluctuation (Morgan, 1984).*

➤ Give positive reinforcement for weight gained rather than amount of food eaten. *Reinforce the outcome goal rather than the means of achieving it.*

Content appearing in this typeface is additional information not included in the NANDA nursing diagnoses.

➤ Avoid power struggles over eating; set firm limits, monitor patient, and institute consequences without a punitive attitude.
    Power struggles only serve to reinforce the patient's need to maintain control through not eating.

➤ Assist patient to experience "control" in ways other than eating; see nursing care plan "Powerlessness" for more interventions on how to increase feelings of power.
    Persons with eating disorders use inappropriate attempts to achieve control through unusual eating behavior and exercise.

➤ Assist patient to recognize and verbalize factors leading to binging (e.g., when patient feels needy or anxious, lack of impulse control) in order to develop alternative ways to nurture self at these times.
    Binging is related to increased anxiety, loneliness, or impulsive behavior (Davies & Janosik, 1991).

➤ Supervise patients closely during and after meals; support patient in dealing with emotional discomfort during meals.
    The patient with an eating disorder had ambivalence regarding food. Attempts to maneuver staff and other patients by talking, crying, delayed or hurried eating, preoccupation with calorie counting, or secretive behavior serve to take focus off eating behavior.

➤ Provide and monitor intake of snacks and supplemental feedings
    to decrease inadequate food intake related to inappropriate food choices and partial consumption of meals.

➤ Institute close one-to-one supervision with bathroom restriction after meals.
    The patient with bulimia is at risk for purging through vomiting, use of laxatives/diuretics, or exercise.

➤ Monitor lab reports (e.g., serum electrolytes, hemoglobin, hematocrit, serum albumin, transferrin or iron-binding capacity, lymphocyte count)
    to evaluate the liver's production of transport proteins and to determine protein status (Blackburn, 1981).

➤ Administer tube feedings, hyperalimentation, or IV feedings as ordered
    to prevent self-starvation and electrolyte imbalances that result in malnutrition, recurrent infections, and cardiac disorders (Reighley, 1988).

➤ Hold staff conferences to discuss and evaluate the plan of care; designate one person as primary therapist to ensure consistency and to minimize manipulation of staff; refer to nursing care plan "Impaired Social Interaction (Borderline Personality Disorder)" for interventions about manipulation.
    Patients with eating disorders tend to use manipulation around the intake of food and purging/binding. Staff cohesiveness is essential in implementing an effective plan of care.

➤ Encourage attendance at all unit group activities
    to decrease feelings of isolation.

➤ Refer to dietician or nutritional support team
    to provide comprehensive dietary management.

➤ Explain all procedures to patient and family
    to reinforce plan of care (Baker, 1984).

➤ Instruct patient regarding basic nutrition
    to ensure that the patient and family possess sufficient knowledge to provide adequate food intake (Suitor & Hunter, 1980).

➤ Reinforce patient's attendance at Overeaters Anonymous or similar community self-help group.
    Facilitating ongoing support after discharge will counteract the denial that is often present with eating disorders.

Charting Components

➤ Abdominal cramping, discomfort
➤ Daily intake (food, fluids) and output
➤ Daily weights; notation of weight loss or gain
➤ Feelings about present status (weight, emotional problems, appearance)
➤ Interest in food
➤ Muscle tone
➤ Nursing action used to enable patient to obtain adequate nutrition
➤ Patient response concerning attitudes toward eating
➤ Patient response to nursing actions
➤ Purging, use of laxatives
➤ Patient/family teaching, response

B. PHYSICAL REGULATION

1. Constipation

Definition

A state in which an individual experiences a change in normal bowel habits characterized by a decrease in frequency/passage of hard, dry stools

Related to

- Diarrhea (irritable bowel)
- Depression
- Anticholinergic effects of psychotropic medications (e.g., antidepressants, antipsychotics)
- Lack of/inadequate dietary fiber
- Inadequate fluid intake
- Decreased activity level
- Stress
- Chronic use of medications and enemas
- Lack of privacy during defecation
- Diagnostic procedures
- Neuromuscular impairment
- Musculoskeletal impairment
- Pain on defecation
- Laxative abuse
- Anorexia

Characteristics/Assessment Findings

- Decreased activity level
- Frequency less than usual pattern
- Hard, formed stools
- Palpable mass
- Reported feeling of pressure in rectum
- Reported feeling of rectal fullness
- Straining at stool

Other Possible Characteristics
- Abdominal pain
- Appetite impairment
- Back pain
- Headache
- Interference with daily living
- Use of laxatives
- Decreased bowel sounds
- Less than usual amount of stool
- Abdominal distention
- Impaction
- Feeling of incomplete bowel evacuation

Expected Outcomes/Goals

The patient will
- establish a program to repattern bowel elimination as evidenced by return of usual pattern of elimination.
- increase intake of fluids and fiber as evidenced by
  - drinking 8 to 10 glasses of water daily
  - eating bran and high-fiber vegetables
- increase activity level as evidenced by
  - walking as often as tolerated
  - performing range-of-motion exercises within tolerance.

Nursing Orders with Rationale

- Assess and monitor for presence/absence/changes in assessment findings outlined above *in order to detect any change in status.*

- Assess patient's usual bowel elimination pattern, routine, and significant factors that brought about the constipation.
  Awareness of the causes of the problem reduces the anxiety associated with the unknown and decreases the potential for recurrence of the problem (Gettrust, Ryan, & Engleman, 1985).

- Assist patient to establish a pattern for elimination:
  - allow a regular time for bowel elimination, preferably at an unhurried hour of the day.
    This body system functions best when a regular schedule is followed (Gettrust et al., 1985).

  - encourage patient to sit on the toilet for approximately 10 minutes following one meal each day, preferably breakfast.
    Mass movement occurs after meals (McFarland & McFarlane, 1989).

  - provide privacy during defecation (e.g., close door, draw curtains, keep room deodorizer available, play TV or radio to mask sounds).
    This will help to create a more relaxed atmosphere (McFarland & McFarlane, 1989).

Content appearing in this typeface is additional information not included in the NANDA nursing diagnoses.

➤ Encourage intake of foods high in fiber and bulk (e.g., fresh fruits and vegetables with skin, bran, nuts/seeds, whole grain breads and cereals); explain importance of maintaining this intake after discharge.

Fiber helps to increase the water content of stool, making it softer and easier to pass. Bulk helps to increase the fluid content in stools, to decrease transmit time in the colon, to increase the weight of stool, and to normalize stool consistency (McFarland & McFarlane, 1989).

➤ Instruct patient/significant other about the importance of drinking 8 to 10 glasses of water every day (including a glass of warm water 30 minutes before breakfast), if not medically contraindicated.

When the body lacks fluids the colon compensates by increasing the amount of water absorbed from stool, making the stool hard and dry (McFarland & McFarlane, 1989).

➤ If patient's life-style is sedentary, instruct on the importance of increasing activity level (e.g., walking).

Activity improves muscle tone, stimulates appetite and peristalsis (Carpenito, 1989).

➤ Collaborate with physician regarding giving a mild laxative or stool softener.

Patients on high doses of psychotropic medications may require a mild, bulk-forming laxative (Haber, Hoskins, Leach, & Sidelau, 1987).

Charting Components

➤ Activity level, frequency
➤ Adherence to bowel management regimen
➤ Appetite; food and fluid intake, amount, type
➤ Effects/side effects of medications
➤ Frequency of bowel movement; stool amount, consistency, color
➤ Patient statements of rectal pressure, rectal fullness, abdominal pain, back pain, headache, straining during defecation
➤ Presence of bowel sounds, abdominal distention, palpable mass
➤ Presence of hemorrhoids
➤ Patient/family teaching, response

C. CIRCULATION

1. Fluid Volume Deficit

Definition

The state in which an individual experiences vascular, cellular, or intracellular dehydration

Related to

➤ Failure of regulatory mechanisms, as in
  ▷ electrolyte balance
  ▷ fever
  ▷ increased metabolic rate
➤ Active loss, as in
  ▷ excessive muscle activity
  ▷ excessive urinary loss
  ▷ vomiting or gastric suction

Characteristics/Assessment Findings

➤ Failure of regulatory mechanisms
  ▷ dilute urine
  ▷ increased urine output
  ▷ sudden weight loss

Other Possible Characteristics
  ▷ possible weight gain
  ▷ hypotension
  ▷ decreased venous filling
  ▷ increased pulse rate
  ▷ decreased skin turgor
  ▷ decreased pulse volume/pressure
  ▷ increased body temperature
  ▷ dry skin
  ▷ dry mucous membranes
  ▷ hemoconcentration
  ▷ weakness
  ▷ edema
  ▷ thirst
➤ Active loss
  ▷ concentrated urine
  ▷ decreased urine output
  ▷ decreased venous filling
  ▷ increased serum sodium
  ▷ hemoconcentration
  ▷ output greater than intake
  ▷ sudden weight loss

Other Possible Characteristics
  ▷ change in mental state
  ▷ decreased pulse volume/pressure
  ▷ decreased skin turgor
  ▷ dry mucous membranes
  ▷ dry skin
  ▷ hypotension
  ▷ increased body temperature
  ▷ increased pulse rate
  ▷ thirst
  ▷ weakness

Expected Outcomes/Goals

The patient will restore/maintain adequate fluid volume as evidence by
➤ decrease in/absence of the initial assessment findings

Content appearing in this typeface is additional information not included in the NANDA nursing diagnoses.

➤ blood pressure, pulse, respirations within normal range
➤ electrolytes (e.g., sodium and potassium) within normal range.

Nursing Orders with Rationale

➤ Assess and monitor for presence/absence/ changes in assessment findings outlined above *in order to detect any change in status.*

➤ Monitor for mental status changes (e.g., confusion, restlessness, anxiety, agitation).
Changes in mental status may indicate increasing dehydration.

➤ Be alert to edema or changes in fluid disposition throughout the body (e.g., increasing abdominal girth).
Extracellular fluid may occur in patients experiencing withdrawal symptoms, particularly if circulatory/hepatic/CHF/pulmonary edema problems coexist.

➤ Monitor and record I&O at least once a shift or prn; notify physician if urine output is less than 30 cc/h or more than 200 cc/h for 2 hours consecutively.
Changes in I&O are early signs of impending dehydration or shock (Caine & Bufalino, 1987).

➤ Monitor specific gravity q2 to 4h; report if greater than 1.025 or less than 1.010.
Specific gravity will be elevated when the urine is hemoconcentrated and when excess water is being lost; both conditions may indicate problems for the patient.

➤ Monitor and record amount and types of fluid losses (e.g., perspiration, number of linen or clothing changes)
to recognize excessive loss of fluid and to intervene as indicated.

➤ Monitor vital signs q1 to 2h or more frequently if unstable; pay particular attention to patient's temperature.
Increased heart rate and temperature reflect an increased metabolic rate associated with withdrawal. Circulatory collapse and hyperthermia are the two leading causes of death associated with delirium tremens (Luckmann & Sorensen, 1987).

➤ Monitor serum electrolytes at least every shift
to recognize signs of related electrolyte imbalances (e.g., hyponatremia, hyperkalemia, hypocalcemia, hypermagnesemia) (Caine & Bufalino, 1987).

➤ Monitor fluid replacement carefully; be alert to indications of fluid overload (e.g., cough, basilar rales, cyanosis, dyspnea, bounding pulse).
Normal adult fluid intake is between 1500 and 2000 cc/day. Patients with withdrawal symptoms frequently have preexisting medical conditions that make it critical to recognize the effectiveness of treatment and the possibility of fluid overload (Brunner & Suddarth, 1988).

➤ Give medications as ordered; evaluate effects/ side effects.
Medications given during withdrawal frequently include sedatives, antiemetics, and antipyretics. Close monitoring can detect any change in status or complications (Brunner & Suddarth, 1988).

➤ Weigh daily at same time, in same clothing, on same scale
to note trends in weight changes.

➤ Provide oral care q4h (e.g., brushing teeth, rinsing mouth)
to prevent drying, cracking, and encrustation of oral mucous membranes (Luckmann & Sorensen, 1987).

➤ Assist with getting out of bed or transferring
to prevent injury as a result of postural hypotension.

➤ Provide cool moist towels for comfort.
Hyperthermia is a problem; placing cool moist towels on the forehead and trunk may help reduce the temperature.

➤ Explain the purpose of all interventions; stress the importance of adhering to medical regimen.

➤ Have suction equipment available if vomiting is likely in an unresponsive patient.

Charting Components

➤ Effects/side effects of medication
➤ I&O
➤ Mental status changes
➤ Signs/symptoms of fluid imbalance
➤ Skin condition: color, moisture, turgor
➤ Urine specific gravity
➤ Vital signs
➤ Weight
➤ Patient/family teaching, response

D. PHYSICAL INTEGRITY

1. Potential for Injury/Trauma

Definition

A state in which the individual is at risk of injury as a result of environmental conditions interacting with the individual's adaptive and defensive resources

Related to

See risk factors below.

Characteristics/Assessment Findings

- ➤ Presence of internal risk factors
  - ➢ biochemical, regulatory function (sensory dysfunction, integrative dysfunction, effector dysfunction, tissue hypoxia)
  - ➢ malnutrition
  - ➢ psychologic factors (affective, orientation)
  - ➢ developmental age (physiological, psychosocial)
- ➤ Presence of individual internal factors
  - ➢ weakness
  - ➢ balancing difficulties
  - ➢ reduced hand-eye coordination
  - ➢ cognitive or emotional difficulties
  - ➢ history of previous trauma
  - ➢ confusion, disorientation
  - ➢ decreased mobility, gait disorder, poor coordination
  - ➢ seizures
  - ➢ syncope
  - ➢ taking psychotropic drugs
  - ➢ vertigo
- ➤ Presence of external risk factors
  - ➢ chemical (e.g., pollutants, poisons, drugs, pharmaceutical agents, alcohol, caffeine, nicotine, preservatives, cosmetics and dyes, nutrients)
  - ➢ physical (e.g., design, structure, and arrangement of building, equipment)
  - ➢ people/provider (e.g., staffing patterns; cognitive, affective, and psychomotor factors)
  - ➢ environmental (e.g., bathtub without hand grip or antislip equipment, entering unlighted rooms, litter or liquid spills on floor)

Expected Outcomes/Goals

The patient will be free from injury from trauma/falls as evidenced by

- ➤ patient/family verbal report
- ➤ absences of fractures, bruises, contusions
- ➤ x-rays.

Nursing Orders with Rationale

- ➤ Assess and monitor for presence/absence/changes in assessment findings outlined above *in order to detect any changes in status.*

For Internal Risk Factors

- ➤ Question patients concerning the use of alcohol or drugs *to identify individuals at risk for injury/trauma as a result of withdrawal symptoms.*

- ➤ Orient patients to the environment with each contact. *Continued orientation to the environment may minimize confusion.*

- ➤ Incorporate fall-prevention strategies into care planning for all patients with confusion, gait disorders, weakness, visual impairment; supervise/assist high-risk patients with transfers or ambulation as needed. *Environmental protective strategies ensure basic safety and security needs of high-risk patients.*

- ➤ Be aware of factors that may alter mobility (e.g., weakness from withdrawal/treatment, medications) *to detect subtle changes that may be warning signs of problems.*

- ➤ Reevaluate the potential for falls any time medication therapy is changed. *Changes in medications may cause the patient to experience disorientation or neuromuscular alterations.*

Content appearing in this typeface is additional information not included in the NANDA nursing diagnoses.

➤ Analyze all falls or near falls for factors that led up to them
>
> *to help develop more effective fall-prevention strategies.*

For External Risk Factors

➤ Use restraints to protect patient from injury; use with caution and concern for the patient's civil liberties; comply with all facility policies/procedures regarding the use of restraints.
>
> *Each facility has specific guidelines for using restraints, which protect both the patient and staff. The least restrictive environment that ensures patient safety is mandated (Sclafani, 1986).*

➤ Explain the purpose of restraints to the patient (e.g., "These restraints are necessary to keep you from hurting yourself. We will remove them when you are able to take control of your behavior.").
>
> *Ensure that the patient knows that the restraints are not designed as punishment.*

➤ Select the type of restraint that will be most effective, yet least constrictive for the patient (cloth vest, cloth wrist/ankle restraints, or leather wrist/ankle restraints).
>
> *A wide variety of restraints is available and the nurse must choose the type that will serve to protect the patient while minimizing the risk of injury associated with the treatment.*

➤ Monitor skin condition and circulation of all tissues surrounding restraints at least q15-min.
>
> *Restraints may interfere with circulation and innervation to tissues surrounding the restraints.*

➤ Offer nourishment and fluids
>
> *to maintain hydration and nutritional status.*

➤ Ensure that patient is in the best possible alignment and posture while restrained, considering the degree of combativeness present.
>
> *Patients may potentially be in one position for an extended period of time.*

➤ Follow hospital protocol when releasing patient from restraints
>
> *to ensure safety of the patient.*

➤ Use crisis team when taking patient to bathroom; do not attempt to assist patient alone.
>
> *Potential for violence decreases when assaultive patient senses she or he can be overpowered (Sclafani, 1986).*

➤ Maintain visual contact with the patient experiencing withdrawal symptoms.
>
> *It is important for staff to observe patients experiencing withdrawal symptoms because these patients are unable to protect themselves.*

Charting Components

➤ Activities to reduce hazards
➤ Amount of assistance needed/given
➤ Dizziness, weakness, disorientation, confusion
➤ Effects/side effects of medication
➤ Explanation to patient/significant others
➤ Nerve and circulatory checks to tissues surrounding restraints
➤ Onset and symptoms indicating detoxification/withdrawal
➤ Purpose of restraints
➤ Release times of extremities, final release of patient
➤ Response to restraints
➤ Type of restraints applied to specific parts of the body

Additional Nursing Orders for THE PATIENT WITH SEIZURES

Before Seizure Begins

➤ Determine previous frequency of seizure activity and the typical length of each seizure.
>
> *Typically patients will describe consistent behaviors during the seizure and a specific duration for the tonic/clonic phase. This information allows the nurse to recognize deviation and to take immediate action (e.g., if the patient's typical seizure lasts for 30 to 45 seconds and the current one is 1 minute, then action can be initiated to prevent status epilepticus).*

➤ Keep side rails up at all times while patient is in bed; maintain bed in low position.
>
> *Seizures are generally unpredictable.*

➤ Pad side rails with pillows if seizure activity is frequent
>
> *to decrease the risk of bruises and contusions to body parts hitting the rails.*

➤ Take only rectal or axillary temperature if seizure activity is frequent; do not use glass thermometers for oral temperatures
>
> *to prevent injury/trauma.*

➤ Keep oral bite block at bedside at all times; avoid using padded tongue blades because the patient may bite improperly made blades in half.
   If there is warning prior to seizure, place bite block or wash cloth in patient's mouth; do not try to place anything in mouth once the seizure has started and the teeth are clenched (Brunner & Suddarth, 1988).

➤ Ensure patient takes medications correctly.
   Maintaining the blood level of anticovulsant medication decreases the possibility of seizure activity.

During Seizure Activity

➤ Note time seizure begins.
   Seizure activity increases the body's oxygen consumption and fatigue. Length of seizure will determine the long-term risk, fatigue, and possible brain damage.

➤ Maintain a calm attitude; instruct onlookers to leave.
   Protecting privacy is essential for the patient's psychosocial health.

➤ Protect patient's head: ease patient to the floor, if standing; position pillow or lap under patient's head, if lying on the floor
   to prevent head injury during seizure.

➤ Position bite block in mouth **only** if mouth is open and teeth are not clenched; avoid causing trauma to mouth and teeth by forcing bite block.
   Biting the tongue and gnashing teeth are common during a seizure. Do not attempt to place anything in patient's mouth once the teeth are clenched (Luckmann & Sorensen, 1987).

➤ Loosen clothing or restrictive items; remove any furniture or other items that may cause injury.

➤ Do not restrain extremities; if possible, pad areas surrounding the patient to prevent bruises and contusions.
   Neuromuscular activity is uncontrolled; physical restraints increase the risk for fractures, bruises, contusions (Brunner & Suddarth, 1988).

➤ Note incontinence of bowel or bladder; observe type of muscular activity.
   Incontinence and type of muscular activity during a seizure can indicate whether the seizure is a result of drug/alcohol intoxication, injury, or is idiopathic in nature.

➤ Monitor length of seizure; notify emergency team if tonic/clonic activity is not resolved within 1 minute or persists longer than normal for patient.
   Prolonged seizure time may indicate patient is developing status epilepticus.

➤ Administer medications as ordered; monitor effectiveness.

After Seizure

➤ Position patient on side; monitor for return of normal respirations
   to promote drainage of blood and secretions that accumulated during the seizure (Brunner & Suddarth, 1988).

➤ Monitor vital signs; if abnormalities exist, continue to monitor q15min until stable.

➤ Assess for bruises, contusions, broken teeth or bones
   to determine if patient sustained any injury.

➤ Monitor level of consciousness; explain previous events to patient.
   Changes in level of consciousness and amnesia about the actual seizure are common once the seizure is over.

➤ Administer medications as ordered; evaluate effects/side effects; teach patient medication self-monitoring skills.
   Nursing observations are critical in determining the effectiveness of any psychiatric medication (Townsend, 1990).

➤ Allow patient to sleep, if possible.
   Fatigue is common because of increased energy expenditure during the seizure. Patient may sleep for 30 minutes to several hours after the seizure.

➤ Ensure call light is accessible at all times.

➤ Observe and report immediately any recurrence of seizure activity.
   Postseizure assessment and monitoring are necessary to ensure patient has a patent airway, rests quietly until fully recovered, and receives treatment for any injury.

Additional Charting Components

➤ Aura or warning
➤ Behavior changes
➤ Effects/side effects of medications
➤ Factors precipitating seizure activity

➤ Incontinence of bowel/bladder
➤ Length and description of seizure
➤ Persons notified
➤ Pupillary changes
➤ Respiratory status, level of consciousness postseizure
➤ Safety measures followed
➤ Visible signs of injury
➤ Vital signs

Additional Nursing Orders for THE PATIENT IN WITHDRAWAL

➤ Determine the type(s) of substance used.
  The withdrawal symptoms and protocols are determined by the substance abused.

➤ Ascertain the amount of the drug ingested and the route by which it was administered.
  The severity of withdrawal will often depend on how much of the drug has been used. Infections and the possibility of HIV are increased by injecting drugs.

➤ Assess how long the individual has been abusing the substance.
  The length of time the person has been abusing the substance will influence the amount and type of associated problems, such as physical deterioration, potential for seizures, financial depletion, family and peer support, dual diagnosis (Caulker-Burnett, 1994).

➤ Initiate prompt treatment of the patient and the specific withdrawal symptoms.
  Serious complications of withdrawal can be avoided with timely treatment. Delayed or untreated alcohol and barbiturate withdrawal is life threatening (Baer & Bradley, 1992).

Alcohol Withdrawal

➤ Determine when the patient had the last drink of alcohol.
  Withdrawal symptoms usually begin 6 to 12 hours after cessation of alcohol use, peak in 2 to 3 days, and subside in 4 to 5 days.

➤ Evaluate the blood alcohol level of the patient.
  A high blood alcohol level with few symptoms of intoxication will be indicative of alcohol dependency. See nursing care plan "Impaired Adjustment Additional Nursing Orders for Patient with Chemical Dependency."

➤ Assess for the following symptoms, which often indicate the onset of alcohol withdrawal syndrome: autonomic hyperactivity, increased vital signs, tremor, insomnia, nausea and vomiting, psychomotor agitation, anxiety, grand mal seizures, tactile or auditory hallucinations or illusions. (*DSM-IV*)
  Alcohol leaves the body rapidly; consequently, withdrawal is short-lived, but very intense. Symptoms of withdrawal may be disguised or prolonged if the patient is a polysubstance abuser.

➤ Administer benzodiazepines as ordered by the physician/protocol or standardized procedure.
  Cross tolerance between alcohol and other CNS depressants represents a combination of cellular and metabolic tolerance.

➤ Assess effectiveness of the administered long-acting benzodiazepine (Librium, Valium, Tranxene).
  The long-acting benzodiazepines provide for a smoother withdrawal course. Valium also acts as an excellent anticonvulsant. Shorter acting benzodiazepines such as Ativan or Xanax can be used if there is decreased metabolism as a result of liver dysfunction (Kuhn, 1994).

➤ Assess for vitamin and mineral deficiencies.
  Ingesting of alcohol results in limited food ingestion and absorption. Deficiencies of the B vitamins, especially B_1, is common. Pyridoxine (B_6) deficiency as well as low B_{12} levels occur because of poor absorption. Conversion of inactive vitamin A to active vitamin A may not occur because of a lack of alcohol dehydrogenase. This can result in night blindness and azoospermia. Liver dysfunction can result in disrupted iron metabolism and may create either a depletion or an idiopathic hemochromatosis (Bennett & Woolf, 1991).

➤ Administer magnesium sulfate as ordered by deep I.M. injection.
  Magnesium deficiency has been associated with seizures. The role of magnesium in preventing delirium tremens has been studied (Fink, 1986).

➤ Initiate seizure precautions. See previous section: "Additional Nursing Orders for the Patient with Seizures."
  Alcohol-induced seizures occur within the first 48 hours after abstinence and may also occur during a prolonged drinking binge.

➤ Adjust lighting to prevent shadows.
  Shadows and ambiguous environmental stimuli may trigger illusions.

➤ Reduce the patient's anxiety level. See nursing care plan "Anxiety."
High levels of anxiety increase psychomotor agitation and the occurrence of seizure and hallucinations.

➤ Monitor the patient's intake and output.
Alcoholic patients may become dehydrated or overhydrated.

➤ Discuss with the patient the type of withdrawal symptoms experienced in the past.
Often the course and type of withdrawal will repeat itself. If a patient experienced seizure in the past, it is more likely that this will happen again.

➤ Offer small appetizing snacks that are low fat, high protein, and high in sugar. See care plan "Nutrition, Altered: less than body requirements."
Gastrointestinal disturbances often prevent eating large portions. Protein is a good source of B vitamins. Low fat is preferred because liver function may be impaired. Foods with a high sugar content help the hypoglycemia, which is often present.

➤ Orient the patient to time, place, and person.
The patient in withdrawal is often confused and disoriented.

➤ Explain that hallucinations are part of the withdrawal syndrome and are not an indication of losing one's mind. See nursing care plan "Sensory/Perceptual Alterations."
Tactile and visual hallucinations can be frightening and the patient may think that this is a symptom of a more serious mental condition.

➤ Monitor environmental stimuli to promote rest. See nursing care plan "Sleep-Pattern Disturbance."
The person in alcohol withdrawal often cannot sleep. When that person does fall asleep, he or she may have frightening dreams that wakes him or her because of REM rebound.

➤ Speak in short, simple sentences that display empathy and caring.
The alcoholic patient may be experiencing a psychosis and not trust caregivers. See nursing care plan "Altered Thought Process."

➤ When discussing the patient's physical symptoms, speak of them as withdrawal symptoms.
Noting that the physical symptoms are part of the withdrawal process helps stop the denial that is often present in alcoholic patients. See nursing care plan "Ineffective Denial."

➤ Be aware that alcoholism is a primary illness, but it can also be a component in a dual diagnosis.
Bipolar disorder, major depression and antisocial personality disorder are the psychiatric disorders that most often accompany alcoholism, but others may also coexist (Wilson & Kneisl, 1996).

➤ Complete a full physical assessment.
All body systems are affected by the ingestion of alcohol, which acts as a poison in the body.

Benzodiazepine Withdrawal

➤ Determine the type of benzodiazepine that has been abused.
Be aware that the withdrawal syndrome varies according to the half-life of the drug.

➤ Be supportive when teaching the patient about the cumulative effects of the benzodiazepines.
Benzodiazepines with long half-lives will accumulate extensively and some patients may have chronic withdrawal symptoms for months and will need extensive emotional support.

➤ Assess how long the patient has been using the medication.
Physical dependency as evidence by withdrawal symptoms has been shown after low-dose and high-dose use. Dependence can occur after therapeutic doses of benzodiazepines have been taken for several months (Baer & Bradley, 1992).

➤ Initiate the withdrawal protocol after collaborating with physician.
The metabolic pathway of benzodiazepines is such that all end up as inactive glucuronide, which is the end product of Ativan and Xanax. By converting over to Xanax and gradually tapering down the dose, a safe and successful withdrawal can take place. This, however, will require a great deal of time and patience depending on the original amount that the patient was accustomed to ingesting (Kuhn, 1994).

➤ Never abruptly stop the patient from taking the medication.
Abrupt withdrawal may precipitate a seizure. The withdrawal protocol calls for a slow tapering off of the drug used or substitute benzodiazepines during acute withdrawal period (Baer & Bradley, 1992).

➤ Assess for symptoms such as anxiety, restlessness, irritability, insomnia.
   Symptoms need to be kept to a minimum so seizures will be prevented and the patient will comply with the withdrawal process. If there is too much subjective distress, the patient may become uncooperative and resort to controlling the unpleasant symptoms through self-medication.

Barbiturate Withdrawal Syndrome

Withdrawal syndrome and treatments are similar to those of the benzodiazepines.

➤ Assess for respiratory depression.
   Patients who overdose on barbiturates and patients who have respiratory insufficiency are prone to respiratory depression and the problems associated with it.

➤ Assess for other CNS depressant medications or alcohol taken concurrently with barbiturates.
   Alcohol and other CNS depressants can potentiate the effects of the barbiturates and lead to death by overdose (Shannon, Wilson, & Steng, 1992).

➤ Observe for signs of overdose and determine the amount of barbiturate taken.
   Tolerance to barbiturates develops quickly. Although the dosage required to give the same effects may be higher, the lethal dose of the barbiturate does not continue to increase; therefore, the addict may continue to increase the dose until the body can no longer compensate with tolerance mechanisms and death can occur.

Opiate Withdrawal Syndrome

➤ Assess for the symptoms of withdrawal: nausea and vomiting, muscle aches, lacrimation, rhinorrhea, piloerection, yawning, fever, insomnia.
   Withdrawal symptoms usually begin within 6 to 12 hours after the last dose.

➤ Use of a matter-of-fact approach in caring for the patient.
   Craving is the most uncomfortable symptom in opiate withdrawal. The withdrawal itself is not life-threatening, but the patient can become highly manipulative in his or her drug seeking behaviors.

➤ Assure the patient that the worst symptoms will subside within three days.
   The withdrawal from opiates is accomplished within 72 hours unless the patient is withdrawing from Methadone, which can take several weeks.

➤ Use withdrawal protocols in collaboration with the physician.
   The Clonidine patch reduces symptoms of autonomic hyperactivity. Naltrexone hastens the withdrawal process and reduces the detoxification time. Naprosyn is used for bone and muscle aches. Bentyl is used for gastrointestinal discomfort.

➤ Use distraction to cope with physical discomfort and withdrawal symptoms.
   Patients will focus less on symptoms if distracted by group interaction and one-to-one interaction.

Stimulant Withdrawal (Cocaine and Amphetamine)

➤ Assess for severity of acute intoxication: tachycardia, pupillary dilation, elevated blood pressure, anxiety, vomiting, psychomotor agitation, chest pain, cardiac arrhythmias, confusion, psychosis, and seizure.
   The intoxication phase of stimulant abuse can be life-threatening as toxic symptoms such as cardiovascular collapse or CNS depression resulting in coma may occur.

➤ Create a calm and accepting atmosphere to decrease grandiosity, hyperactivity, and psychomotor agitation that might escalate into acting out behaviors. Refer to nursing care plan "Potential for Violence: Directed at Others." For additional orders for the psychosis accompanying stimulant intoxication and withdrawal, refer to nursing care plans "Altered Thought Processes" and "Alteration in Perception."

➤ Assess for the degree of acute withdrawal symptoms present: emotional instability, suicidal ideation, depression, fatigue, craving, increased appetite, psychomotor retardation or agitation.
   Acute withdrawal symptoms usually begin within one hour after the drug is stopped and may last up to 10 days. In some cases of chronic abuse, anhedonia may persist.

➤ Initiate withdrawal protocol in collaboration with the physician: dopamine agonists (Bromocriptine, amantadine), low dose of benzodiazepine for agitation, Haldol for psychosis, antidepressants for depressive symptoms.
   Using medications that might lessen the intense craving and depression associated with withdrawal from stimulants has decreased recidivism.

➤ Initiate suicide precautions. See nursing care plan "Potential for Violence: Self-Directed."

II. Communicating

A. COMMUNICATION

1. Impaired Verbal Communication

Definition

The state in which an individual experiences a decreased or absent ability to use or understand language in human interaction

Related to

➤ Decrease in circulation to brain
➤ Physical barrier (e.g., brain tumor, tracheostomy, intubation)
➤ Anatomical defect, cleft palate
➤ Psychological barriers (e.g., psychosis, lack of stimuli)
➤ Cultural differences
➤ Developmental or age-related factors (inability to express concerns/needs)
➤ Altered thought processes (e.g., psychosis, confusion, cognitive deficits)
➤ Brain injury to speech/language centers (e.g., aphasia)
➤ Hearing impairment
➤ Inability to read, write
➤ Inability to speak, read, or write dominant language or caregivers' language
➤ Neurological damage resulting in loss of control of muscles involved in speech (e.g., dyspraxia, apraxia)
➤ Severe anxiety

Characteristics/Assessment Findings

➤ *Inability to speak dominant language
➤ *Speaks or verbalizes with difficulty
➤ *Does not or cannot speak
➤ Stuttering
➤ Slurring
➤ Difficulty forming words or sentences
➤ Difficulty expressing thoughts verbally
➤ Inappropriate verbalization
➤ Dyspnea
➤ Disorientation
➤ Speech impairments
  ➣ abnormalities of fluency, rate, pattern
  ➣ abnormalities in voice quality (e.g., pitch or volume variations beyond normal)
  ➣ absence of speech or attempts at speech
  ➣ difficulty in finding the right word
  ➣ inability to form and speak words clearly
  ➣ inability to repeat words
  ➣ lack of meaningfulness in content of speech
➤ Impaired comprehension
  ➣ inability to respond accurately to "yes/no" or other simple questions
  ➣ inability to point to objects, body parts when directed to do so
  ➣ inability to follow simple directions
  ➣ echolalia, neologism, word salad
  ➣ clang associations
➤ Inability to read, write
  ➣ inability to answer simple written questions with a yes/no
  ➣ inability to write simple words
  ➣ inability to point to words for everyday objects

Content appearing in this typeface is additional information not included in the NANDA nursing diagnoses.

*Critical.

➤ Absence of assistive devices (e.g., clean glasses, functional hearing aid, speech-therapy devices)
➤ Decreased cognitive function and awareness, mental status (e.g., somnolence, lethargy)
➤ Confusion
➤ Anxiety
➤ Willingness/unwillingness to work at developing alternative systems of communication
➤ Frustrated response to difficulties in communication (e.g., agitation, withdrawal, refusal to try again)

Expected Outcomes/Goals

The patient will
➤ improve communication as evidenced by
  ▷ ability to communicate basic needs, simple needs
  ▷ ability to follow simple directions
  ▷ appropriate response to visual and verbal language stimuli
  ▷ normal tone, rate, rhythm of speech.
➤ demonstrate meaningful communication with others (in relation to content, feeling, ideas) as evidenced by
  ▷ interactions with staff, visitors
  ▷ sense of comfort and peace that needs are met.

Nursing Orders with Rationale

➤ Assess and monitor for presence/absence/ changes in assessment findings outlined above
  in order to detect any change in status.

➤ Identify available communication skills and patient's willingness to use them (e.g., able to write if cannot talk).
  Such information provides a baseline for planning successful interventions.

➤ Express empathy for the frustration expressed regarding attempts to communicate; ask patient what would be less frustrating.
  Sensitivity to what patient is experiencing acknowledges awareness of patient's feelings, helps to elicit expression of feelings (Carpenito, 1989).

Content appearing in this typeface is additional information not included in the NANDA nursing diagnoses.

➤ Develop alternative modes of communication (e.g., flash cards, pantomime, pencil and paper, eye blinks, alphabet letters); communicate strategies to all who care for patient.
  This will allow patient to communicate regarding basic needs and care (Menikheim & Loen, 1983).

➤ Incorporate specialist findings (e.g., speech therapist, psychiatrist/psychologist) into interventions.
  The expertise of other professionals can bring new skills and information that will individualize approaches to care (Pimental, 1986).

➤ Keep choices to a minimum with delirious patients; using orienting phrases such as "here in the hospital" or "now in April"; use simple direct statements.
  These patients will not be able to think of alternatives and choose priorities. Patients who are having difficulty processing information need clear messages and instructions from others. Orientation to time and place are reassuring (Davies & Janosik, 1991).

➤ Identify those who can speak "for" the patient with accuracy; involve them in care.
  Including significant others facilitates more meaningful interpretations of patient's needs.

Charting Components

➤ Ability to communicate basic needs
➤ Interactions with staff, family visitors
➤ Family involvement, response
➤ Referrals made
➤ Signs of frustration/agitation in response to communication problems
➤ Techniques used to enhance communication; patient's response and success
➤ Patient/family education, response

Additional Nursing Orders for THE PATIENT WITH DEMENTIA

➤ Begin each conversation by identifying yourself and calling the person by name.
  Recent memory loss is a feature of dementia.

➤ Approach the patient with feelings of calmness, acceptance, and willingness to be with the person.
  The attitude of the nurse can have a calming effect and decrease the patient's disruptive behavior.

➤ Identify your feelings about caring for the demented elderly person; discuss feelings of resentment, anger, disgust, and frustration with other staff.

According to Sullivan theory, an advanced-demented elderly person, like an infant, is unable to understand language, but experiences in a parataxic sense the feelings of the caregiver (Whall, 1989).

➤ Communicate with patient using explanations of what you are doing and how you are doing it; orient to nursing care situations even though she or he has lost the ability to communicate with language and other symbols.

Talking to patients even when they do not seem to understand conveys respect and kindness.

➤ Ask how patient is feeling and whether she or he wishes you to proceed, even though the person may not be able to respond.

The patient can understand the intent and feelings of the nurse in a parataxic sense (Whall, 1989).

➤ Do not expect the patient to understand or participate in complex activities or conversations.

With Alzheimer's dementias there is progressive aphasia, apraxia, agnosia, and mnemic disturbances. It becomes increasingly difficult to find the correct word, to reproduce pictures in perspective, to recognize pictures and objects, and to remember recent events (Wolanin & Phillips, 1981).

➤ Accompany all nonverbal activity with appropriate verbal direction; give constant reminders during an activity (e.g., eating, bathing) on what is expected.

The teaching that nurses find successful with others does not work with the patient suffering from dementia (Wolanin & Phillips, 1981).

➤ Test by asking a simple question, then wait for the answer until you are sure that the patient has gone on to something else.

Impatient nurses are more likely to act quickly and perform the action themselves, instead of giving the patient a chance to be involved (Wolanin & Phillips, 1981). The patient may be able to respond appropriately, but take a long time to organize a response. Patients who feel hurried may not try to respond.

➤ Study the eyes of the patient for clues to feelings of discomfort, pain, anger, hostility, misunderstanding; observe body movements for signs of frustration and anger.

Patients will use nonverbal substitution for the words that no longer come easily. They will use body position and eye expressions to indicate their feelings (Bartol, 1979).

➤ If the patient does not give you his or her full attention, stop and try later.

An important aspect of the patient's nonverbal behavior is his "nonlistening" behavior. Nonreceptive behaviors of the patient tell the nurse to go away (e.g., walks away, closes eyes, other avoidance behavior) (Bartol, 1979).

➤ Simplify communication to patient (e.g., say one idea at a time; use short statements, "yes/no" questions, common words); use short words and no pronouns.

This type of communication gives limited input and thereby omits opportunities for misinterpretation. Asking for a limited response makes it easier for the patient to respond (Pimental, 1986).

➤ Don't shout or "talk down" to patient; if you increase your speech volume, lower the tone.

While the patient does not understand what is said, brain injury leading to aphasia does not mean that the patient is retarded or deaf.

➤ Decrease environmental distractions (e.g., noise from outside room, radio, TV, other persons).

Brain injury causing the aphasia may make the patient less able to separate your verbal communication from other auditory stimuli in the environment.

➤ Use gestures; avoid abstract ideas or very emotional content; use overemphasis and exaggerated facial expression to emphasize your point.

Gestures give additional meaning to words. When there is high emotional content or great abstraction, it may be harder for the patient to understand or organize speech (Carpenito, 1989).

➤ Repeat as necessary but use exact same words each time.

Using similar, but different, words only confuses the patient more.

➤ Accompany verbal stimuli with written stimuli.

Stimulating two senses increases the likelihood of being understood (Menikheim & Loen, 1983).

➤ Listen attentively; restate message to convey understanding; ask for a repeat of the statement if you don't understand; offer your best guess and continue until there is a resolution.

This demonstrates that the nurse wants to understand instead of just letting something go by. The request for the message to be repeated can be accompanied by reassurance that the nurse wants to understand (Davies & Janosik, 1991).

➤ If speech is not understandable, respond to feeling, tone, context of message.

If the nurse can indicate understanding of the feelings being expressed, the patient will experience some success.

➤ Do not pressure or tire patient; if you have not succeeded in 5 minutes or less, it is better to leave and return later.

Symptoms increase with fatigue, anxiety.

➤ Chart all phrases and nonverbal techniques used that consistently "get through" for the patient in different situations.

Documentation allows other staff to use successful techniques and saves frustration for both the staff and patient (Davies & Janosik, 1991).

➤ Refer to nursing care plan "Chronic Confusion for Additional Nursing Orders."

Patients with dementia suffer from confusion.

Additional Charting Components

➤ Responses from patient
➤ Specific ways patient communicates
➤ Successful phrases and nonverbal techniques
➤ Time needed for patient to respond
➤ Toleration of frustration, attempts to respond

Additional Nursing Orders for
THE PATIENT WITH SCHIZOPHRENIA

➤ Respond to symbolic messages by action or reassurance, rather than sharing an interpretation.

Bringing unconscious material into awareness can create high anxiety and panic, leading to a loss of control.

➤ Respond to symbolism with an interpretation only after careful consideration of what the patient is trying to convey; assess if patient can handle an interpretation of the meaning.

The patient is speaking indirectly for a reason; the symbolism may screen thoughts and feelings that would be difficult to handle if stated directly (Stuart & Sundeen, 1987).

➤ Ensure that communication is congruent between verbal and nonverbal messages.

Patients are very sensitive to nonverbal behavior and whether the nonverbal supports the verbal message.

➤ Model expression of feelings by interacting with other staff members in the presence of the patient and then discussing the situation with the patient.

Schizophrenics take time to reach a level of trust where they can tolerate feelings directed from the nurse toward them. They need to see that nothing devastating happens when feelings are expressed (Stuart & Sundeen, 1987).

➤ Be sensitive to the behaviors that indicate a resistance to closeness (e.g., withdrawal, verbal threats, rejection, symbolic gestures) and reduce the level of anxiety by assuring the patient that you will not demand more than she or he can tolerate.

The threat of closeness can result in many behaviors that are indicative of the patient's resistance. Interpersonal anxiety may lead to obscene language to drive the nurse away.

➤ Use touch very carefully, if at all.

Casual touch may be perceived as an invasion, a heterosexual or homosexual advance, which may precipitate a panic reaction.

➤ Use words "I" and "you" rather than "we" and "us" to avoid confusing the patient who does not know where his or her self ends and the nurse's begins.

Ego boundaries may be reinforced by clearly separating self from other in communication.

Additional Charting Components

➤ Gains in trust level
➤ Level of anxiety
➤ Practice sessions expressing feelings
➤ Reactions to interpretations
➤ Resistive behaviors to interpersonal closeness
➤ Symbolic gestures, statements expressed

III. Relating

A. ALTERED SOCIALIZATION

1. Impaired Social Interaction

Definition

The state in which an individual participates in an insufficient or excessive quantity or ineffective quality of social exchange

Related to

- Knowledge/skill deficit about ways to enhance mutuality (e.g., as associated with mental retardation or organic disorders)
- Communication barriers (e.g., with hearing, visual, or speech impairments or language/cultural barriers)
- Self-concept disturbance (associated with chronic depression, anxiety)
- Absence of available significant others or peers
- Limited physical mobility
- Chronic therapeutic isolation from others
- Sociocultural dissonance
- Environmental barriers
- Altered thought processes
- Unconscious conflicts associated with chronic lack of trust and abandonment experiences
- Inadequate personal resources

Content appearing in this typeface is additional information not included in the NANDA nursing diagnoses.

Characteristics/Assessment Findings

Severe
- Verbalized or observed discomfort in social situations
- Verbalized or observed inability to receive or communicate a satisfying sense of belonging, caring, interest, shared history
- Verbalized or observed use of unsuccessful social interaction behaviors
- Dysfunctional interactions with peers, family, or others
- Observed impact of life functioning (e.g., loss of job, record of police contacts due to poor impulse control)
- Disorganized thinking/inability to concentrate
- Inability to control effects of rage, envy, hate when with others
- Pervasive and extensive lack of self-care skills

Moderate
- Severe/chronic anxiety
- Lack of or chaotic motivation without ability to accomplish simple daily goals
- Delay in accomplishing developmental tasks
- Eccentric behaviors (e.g., refusal to answer door/telephone)
- Inability or refusal to follow cultural norm as to dress, bathing, other self-care behaviors
- Preoccupation with own thoughts/feelings
- Passive expression of anger (e.g., pouting, procrastinating, forgetting, obstructing)

Low
- Reports by family/others of change in style or pattern of interactions (e.g., "John seems 'different' or 'eccentric.'")
- Tendency to blame others
- Numerous superficial relationships
- Chronic experience of self as different from others

➤ Immature interests
➤ Exhibits behavior unaccepted by dominant cultural group

Expected Outcomes/Goals

The patient will

➤ acknowledge difficulty that impaired social interactions create in own life as evidenced by
  ▷ verbalizing personal losses associated with interaction deficits
  ▷ listing causes associated with (reasons for) interaction handicaps.
➤ set and achieve small daily goals related to increased socialization as evidenced by
  ▷ attending individual/group unit meetings within therapeutic milieu
  ▷ evaluating changes in own socialization behavior
  ▷ self-report of feeling of connection/trust (feeling of being heard and understood) with one other person
  ▷ statements that all people have both bad and good qualities.
➤ initiate and maintain appropriate social interactions as evidenced by
  ▷ self- and family reports of increased predictability/stability and meaningfulness in social interactions
  ▷ self- and family reports of decreased extreme splitting/blaming behaviors
  ▷ effecting stability in a variety of social contacts
  ▷ putting feelings into words rather than actions
  ▷ accepting responsibility for own behavior.

Nursing Orders with Rationale

➤ Assess and monitor for presence/absence/ changes in assessment findings outlined above
  in order to detect any change in status.

➤ Help patient to assess/monitor the cause/meaning of current isolation.
  Patient involvement is needed to obtain accurate assessment data (Arnold & Boggs, 1989).

➤ Assess for the presence of hallucinations and delusions; if present, refer to nursing care plans "Altered Thought Processes" and "Sensory/Perceptual Alterations."
  Hallucinations/delusions may be interfering with the patient's ability to socialize with others.

➤ Provide self as a role model of person in meaningful social interactions with patients/peers.
  Patients will model behavior that they see exhibited by their nurses (Hill & Smith, 1990).

➤ Introduce alternative holistic nursing approaches (e.g., pet therapy).
  The opportunity to touch and attach self to a pet provides practice in trusting and relating. This is often the first step toward meaningful human interaction (Davis, 1988).

➤ Work with patient to set at least one daily goal (e.g., attend group sessions, participate at least once in session).
  Making initial goals low enough so patient can achieve a degree of success that will enhance patient's self-esteem.

➤ Include exercise, physical therapy, and massage in treatment milieu.
  For chronically emotionally deprived people, connection with and awareness of own physical body is helpful in building trust and beginning relationships with others (Taylor, Lillis, & LeMone, 1989; White, 1988).

➤ Use role playing and videotape feedback to provide patient with information as to quality, style, specific progress of his or her interactions with others.
  Videotape feedback provides patients with immediate and concrete information as to how they are interacting with others. Changes can be measured through review of past tapes in comparison/contrast with current ones.

➤ Teach and role model basic communication/conversation skills.
  Isolated patients benefit from basic training in how to talk to others (Goodman & Esterly, 1990).

➤ Teach and role model basic anxiety-management skills and assertive-behavior approaches.
  Skills in behavioral management of anxiety are essential for isolated patients (Arnold & Boggs, 1989).

Content appearing in this typeface is additional information not included in the NANDA nursing diagnoses.

➤ Observe for and document resistant behaviors (e.g., ineffective actions, silent treatment, slamming doors).

> *This helps to assess if the patient has established a passive-aggressive pattern in relating to others.*

➤ Use of matter-of-fact approach when confronting patient exhibiting resistant behavior or covert expression of anger.

> *This approach helps to avoid a power struggle.*

➤ Define clear limits of acceptable behavior and encourage feedback from the patient; discuss possible alternative behaviors; encourage open, genuine expressions of anger.

> *The passive person must be helped to recognize that she or he can actively participate and problem solve; the patient needs to learn that overt expressions of anger are acceptable.*

➤ Administer medications as ordered; evaluate the effects/side effects; teach patient medication self-monitoring skills.

> *Nursing observations are critical in determining the effectiveness of any psychiatric medication (Townsend, 1990).*

➤ Help patient identify positive reinforcers for progressive healing interactions.

> *To be effective, reinforcers must be chosen by the patient (not by nurses) (Sundeen, Stuart, Rankin, & Cohen, 1989; Hill & Smith, 1990).*

➤ Provide continual assessment/evaluation of suicide risk.

> *Severely isolated patients often do not make their suicidal feelings known to others (Aguilera, 1990).*

➤ Develop an alliance with family; involve them in assessment and ongoing evaluation of patient's social interactions; evaluate themes of family symbiosis, blaming, splitting.

> *Many chronically ill people return to their family after hospitalization (Carpenito, 1989).*

➤ Refer patient/family to self-help community group for specific type of isolation difficulty.

> *Self-help groups provide the most effective and least expensive therapeutic assistance for isolated patients (Katz & Bender, 1990; Roth, Stone, & Kibel, 1990).*

Charting Components

➤ Behaviors implemented by the nurse that encourage appropriate social interactions
➤ Duration, frequency, type of interactions with others
➤ Effects/side effects of psychotropic medications
➤ Indications of substance use/abuse
➤ Patient report of comfort/discomfort in social interactions; improved concentration; decreased interference from hallucinations, delusions, distortions
➤ Patient statements of reasons for/impact of impaired social interactions
➤ Quality of attachment/interaction with staff members
➤ Quality of basic self-care activities, general appearance of patient
➤ Subjective reaction/reports of staff/family/other patients as to level and observed changes in patient's social interaction
➤ Suicidal assessment, findings
➤ Verbalizations related to self-esteem, self-concept
➤ Willingness to use family, community resources

Additional Nursing Orders for THE PATIENT WITH A BORDERLINE PERSONALITY DISORDER

➤ Provide empathy in context of clear, firm limits on splitting and projecting behaviors.

> *This response conveys staff's strong, consistent stand against destructive behavior (Haber, Hoskins, Leach, & Sideleau, 1987).*

➤ Develop shared "language" to describe intense affects in preference to acting out rage, humiliation.

> *These patients often lack "words" to describe their extreme upset state and vulnerability. Emotional progress cannot proceed without a way for them to talk about their internal experiences (Winnicott, 1988).*

➤ Involve family/significant others in the plan of care

> *to prevent the patient from setting staff and family at odds with each other.*

➤ Be aware that anger is a natural response to being manipulated; deal with your own feelings of anger and those of other staff members

> *to prevent staff from being punitive with the patient.*

➤ Monitor staff reactions to patient.
  Careful monitoring will identify staff splitting and dissension that results from having a manipulative patient on the ward (Davies & Janosik, 1991).

➤ Establish firm rules that are rigidly interpreted and consistently enforced.
  Consistent rules will decrease manipulation of staff and other patients.

➤ Identify and confront patient with his or her failure to comply with set rules and limits; enforce agreed-upon restrictions and consequences immediately without anger.
  There must be an expectation that the patient will meet standards of healthy behavior (Stuart & Sundeen, 1987).

➤ Communicate frequently with other staff members about the patient's status.
  Shared information will prevent manipulative patients from attributing blame and responsibility to others instead of to themselves (Haber et al., 1987).

➤ Examine your own level of involvement and seduction by charm with the manipulative patient; seek supervision for impulses to rescue, hurt, or admire the patient.
  These patients have little tolerance for intimacy; their maneuvering of others is an effective way of keeping them at a safe distance (Stuart & Sundeen, 1987).

➤ Use behavior techniques to modify antisocial behavior:
  ▷ use concrete and readily available reinforcers (e.g., cigarettes, pass for the weekend).
  ▷ avoid response to an undesirable behavior if possible.
  ▷ maintain matter-of-fact attitude in implementing consequences.
  ▷ remove patient from contact with others for a period of time.
    Behavior-modification techniques may be helpful in decreasing antisocial behavior (Haber et al., 1987).

➤ Refer to nursing care plan "Self-Mutilation" for additional nursing orders.
  Borderline patients often demonstrate self-mutilating behavior as a means to relieve tension and anger.

Additional Charting Components

➤ Consequences applied and patient's reaction
➤ Degree of compliance to limits
➤ Limits and rules set for the patient
➤ Staff's/other patients' reaction to patient behavior

2. Social Isolation

Definition

Aloneness experienced by the individual and perceived as imposed by others and as a negative or threatened state

Related to

➤ Factors contributing to the absence of satisfying personal relationships
  ▷ delay in accomplishing developmental tasks
  ▷ immature interest
  ▷ alterations in physical appearance (e.g., severe depression, thought disorder)
  ▷ alterations in mental status
  ▷ unaccepted social behavior
  ▷ unaccepted social values
  ▷ altered state of wellness
  ▷ inadequate personal resources
  ▷ inability to engage in satisfying relationships
➤ Communicable diseases (e.g., AIDS)
➤ Sensory/motor impairment
➤ Recent exposure to traumatic event (e.g., rape, financial ruin, plane crash)
➤ Emotional handicaps (e.g., extreme anxiety, depression, paranoia, phobias)
➤ Drug or alcohol dependency
➤ Recent divorce, family death, cultural alienation

Content appearing in this typeface is additional information not included in the NANDA nursing diagnoses.

Characteristics/Assessment Findings

Objective

➤ *Absense of supportive significant other(s)
➤ Sad, dull affect
➤ Inappropriate or immature interest/activities for age
➤ Uncommunicative, withdrawn, no eye contact
➤ Preoccupation with own thoughts
➤ Repetitive meaningless actions
➤ Projects hostility in voice, behavior
➤ Seeks to be alone, or exists in a subculture
➤ Evidence of physical/mental handicap or altered state of wellness
➤ Shows behavior unaccepted by dominant cultural group
➤ Physical or verbal underactivity
➤ Increased signs and symptoms of physical/ mental illness
➤ Refusal to drive, go to market, etc.
➤ Undue dependence on telephone/mail for outside contact

Subjective

➤ *Expresses feelings of aloneness imposed by others
➤ *Expresses feelings of rejection
➤ Experiences feelings of difference from others
➤ Inadequacy in or absence of significant purpose in life
➤ Inability to meet expectations of others
➤ Insecurity in public
➤ Expresses values acceptable to the subculture but unacceptable to the dominant cultural group
➤ Expresses interests appropriate to the developmental age/state
➤ Expresses feelings of unexplained dread or abandonment
➤ Desire for more contact with people
➤ Extreme fear of public places
➤ Ritualistic, meaningless approaches to daily life that interfere with needs of self/family
➤ Feelings of uselessness
➤ Inability to concentrate and make decisions
➤ Blaming others for own insecurity
➤ Primary identification with subculture; exists on fringe of subculture

*Critical.

Expected Outcomes/Goals

The patient will

➤ identify new skills for engaging/maintaining social relationships as evidenced by
  ▷ demonstrating improved communication skills
  ▷ completing a self-contract for daily contact with others
  ▷ spending part of each day with thoughts/activities not centered on self and own symptoms.
➤ report a sense of comfort with current social contacts as evidenced by decreased panic reactions, improved sleep patterns, a general sense of improved health.
➤ identify continuing interaction goals for self as evidenced by
  ▷ setting future goals for self such as attending a class or participating in a group sport
  ▷ identifying a small support network available for ongoing contacts
  ▷ agreeing to participate in a self-help support group for people with isolated/isolating lifestyles.

Nursing Orders with Rationale

➤ Assess and monitor for presence/absence/ changes in assessment findings outlined above *in order to detect any change in status.*

➤ Assess isolation behaviors within a cultural context. *Some behaviors may be culturally syntonic and not problematic to patient/family (Funkhouser & Moser, 1990).*

➤ Assess elderly patients carefully for hearing, vision, ambulation, and other sensory deficits that could account for isolating symptoms. *The elderly are particularly at high risk for social isolation (Carpenito, 1989).*

➤ Establish a trusting relationship with the patient:
  ▷ initiate a contract that is mutually agreed on by the patient and nurse.
  ▷ provide for privacy and comfort during interactions.
  ▷ be accessible and consistent in behavior.
  ▷ develop mutual long- and short-term goals with patient.
    Learning to trust someone allows the patient to take interpersonal risks (Davies & Janosik, 1991).

Content appearing in this typeface is additional information not included in the NANDA nursing diagnoses.

➤ Look directly at patient when greeting him or her; lean toward patient but maintain a comfortable distance; use gentle touch if appropriate.

> *An attitude of concern, but not intrusive interest, allows the patient to control the pace of the development of closeness (Davies & Janosik, 1991).*

➤ Spend time in silence with the withdrawn patient; ask open-ended questions followed by pauses.

> *Constant chatter conveys to the patient the message there is no expectation for him or her to verbalize (Davies & Janosik, 1991).*

➤ Approach long-term goals with a series of short-term goals:
  ▷ establish daily contact with patient for a few days before initiating other goals.
  ▷ have patient attend one group meeting with nurse.
  ▷ have patient participate in one activity after two group observation sessions.
  ▷ have patient attend group session alone after four meetings with nurse present.

> *This kind of stepwise program gradually exposes the patient to more complex interactions and decreases involvement with the nurse (Davies & Janosik, 1991).*

➤ Provide ongoing feedback/reinforcement to patient for each successful step toward social involvement.

> *Feedback from others is crucial to the change process. Socially isolated people usually have been alienated from family/peer feedback (Davies & Janosik, 1991).*

➤ Help patients to identify causes/issues related to isolation and anxiety by exploring
  ▷ degree of trust/mistrust concerning others and self
  ▷ economic, transportation, and knowledge deficits
  ▷ isolation factors within cultural context
  ▷ family's level of involvement and perceptions of patient.

> *An accurate nursing assessment must include exploration of all factors of the patient's life (Taylor, Lillis, & LeMone, 1989).*

➤ Assist patient to eliminate above factors by referring to community resources for support, information, and financial aid; plan family meetings to explore ways to increase family connections.

> *Environmental manipulation of isolating factors can increase the individual's sense of community and family support.*

➤ Assess interest and use of leisure activities during an interdisciplinary team meeting for inclusion on Axis V.

> *Depressed patients have restricted interest in leisure activities, which contributes to performance dysfunction and isolation (Bonder, 1990).*

➤ Teach patient to evaluate effectiveness of own communication skills, social appropriateness, and efforts at renewed socialization.

> *Self-evaluation is a crucial part of any behavior change program (Hill & Smith, 1990).*

➤ Role model and teach patient effective communication skills:
  ▷ use congruent verbal and nonverbal communications.
  ▷ validate the mean of communications with patient.
  ▷ share perceptions and reactions to the patient.
  ▷ give empathic responses to expression of feelings.
  ▷ set limits in a clear and consistent manner.

> *Effective expression of one's feeling/needs is the first step in behavior change (Goodman & Esterly, 1990).*

➤ Help to increase support system:
  ▷ review availability of current support systems and resources (e.g., family, friends, self-help groups, community).
  ▷ provide information regarding supports/resources (e.g., self-help groups, books, clubs).
  ▷ provide opportunities to enhance contacts with new supports (e.g., most supportive person).
  ▷ refer to desired resources.

> *Increase supportive relationships, resources, and guidance through individual or group experiences that facilitate coping (Kinney, Mannetter, & Carpenter, 1985).*

➤ Implement a program of regular exercise into the patient's daily schedule.

> *Regular exercise, especially aerobic exercise, three times a week for 45 minutes improves well-being and lifts mood.*

➤ Help patient to create self-contract for general self-care in areas of exercise, nutrition, relaxation, and environmental awareness.

> *When patients begin to take responsibility for their general health and self-care they will also feel more empowered to improve their emotional health (Hill & Smith, 1990).*

➤ Teach empowerment (refer to nursing care plan "Powerlessness" for interventions) and assertiveness skills.
These skills will help to decrease feelings of powerlessness and hopelessness associated with social isolation (Arnold & Boggs, 1989).

➤ Help patient to grieve losses associated with onset of social isolation (e.g., severe illness, traumatic event); refer to nursing care plans "Anticipatory Grieving" and "Dysfunctional Grieving."
When patients are able to grieve appropriately they can usually proceed with health development that was only temporarily blocked (Winnicott, 1988).

➤ Use peer counseling by former patients or refer to a self-help group such as Emotional Health Anonymous
to improve interpersonal competence, provide positive role models, and reduce isolation and alienation that come from social stigma to mental illness (McGill & Patterson, 1990).

Charting Components

➤ Ability to role play successful interactions with others
➤ Additional support developed/used
➤ Attendance and participation in group activities
➤ Behaviors implemented by the nurse that decrease patient's social isolation
➤ Friendships established, number of visitors
➤ General appearance and self-care activity
➤ Nurse's subjective experience/feelings when with patient
➤ Patient's self-report of anxiety level in general and in key phobic situations, sleep patterns
➤ Patient's self-report of decreased loneliness
➤ Subjective reaction/reports of staff/family/other patients as to level and observed changes in patient's social isolation
➤ Support system available, used

Additional Nursing Orders for THE PATIENT WITH SOCIAL PHOBIAS AND AGORAPHOBIA

➤ Alleviate high levels of interpersonal anxiety:
  ▷ maintain a calm, supportive manner.
  ▷ minimize environmental stimuli.
  ▷ explain events that are going on, who everyone is.

  ▷ recognize defensive behaviors and point them out to patient.
  ▷ promote structured, time-limited sessions with self and others.
  Severe levels of anxiety and panic interfere with relationships.

➤ Administer medications as ordered; evaluate effects/side effects; teach patient medication self-monitoring skills.
Nurse observations are critical in determining the effectiveness of any psychiatric medication (Townsend, 1990).

➤ Employ systematic desensitization and behavioral rehearsal to extinguish phobic reactions within therapeutic milieu; see nursing care plan "Fear (The Patient with Phobias)" for exact steps.
Behavioral approaches are often a first line of attack against phobic symptoms (Haber, Hoskins, Leach & Sideleau, 1987).

➤ Teach and model deep breathing, relaxation, imagery, and visualization to decrease anxiety and to provide an increased sense of control.
The ability to relax and to "imagine" success in interactions with others does not come naturally but must be provided as an integral nursing intervention (Mast, 1986; Titlebaum, 1988).

Additional Charting Components

➤ Change in phobic reactions
➤ Effects/side effects in psychotropic medications
➤ Participation in relaxation exercises, ability to relax
➤ Patient's level of anxiety

Additional Nursing Orders for THE PATIENT WITH SUSPICION

➤ Foster trust:
  ▷ follow through on commitments made to the patient.
  ▷ plan several brief contacts spaced throughout the day.
  ▷ inform the patient when you will be talking to him or her.
  ▷ give careful explanations for treatments and medications.
  Nurses demonstrate trust by making themselves accessible to the patient both physically and emotionally.

➤ Warn the patient that you are approaching *to avoid startling the suspicious patient.*

➤ Allow the patient to control the amount of self-revelation that takes place in the interaction. *A probing approach will only alienate the patient and retard the development of trust (Stuart & Sundeen, 1987).*

➤ Designate one or two people to work consistently with the suspicious patient. *Consistency in staffing helps promote trust.*

➤ Inform the patient of plans to meet with family; discuss the issue of confidentiality with patient and family; include patient in family meetings. *Families of suspicious families often abound with family secrets. The nurse should not become involved in this pattern (Haber et al., 1987).*

Additional Charting Components

➤ Behaviors indicating willingness to trust

B. ROLE

1. Sexual Dysfunction

Definition

The state in which an individual experiences a change in sexual function that is viewed as unsatisfying, unrewarding, inadequate

Related to

➤ Biopsychosocial alteration of sexuality
  ▷ ineffectual or absent role models
➤ Physical abuse
➤ Psychosocial abuse (e.g., harmful relationships)
➤ Vulnerability
➤ Values conflict
➤ Lack of privacy
➤ Lack of significant other
➤ Altered body structure or function, e.g.
  ▷ pregnancy
  ▷ recent childbirth
  ▷ drugs
  ▷ surgery
  ▷ anomalies
  ▷ disease process
  ▷ trauma
  ▷ radiation
➤ Misinformation or lack of knowledge
➤ Low self-esteem
➤ Altered body image
➤ Anxiety
➤ Excessive guilt
➤ Substance abuse
➤ Alteration in mood
➤ Alteration in sexuality patterns
➤ Relationship discord
➤ Cognitive disorders

Content appearing in this typeface is additional information not included in the NANDA nursing diagnoses.

Characteristics/Assessment Findings

➤ Verbalization of problem
➤ Alterations in achieving perceived sex role
➤ Actual or perceived limitation imposed by disease or therapy
➤ Conflicts involving values
➤ Alteration in achieving sexual satisfaction
➤ Inability to achieve desired satisfaction
➤ Seeking confirmation of desirability
➤ Alteration in relationship with significant other
➤ Change of interest in self and others
➤ Exacerbation of psychiatric symptoms
➤ Past sexual difficulties
➤ Reaction of significant other
➤ Onset of dysfunction (gradual or abrupt)
➤ Past traumatic sexual events
➤ Global or specific to situations or partners
➤ Preoccupation with sexual performance
➤ Length of time since dysfunction noticed (acute or chronic)
➤ Compulsive sexual behavior

Expected Outcomes/Goals

The patient will report decreased conflict/anxiety regarding sexual functioning as evidenced by
➤ verbalizing knowledge of the sexual response cycle
➤ identifying stressors that contribute to the dysfunction
➤ stating alternative sexual practices that enhance sexual expression
➤ demonstrating effective communication skills when discussing sexuality
➤ acknowledging need for complete physical examination by a practitioner to aid in assessment
➤ accepting referral to an individual trained in human sexuality for more specific therapy regarding the dysfunction
➤ acknowledging need for psychotherapy when sexual dysfunction is compounded by other psychosocial issues.

Nursing Orders with Rationale

➤ Assess and monitor for presence/absence/ changes in assessment findings outlined above *in order to detect any change in status.*

➤ Refer to nursing care plan "Altered Sexuality Patterns" for guidance in establishing a therapeutic relationship with patient before initiating a sexual history.

➤ Be direct, honest, and genuine in your approach with the patient; use open-ended questions (e.g., "Tell me about any concerns you have above your illness or treatment that may affect your relationships. How do you feel this may affect the way you fell or respond sexually?").
   Therapeutic communication techniques encourage the patient to express thoughts and feelings.

➤ Determine if the patient has had successful intercourse in the past.
   Finding out if the dysfunction is primary (never achieved successful coitus) or secondary (lost a former ability) is essential for beginning assessment on sexual functioning.

➤ Gather baseline data on the patient's usual sexual functioning and practices.
   The goal of overall therapy is to return a patient to his or her previous level of functioning. Though patients may wish to enhance their former sexuality, it is important to understand what had worked for them prior to the dysfunction.

➤ Review professionally accepted terminology for sexual dysfunction with patient (e.g., general sexual unresponsiveness, dyspareunia, vaginismus, orgasmic dysfunction, erectile dysfunction, premature or early ejaculation, retarded ejaculation).
   This will cut down on confusion when patient confers with other professionals on the health-care team regarding own concerns or possible dysfunction.

➤ Use therapeutic communication when eliciting information for the sexual history; gather detailed information in the following areas:
   ▷ description of current problem
   ▷ onset (age, gradual or sudden precipitating events)
   ▷ course (changes over time: increase, decrease, fluctuation in severity, frequency, intensity)
   ▷ patient's concept of the cause and maintenance of the problem

▷ past treatment and outcome
▷ medical evaluation (specialty, dates, form of treatment, results, current or past medications)
▷ professional help (specialty, date, form of treatment, results)
▷ self-treatment (type, results)
▷ current expectancies, goals of treatment (concrete or ideal).
   Sexual difficulties that come on gradually, seem to have no precipitating psychosocial event, and do not fluctuate situationally often have an organic basis.

➤ Provide information on the human sexual response cycle—excitement, plateau, orgasm, resolution.
   Specific dysfunctions may interfere with one or more of the phases.

➤ Offer information about the role the autonomic nervous system plays in the stages of the human sexual response cycle (the parasympathetic nervous system influences the first two stages; the sympathetic nervous system influences the last two stages).
   Patients who have this information may gain a better understanding of how specific diseases or medications affect their sexuality.

➤ Give specific information on medications that can affect sexual responsiveness (e.g., antidepressants, antihypertensives, neuroleptics, other CNS depressants).
   Adrenergic (sympathetic) action of the autonomic nervous system produces ejaculation and orgasm while cholinergic (parasympathetic) action controls penile erection and vasocongestion. Blockage of either system by drugs can interfere with sexual functioning. Ganglionic blocking agents interfere with both sympathetic and parasympathetic responses. CNS depressants may interfere with desire as well as cause disruption within the limbic system. Often, changing medications within a class of drugs or decreasing the dosage enhances sexual responsiveness (Harris, 1988).

➤ Provide referral and specific information to male patients who are experiencing chronic erectile dysfunction due to organic causes (e.g., chronic diabetes, radical prostatectomy, atherosclerosis, neurological disorders).

Evaluation for a penile implant for the use of papaverine injections is usually done by a urologist. Intravenous injections of papaverine have been successful with patients who have a variety of disorders that contribute to impotence, including selected patients with vasculogenic diseases (Mooradian et al., 1989).

➤ Provide information on the effects of consuming alcoholic beverages and using recreational drugs on sexual responsiveness.

While small quantities of alcohol may help patients become more uninhibited in their sexual expression, moderate amounts interfere with sexual performance in both males and females. Recreational drugs alter individual perception and distort sexual performance.

➤ Discuss the concept of anxiety and how it might interrupt the sexual response cycle; refer to nursing care plan "Anxiety."

Mild anxiety is often associated with orgasm and ejaculation dysfunction. Moderate anxiety tends to disrupt the excitement phase, thus blocking erection and general sexual excitement. Severe anxiety interferes with the desire phase and contributes to inhibited sexual desire.

➤ Explore with the patient how fear of failure in sexual performance contributes to anxiety and lack of sexual enjoyment.

"Spectatoring" (patient watches own sexual performance critically as though she or he were a third person) often results in erectile and orgastic failures. This is often created by performance anxiety that occurred after a perceived sexual failure. Direct behavioral intervention by a therapist during short-term counseling has been quite successful. The individual must learn abandonment to erotic impulses rather than be controlled by obsessive ideas. In some cases, spectatoring may have its roots in deeper characterologic or marital problems that require more intensive psychotherapy (Kaplan, 1974).

➤ Teach patient relaxation exercises and the use of fantasy to promote relaxation and to increase erotic pleasure.

The tendency to intellectualize or to be overly concerned about pleasing one's partner is a major source of anxiety for many people.

➤ Provide patient with information regarding masturbation and the need to identify what is sexually pleasing to his or her own body; give permission to use masturbation as a means of finding out about self sexually as well as a way of finding sexual gratification when a partner is unavailable; be sensitive to cultural and religious beliefs that may interfere with this practice.

Many patients have misconceptions about the value of self-stimulation in overcoming sexual inhibition. Often, individuals are unaware of what pleasures them or what type of touching is stimulating.

➤ Evaluate patient's self-esteem; refer to nursing care plans "Chronic Low Self-Esteem" and "Situational Low Self-Esteem."

A disturbance in self-esteem can contribute to sexual dysfunction as well as stem from sexual difficulties. A vicious cycle can begin in which the individual's sexual difficulties can compound the view of self as inadequate or undesirable.

➤ Refer the patient who reports transient erectile difficulties, problems with ejaculation, or inability to achieve orgasm to a medical specialist.

Many conditions can contribute to disturbed sexual functioning. Often, the problem is complex in that a transient physical condition may have set up performance anxiety. Absence of sleep-related erections, loss of the ability to achieve orgasm, and difficulty with ejaculation are indications that some organic factor may be operating to maintain, or may have initiated, the dysfunction.

➤ Collaborate with the physician and patient when the patient expresses interest about resuming sexual activity after a medical or surgical condition has necessitated abstinence.

Many medical or surgical conditions require patients to refrain from sexuality during recuperation. They may need reassurance from both the physician and nurse in order to feel safe in resuming sexual activity. Sexual dysfunction can be prevented if the patient's anxiety is discussed (Lion, 1982).

➤ Encourage patient to have significant other involved in the assessment process.

The nurse may get a better picture of the presenting problem when the couple is present and both people can state what they feel is causing them difficulty in their sexual relationship.

➤ Discuss using alternate positions or sexual practices with patients who are experiencing physical discomfort or fatigue during sexual activity.

Open communication and creativity can help eliminate discomfort during coitus, enabling couples to resume satisfactory sexual activity. Prolonged sexual abstinence can predispose a couple to sexual dysfunction.

➤ Acknowledge the importance of giving sensual/sexual physical pleasure that does not involve intercourse when the couple is experiencing a dysfunction in the excitement phase of the sexual response cycle.

Touching and caressing promote physical intimacy and can bring about closeness that is not viewed as sexually demanding when intercourse is forbidden. Verbal communication is enhanced when couples tell each other what is physically pleasing.

➤ Focus on the feelings that the couple share; facilitate open discussion between partners.

Sexual difficulties in a relationship may be a major source of emotional pain for the couple and block closeness and emotional intimacy. Sexual dysfunction may be the major source of distress or may signal deeper marital discord.

➤ Explore with the couple the option of seeing a marriage counselor who has expertise in human sexuality.

It is beyond the scope of practice for the nurse generalist to initiate marital counseling. A therapist with training in human sexuality can help the couple decide if they need conjoint therapy, which may also include specific sex therapy or more traditional marital counseling.

➤ Promote good will between partners by removing blame and sharing information about the system's approach to sexual dysfunction.

Systems theory proposes a reciprocal and mutual causation of sexual dysfunction. The focus is on elucidating the role that sex plays in maintaining equilibrium in the marital relationship.

➤ Become knowledgeable in specific behavioral techniques that may be employed during sex

therapy (e.g., sensate focus exercises, squeeze technique, self-stimulation).

The nurse who understand these concepts can often help clarify what is involved in sex therapy and correct misconceptions. The patient may have already had some previous treatment and wish to discuss past difficulties.

➤ Give the patient/couple basic information about the potential use of papaverine and phentolamine intravenous injections as an aid in treating psychogenic erectile dysfunction.

Self-administration of a combination of papaverine and phentolamine has proven to be an adjunct to sex therapy. Increased frequency of intercourse and sexual satisfaction has been reported. The injections appear to be safe when self-administration has been properly taught. Anxiety and depression appear to decrease and patients report an increase in self-esteem. However, performance anxiety may not be removed and the patient may come to depend on injections for intercourse (Turner et al., 1989).

➤ Ascertain if a major depression is contributing to the sexual dysfunction; work closely with the psychiatrist and mental health team in sharing data.

Sexual dysfunctions can either be the cause of depression or appear as the result of preexisting depression; the clinician must distinguish between these two sequential relationships. Sexual therapy is usually not advised while the patient is in the acute phase of a depressive disorder, but reactive depression tends to diminish when the sexual symptom is relieved (Kaplan, 1974).

➤ Collaborate with other mental health team members when sexual issues become apparent in a patient who is schizophrenic.

It is important to ascertain the role that the sexual symptom is playing in the schizophrenic patient's psychic structure. If it appears that the sexual symptom is a defense against emergence of frank psychopathology, treatment is deferred until the deeper sources of anxiety have been resolved. Many schizophrenics who are in remission of their acute symptoms, however, can benefit from sex therapy if a sexual dysfunction exists. Problems in relating intimately often leave the patient without a partner or afraid to get close to others (Kaplan, 1974).

- Offer support and convey empathy for the patient who is expressing guilt or shame regarding own sexual activity.

  Sexual addiction is not uncommon in this culture. Patients who have a sexual addiction feel isolated and ashamed of their compulsive rituals. Many patients feel powerless to stop their sexual acting out and experience intense guilt (Carnes, 1989).

- Refer patients who express a need for help with either a sexual deviation or sexual addiction for psychotherapy and or to a self-help group such as Sex Addicts Anonymous.

  Sexual disorders that are found in the DSM-IV (e.g., those who have deviant sexual practices, sexual offenders) can expect relief from their sexual acting out through a combination of intensive psychotherapy and belonging to a 12-step program.

Charting Components

- Current medications
- Course of the problem
- Degree of psychosocial distress
- Onset of the problem
- Past treatment(s) of sexual problem(s)
- Patient's concept of the cause of the dysfunction
- Patient's mood
- Presence of specific physical disorders
- Presence/availability of significant other
- Referrals made
- Results of treatment(s)
- Self-treatment(s)
- Significant other's concerns, perception of the problem
- Specific description of the problem
- Use of alcohol/recreational drugs
- Patient/significant other teaching, response

2. Altered Family Processes

Definition

The state in which a family that normally functions effectively experiences a dysfunction

Reltated to

- Situation transition or crisis
  - illness or hospitalization of family member
  - financial constraints
  - time constraints (e.g., disruptions due to treatments)
  - coping strategies

- economic status, work history
- external/internal sources of stress
- family strengths, limitations
- health practices
- inability of members to meet physical/emotional/spiritual needs
- relationship patterns
- religious, ethnic background
- support systems, resources available
- Developmental transition or crisis
  - loss of family member
  - new family member
  - perceived/actual change in the functional level of individual family members
  - perceived/actual change in role of family member
  - separation from family

Characteristics/Assessment Findings

- Family system unable to meet
  - emotional needs of its members
  - physical needs of its members
  - spiritual needs of its members
- Parents do not demonstrate respect for each other's views on child-rearing practices
- Inability to
  - accept/receive help appropriately
  - express/accept wide range of feelings
  - express/accept feelings of members
  - relate to each other for mutual growth and maturation
- Rigidity in function and roles
- Family
  - failure to accomplish current/past developmental task
  - not demonstrating respect for individuality and autonomy of its members
  - uninvolved in community activities
  - inability to adapt to change/deal with traumatic experience constructively
  - inability to meet security needs of its members
- Unhealthy family decision-making process
- Failure to send and receive clear messages
- Inappropriate boundary maintenance
- Inappropriate/poorly communicated family rules, rituals, symbols
- Unexamined family myths
- Inappropriate level and direction of energy

Content appearing in this typeface is additional information not included in the NANDA nursing diagnoses.

Expected Outcome/Goals

The family will

➤ retain/maintain open lines of communication as evidenced by members sharing feelings with each other.

➤ adapt to the changes within the family as evidenced by each member sharing responsibilities.

➤ respect the individuality of each member as evidenced by encouraging self-care activities.

➤ participate in the care of the patient as evidenced by

  ▷ assisting with the medical regimen

  ▷ seeking resources as needed.

Nursing Orders with Rationale

➤ Assess and monitor for presence/absence/ changes in assessment findings outlined above
  in order to detect any change in status.

➤ Identify the family dysfunction (e.g., denial of the problem, separation, exploitation, no negotiation), the most distressing aspects of the current situation.
  Successful coping with illness requires that the family acknowledge the problem and seek help to adjust to the changes (Friedman, 1981).

➤ Orient family to environment (e.g., visiting hours, cafeteria, lounge) and to the schedule of patient's daily activities.
  Familiarity and knowledge decrease anxiety.

➤ Assess the interactions between family members; monitor for dysfunctional behaviors (e.g., poor communication, power struggles); discuss behaviors identified with the family.
  Communication patterns of the family determine the quality of the family life (Carpenito, 1989).

➤ Assess the impact of the patient's illness on the family's stability and functioning; explore potential problems and family's coping abilities.
  Each family member influences the family unit, so illness of a member will influence the functioning of the family (Carpenito, 1989).

➤ Listen attentively to all members; maintain nonjudgmental attitude; convey realistic hope.
  Active listening conveys caring and understanding, and allows family members to express their concerns.

➤ Encourage members to express thoughts/feelings/perceptions such as guilt, anger, fear; give permission for family to have a wide range of emotions.
  Release of emotions helps people to accept the current situation and prevents prolonged grieving.

➤ Schedule family conferences
  to assist family to gain a realistic perspective of the situation and to make choices based on discussion of all the alternatives (Caine & Bufalino, 1987).

➤ Keep family members informed of progress; explain all test/procedures in simple terms
  to decrease fear and anxiety.

➤ Discuss with the family how the illness is affecting the patient's mood, activity level, stress level, and degree of comfort.
  This helps the family accept the patient's disabilities and make necessary accommodations.

➤ Determine the desire of each member to participate in the care of the new/ill family member; develop a plan to incorporate each member in the care activities.
  The family may be viewed as a system; each member's contribution affects the total functioning (Miller & Winstead-Fry, 1982).

➤ Support role-playing activities; support acceptable methods of ventilation; reinforce positive coping mechanisms
  in order to assist family members to appreciate each other's feelings and point of view.

➤ Help to explore new coping strategies (e.g., greater reliance on each other, humor, sharing feelings, use of resources and support systems); support acceptable methods of ventilation; reinforce positive coping mechanisms.
  Constructive coping assists the family to adjust to member's illness and the necessary changes to be make (Friedman, 1981).

➤ Inform all members of the importance of taking care of themselves; assist to balance daily activities with self-fulfilling activities.
  Self-care of each member is critical so no one else becomes sick during a time of crisis.

➤ Identify resources (e.g., professional and self-help groups, financial, housekeeping) available
  to assist with the adaptation to new/altered roles.

➤ Discuss possible role changes, necessary adaptations, and potential changes in ill family members; explore feelings; develop a plan to cope with change in family structure.

Within one family, members interact in a variety of roles. Illness of one member may cause great role changes, making the family at high risk for maladaptation (Fife, 1985).

Charting Components

➤ Behaviors and stated feelings of family members
➤ Interventions made with family to facilitate communication, problem solving, adaptation to role changes
➤ Participation in care of patient
➤ Plan of health team
➤ Potential/actual problems created by illness of family member
➤ Referrals made
➤ Responsibilities shared
➤ Resources identified

3. Altered Family Processes: Alcoholism

Definition

The state in which the psychosocial, spiritual, and physiological functions of the family unit are chronically disorganized, leading to conflict, denial of problems, resistance to change, ineffective problem solving, and a series of self-perpetuating crises

Related to

➤ Abuse of alcohol
➤ Family history of alcoholism
➤ Resistance to treatment
➤ Inadequate coping skills
➤ Genetic predisposition
➤ Addictive personality
➤ Lack of problem-solving skills
➤ Biochemical influences

Characteristics/Assessment Findings

Feelings
➤ Decreased self-esteem/worthlessness
➤ Anger/suppressed rage
➤ Frustration, powerlessness
➤ Anxiety/tension/distress
➤ Insecurity
➤ Repressed emotions
➤ Responsibility for alcoholic's behavior
➤ Lingering resentment
➤ Shame/embarrassment
➤ Hurt, unhappiness, guilt
➤ Emotional isolation/loneliness
➤ Vulnerability, mistrust
➤ Hopelessness, rejection

Roles and Relationships
➤ Deterioration in family relationship, disturbed, family dynamics
➤ Ineffective spouse communication, marital problems
➤ Altered role function, disruption of family roles
➤ Inconsistent parenting, low perception of parental support
➤ Family denial
➤ Intimacy dysfunction
➤ Chronic family problems
➤ Closed communication systems

Behaviors
➤ Expression of anger inappropriately
➤ Difficulty with intimate relationships
➤ Loss of control of drinking
➤ Impaired communication
➤ Ineffective problem-solving skills
➤ Enabling to maintain drinking
➤ Inability to meet emotional needs of family members
➤ Manipulation
➤ Dependency
➤ Alcohol abuse
➤ Broken promises
➤ Rationalization/denial of problems
➤ Refusal to get help, inability to accept and receive help appropriately
➤ Inadequate understanding or knowledge of alcoholism
➤ Stress related illnesses
➤ Substance abuse other than alcohol

Expected Outcomes/Goals

The family will
- Establish a functional equilibrium as evidenced by
  - communicating effectively
  - correcting distorted perceptions about alcoholism
  - understanding the disease concept of alcoholism
  - believing that alcoholism is a family illness
  - discussing feelings openly
  - establishing functional roles
  - making a genogram
  - attending appropriate 12-step programs
  - facilitating each member to maintain a self-focus and self-care
  - establishing personal and intergenerational boundaries
  - implementing effective problem solving
  - contacting community/school resources
  - understanding the process of intervention.

Nursing Orders with Rationale

- Assess and monitor for presence/absence/changes in assessment findings outlined above *in order to detect any change in status.*

- Assess family coping strategies and support systems.
  Many family systems in which there is chemical dependency are closed systems that are cut off from community support as well as from the emotional support of each other.

- Assure confidentiality and assist the family members in discussing how alcoholism has affected them individually and as a family.
  Open discussion of toxic issues in a safe environment inhibits denial and encourages the giving up of family secrets (Lewis, Dana, & Blevins, 1988).

- Provide factual information on addictions and the disease concept of alcoholism.
  Knowledge can instill hope and help dispel stigma thus reducing the amount of guilt and shame felt within the family.

- Observe for signs of physical abuse, incest, or other maladaptive behaviors that may be acted out within the family.
  Violence and incest have been identified as problematic in homes with addictions (Yegidis, 1992).

- Report child, elder, or spousal abuse to proper authorities.
  Nurses are mandatory reporters of sexual abuse, and child, elder, and dependent adult abuse.

- Educate the family concerning the belief that alcoholism is a family illness in which all members have been affected.
  Family members are often so involved and focused on the chemically dependent member that they are unable to see how they will also need support in changing dysfunctional patterns that may have perpetuated the disease.

- Encourage the family to label and verbally express their feelings.
  Family members may not have access to their feelings because of the amount of stress the family system is undergoing. Often family members have ambivalent and conflicting feelings that can be painful to experience and difficult to identify.

- Inform the family about the three C's: They didn't *cause* alcoholism, they can't *cure* alcoholism, and they can't *control* alcoholism.
  This knowledge will help reduce the shame and guilt within the family.

- Attempt to include the extended family in the counseling sessions.
  Alcoholism is often multigenerational. A genetic predisposition may exist (Blum, Noble, and Sheridan, 1991).

- Assist family members to identify triangles and unhealthy coalitions within the system *to establish healthy boundaries between generations (Coleman, 1987).*

- Assess pursuing/distancing patterns used by the family in retreating from personal interactions and intimacy (Bowen, 1978).
  Excessive consumption of alcohol makes people unavailable, thus the dynamic of pursuit is triggered when the alcoholic distances.

- Reinforce the concept of detachment and support the family in attending Al-Anon or other appropriate 12-step programs.
  This will help modify the behavior of the pursuer and will give the family additional needed support.

➤ Assess the dysfunctional role behaviors within the family.
Roles such as chief enabler, family hero, scapegoat, lost child, and mascot have been identified in chemically dependent homes and help defend against anxiety and feelings of inadequacy (Wegscheider, 1979).

➤ Observe for overfunctioning/underfunctioning patterns within the family dyad.
This will help identify the role of the enabler who is unconsciously assisting in the dysfunctional process.

➤ Help the family to create a genogram for the past three generations.
This will help the family to discover dysfunctional patterns and address interdependencies. The overfunctioning spouse can refocus on discovering patterns within the family (Bennett & Woolf, 1991).

➤ Help the codependent to distinguish between enabling behaviors and caring.
Codependents display resistance to change and often focus on blame rather than on changing their reactions and behaviors.

➤ Explore with the codependent how that person has coped with the alcoholic's behavior in the past.
The chemically dependent person relies on others to cover up destructive behaviors, thus they remain powerless.

➤ Help the individual family members to maintain self-care, socialize, and participate in outside hobbies and interests.
Many times, family members in alcoholic homes lose touch with their own needs and wants while they focus on the problematic behaviors of the chemically dependent person.

➤ Facilitate the discussion of behaviors used to reduce family stress.
The family with chemical dependency develops exaggerated defenses that protect them from pain and that create the least amount of personal distress.

➤ Assist the family to identify activities that will reduce stress and provide for recreational needs.
This will support the family in maintaining adaptive ways to function.

➤ Explain the concept of *intervention* to the family.
Family intervention is an event and a process designed to motivate a chemically dependent person to use professional help. The chemically dependent person is confronted with accurate data concerning the disease of alcoholism by a group of concerned others. Concerned others are involved in a series of preparatory and follow-up stages to enable them to participate in the family intervention event.

➤ Assess the family's readiness for an intervention.
The family must be willing to cooperate with each other and recognize the need for outside help and support before an intervention can be effective.

➤ Determine with the family a plan for referral and follow-up services.
The family may need assistance in contacting an intervention counselor/facilitator or appropriate treatment for the chemically dependent person.

Charting Components

➤ Authorizing consents for treatment for minors
➤ Community resources contacted
➤ Feelings expressed
➤ Roles and behavior patterns identified
➤ Family teaching completed
➤ Effective coping strategies used

C. SEXUALITY PATTERNS

1. Altered Sexuality Patterns

Definition

The state in which an individual expresses concern regarding his or her sexuality

Related to

➤ Knowledge/skill deficit about alternative responses to health-related transitions, altered body function or structure, illness
➤ Lack of privacy
➤ Lack of significant other
➤ Ineffective or absent role models
➤ Conflicts with sexual orientation or variant preferences
➤ Fear of pregnancy or of acquiring a sexually transmitted disease
➤ Impaired relationship with a significant other
➤ Altered self-concept from change in appearance
➤ Altered self-concept from change in functional role(s)
➤ Anxiety, guilt
➤ Fatigue, pain
➤ Fear of sexual failure
➤ Ineffective coping
➤ Medications (e.g., antihypertensives, psychotropics)
➤ Substance abuse
➤ Alteration in mood
➤ Cognitive dysfunction
➤ Shame regarding sexual practices
➤ Menopause
➤ Aging

Content appearing in this typeface is additional information not included in the NANDA nursing diagnoses.

Characteristics/Assessment Findings

➤ Reported difficulties, limitations, or changes in sexual behaviors or activities
➤ Anticipated body function changes resulting from medical/surgical treatment (e.g., mastectomy, colostomy)
➤ Presence of illness or medical problem likely to require an adjustment in sexuality patterns (e.g., neurological, gynecological, urological, cardiac, endocrine problems)
➤ Presence of psychiatric illness resulting in loss of impulse control (e.g., bipolar disorder, organic mental disorder)
➤ Loss of social judgment regarding appropriateness of sexual expression (e.g., cognitive disorders, personality disorders)
➤ Loss of sexual desire as found in depressive disorders

Expected Outcomes/Goals

The patient will reestablish satisfactory (to him or her) sexual functioning as evidenced by
➤ positive self-report
➤ positive report from partner
➤ verbalized willingness to explore solutions to perceived difficulties
➤ verbalized report regarding acceptance of sexual practices
➤ verbal willingness to contact professional support if the need for more intensive therapy has been identified

Nursing Orders with Rationale

➤ Assess and monitor for presence/absence/changes in assessment findings outlined above *in order to detect any change in status.*

➤ Explore own attitudes, values, and feelings regarding sexuality.
   Until the nurse is comfortable discussing sexuality openly, free discussion of sensitive issues will be impossible. Values clarification is necessary so that the nurse does not project own beliefs onto the patient.

➤ Establishing a trusting relationship with patient
  to build trust and rapport, making it easier to discuss intimate issues (Carpenito, 1989).

➤ Gather information about the patient's usual sexual functioning
  to determine realistic approaches to current sexual needs.

➤ Assess patient's perception of the actual or potential problem
  to determine if it is realistic.

➤ Assess if the patient has had sexual difficulty in the past; if so, what the specific problem was and how it was resolved; refer to nursing care plan "Sexual Dysfunction."
  A more detailed assessment is carried out once a problem is acknowledged or assistance is requested.

➤ Assess frequency of sexual activity either with a partner or through masturbation.
  Most individuals think that a certain frequency of sexual activity is normal; the nurse can provide information concerning the wide range of frequency. Many individuals think that masturbation is unhealthy or immoral. Reassurance that masturbation is natural and can enhance a person's sexual sensitivity is valuable. Masturbation is also used to reduce stress and tension.

➤ Ensure privacy and confidentiality; approach patient with an open, nonjudgmental attitude; move at patient's pace, allow patient to refuse to discuss topic; be aware of age, gender, and cultural differences between nurse and patient.
  Most patients will be reluctant to discuss sexual matters. Nurses need to create a climate that facilitates, not forces, discussion of these topics. Communication needs to be clear, confident, and reassuring (Caine & Bufalino, 1987).

➤ Begin sexual assessment in areas that are least sensitive.
  Adapt your discussion to the patient's life-style and stated needs. Use the patient's terminology to decrease embarrassment (Katzin, 1990).

➤ Explore patient's knowledge of birth control.
  When discussing birth-control measures the nurse must remain sensitive to the culture, religious, and economic background of the patient.

➤ Assess patient's self-esteem, how patient feels about own looks, body, achievements, relationships.
  Positive self-esteem and body image are characteristic of a sexually healthy person (Lion, 1982).

➤ Assess how the patient's role performance has affected own sense of being sexually attractive.
  When a patient is forced to give up a role or function that is linked to his or her sex role, actual sexuality or the perception of being an acceptable partner is often threatened.

➤ Ascertain if patient perceives that illness, treatments, etc., are interfering with usual sexual functioning.
  Studies have indicated that about half of medical-surgical patients thought their illness might interfere with usual sexual functioning (Wilson, 1987).

➤ Encourage patient/partner to verbalize thoughts and feelings regarding anticipated/actual sexual changes (e.g., imagined responses of partner, fear of rejection).
  Patients may need to be given "permission" to discuss sexual concerns. The nurse may need to initiate the discussions (Carpenito, 1989).

➤ Provide information regarding the possible effects that treatment, illness, and medication can have on sexual desire and functioning.
  Knowledge of potential problems decreases feelings of fear, shame, and embarrassment. This discussion lets the patient know that the nurse is knowledgeable and available to talk about sexual concerns.

➤ Discuss the effect of psychotropic medication on sexual desire and performance.
  Almost all psychotropic medication affects sexuality by either increasing desire, decreasing interest, or interfering with the sexual response cycle. The nurse needs to know the specific effects that the prescribed medication can produce (Harris, 1988).

➤ Assess attitudes concerning sexual variations, knowledge of anatomy and physiology, and knowledge of the human sexual response cycle
  to establish what is possible for the patient and what needs to be taught.

➤ Assess for neurovegetative changes in functioning that can often be associated with menopause or hysterectomy.
  Fatigue, insomnia, constipation, changes in eating patterns, and decreased interest in sex indicate the presence of depression rather than an endocrine imbalance. Depression that results from grief is often associated with loss of menstruation or alteration in body functioning. These losses are highly symbolic for many women as well as men (Barry, 1984).

➤ Assess for emotional responses of guilt, anxiety, or avoidant reactions to sexuality.

Many incest survivors have severe guilt because they believe they did not resist the incestual relationship, derived physical pleasure from the experience, or because of the rewards or privileges bestowed upon them by the perpetrator (Urbanic, 1989).

➤ Be alert for underlying issues regarding childhood incest or abuse when working with patients who are self-destructive or who discuss child-rearing problems.

There is a high incidence and lingering traumatic effects of childhood incest among women who seek treatment at psychiatric and mental health facilities (Urbanic, 1987).

➤ Encourage patient to share his or her incest "secret" with a trusted professional.

Sharing the secret provides an opportunity for an emotional cleansing or catharsis (Urbanic, 1989).

➤ Provide information regarding incest in a matter-of-fact manner that also offers support and reassurance; refer to support group or for intensive psychotherapy as indicated.

The adult is always responsible for the sexual behavior as the child lacks an adult concept of sexuality and seductiveness.

➤ Have patient complete a questionnaire that covers sexual myths, practices, and beliefs.

Using an objective questionnaire allows patient time to think through issues in privacy and helps generate questions for future discussion.

➤ Discuss with the patient/couple what is considered adaptive sexuality.

The criteria for adaptive sexuality are that it be between two consenting adults, mutually satisfying, not psychologically or physically harmful, lacking in force or coercion, and conducted in private. According to the American Psychological Association, homosexuality is not deviant sexual behavior.

➤ Reassure that the patient's sexual practices are adaptive.

Permission by a professional can often prevent the escalation of a major problem.

➤ Provide information to dispel anxiety over myths, body parts, and types of sexual contact.

Giving limited information in such areas as breast and penis size, masturbation, intercourse during menstruation, oral-genital contact, sexual frequency, and use of fantasy often relieves anxiety and enhances self-esteem.

➤ Encourage frank discussion between partners; allow private time; help patient view and share body changes with partner if appropriate; refer to nursing care plan "Body-Image Disturbance" as necessary.

Emphasizing the importance of telling each other personal concerns and fears can avoid many problems. Often, partners will try to protect each other or avoid making demands and the message is interpreted as, "I am not attractive or desirable any longer."

➤ Emphasize the emotional aspects of sex, especially if major physical change prohibits successful coitus.

Nonphysical avenues of sexual expression and noncoital activities can be satisfying.

➤ When discussing sexual difficulties or changes in sexuality with a couple, do not focus on just one partner as the individual who has a problem, but rather present the attitude that sexual problems are solvable together.

If one partner is identified as having the problem, blame and guilt are enhanced and the couple will not be able to mutually support each other. Major sexual dysfunction may result if one partner assumes all the responsibility.

➤ Indicate to the couple that specific sexual difficulties do not mean that the couple is having other serious relationship problems.

Though difficulty with intimacy may underlie sexual problems, just increasing intimacy and communication may not solve the actual sexual difficulty. Approximately 75% of couples seeking marital counseling have significant sexual problems (Wilson, 1987).

➤ Discuss with the patient the effect of cigarette smoking and the consumption of alcoholic beverages on sexuality.

One of the first suggestions made to males who are having difficulty maintaining erections is to decrease the use of tobacco and alcohol. Nicotine restricts blood flow and can cause subtle neurologic changes. Alcohol decreases the amount of testosterone and can even produce female secondary sex characteristics.

➤ As patient desires, discuss methods to facilitate sexual functioning or alternate methods if needed (e.g., analgesics, relaxation techniques, erotic materials, massages, alternative positions, time of day, or techniques).

Depending on the cause of the alteration, a variety of methods may need to be employed temporarily or permanently. Fatigue and pain can be minimized.

➤ Foster and assist the patient to maintain personal appearance (e.g., by using perfumes or aftershave lotion, wearing jewelry).

Looking attractive contributes to feeling sexy and desirable (Lion, 1982).

➤ Include discussion of sexual concerns with all age groups.

Sexuality is not restricted to the young and healthy; sexual expression is important for all age groups.

➤ Provide information regarding sexuality and the aging process; assure patients that sexual capability can be maintained throughout the life span.

An extremely important variable affecting altered sexuality of older persons is prolonged abstinence. The older female who abstains from sexual activity may have shrinkage in the size of her vagina; the older male who abstains may experience difficulty with erections.

➤ Discuss physiological changes that may occur in the older male.

To prevent sexual dysfunction both men and women need to know the normal physiological changes that occur in male sexuality (e.g., needing more direct genital stimulation to achieve erection, decreased firmness of erections, less intensity during ejaculation, a greater refractory time between ejaculations).

➤ Discuss changes that may occur during menopause; provide information to patients that may decrease symptoms.

Vaginal dryness, depression, anxiety, flushes, insomnia are related to decreased levels of estrogen. Hormone replacement therapy needs to be discussed with the patient's physician. The use of a water-soluble lubricant facilitates intercourse. Remaining sexually active either with a partner or by masturbation aids sexual functioning (Sarrel & Sarrel, 1986).

➤ Discuss with the patient and sexual partner the effect of mood on sexual desire.

Severe depression often results in decreased interest in sexuality while mania can create hypersexuality.

➤ Observe for behaviors that are sexually acted out.

Sexual acting out occurs in a variety of psychiatric disorders. Inappropriate expression of sexuality can be a sign of low self-esteem or loss of impulse control.

➤ Decrease patient's inappropriate expressions of sexual feelings and behavior:
  ▷ set limits on patient's sexual behavior.
  ▷ decrease environmental stimuli.
  ▷ assign a mature, experienced nurse as the patient's primary caregiver.
  ▷ use a calm and matter-of-fact approach.
  ▷ convey caring for the individual.
  ▷ positively reinforce appropriate interactions.

The manic patient can become the brunt of jokes by both staff and other patients. Patients are often ashamed of their behavior once the mania is controlled. A total team approach is necessary in decreasing hyperactivity (Brenners & Weston, 1987).

➤ Explore the meaning of the patient's behavior.

Sexually inappropriate or aggressive behavior may mask many other needs. Until the nurse and patient set limits and engage in a therapeutic relationship, much valuable data may be missed. Patients often use the sexual arena to gain attention and caring. Many patients who have cognitive impairments are unaware that their behavior is inappropriate. Other patients are suffering from low self-esteem.

➤ Respect patient's boundaries.

Patients who have cognitive impairment or who are hypersexual may misperceive the nurse's use of touch.

➤ Maintain a caring and professional attitude while assessing for the presence of sexually transmitted diseases.

Guilt and shame that can result from contracting a sexually transmitted disease may decrease self-esteem and cause an individual to feel undesirable.

➤ Offer health teaching regarding sexually transmitted diseases.

> *Giving specific information on how the disease is contracted and transmitted will help reduce anxiety.*

➤ Assist patient to see the illness as separate from the self.

> *Fear of rejection is a common feature of individuals who have been infected with a sexually transmitted disease. Patients need to learn to separate the illness from the self in order to have a healthy self-image.*

➤ Offer information concerning genital herpes; refer to a physician for medical treatment as necessary.

> *Surveys have shown that individuals with genital herpes report reduced intimacy and sexual pleasure, inhibited sexual freedom, and increased impotence and other sexual problems (Chenitz & Swanson, 1989).*

➤ Provide resources and referrals for emotional support.

> *A more adaptive adjustment to herpes has been correlated with positive social support (Chenitz & Swanson, 1989).*

➤ Refer to appropriate therapist or group for more intensive counseling if giving "permission," giving "limited information," giving "specific suggestions," or helping the patient contain his or her behavior has proved ineffective.

> *Sexual counseling may be outside the scope of the nurse's expertise or level of comfort. Patients need to know that help is available and can be accessed (Kim, McFarland, & McLane, 1987).*

Charting Components

➤ Ability to describe current problem, onset, course over time
➤ Change in sexual attitudes/behavior
➤ Concerns expressed
➤ Counseling strategies employed by the nurse
➤ Patient's concept of the cause of the problem
➤ Patient's report of increased sexual satisfaction
➤ Referrals made
➤ Significant other's concerns, perception of the problem
➤ Patient/significant other teaching, response

Additional Nursing Orders for THE PATIENT AT RISK FOR A POSITIVE HIV TEST

➤ Provide a nonjudgmental attitude with care and support.

> *Nurses must be aware of their own feelings, fears, and prejudices. Support groups for healthcare providers are essential (Van Devanter, Grisaffi, Steilen, Scarola, & Shipton, 1987).*

➤ When discussing sexuality, be sensitive to expressions of anxiety related to powerlessness and stigma; refer to nursing care plan "Powerlessness" as needed.

➤ Present facts, but also try to convey a sense of hopefulness.

> *Carrying the virus is not the same as having AIDS or other complications that the virus can cause. Teach health-promotion activities and discuss safe sex practices (Van Devanter et al., 1987).*

➤ Use a crisis-interventional approach to the newly diagnosed HIV patient.

> *Learning of a positive antibody test confronts a person with an overwhelming sense of loss. Initial reactions vary depending on personality, coping style, and support available (Van Devanter et al., 1987).*

➤ Explore the range of creative sexual possibilities that exist once the shock of a positive test has subsided.

> *Offering support, opening up communication options and alternatives reduces the sense of loss.*

Additional Charting Components

Before charting information concerning sexually transmitted diseases, know the laws in your state.
➤ Interventions used, response
➤ Patient's response to positive test

IV. Valuing

A. SPIRITUAL STATE

1. Spiritual Distress

Definition

Disruption in the life principle that pervades a person's entire being and that integrates and transcends one's biological and psychosocial nature

Related to

- Separation from religious/cultural ties
- Challenged belief and value system (e.g., caused by moral/ethical implications of therapy, intense suffering)
- Death of a significant other
- Hopelessness
- Illness
- Lack of purpose and meaning in life
- Life changes
- Questioning personal belief and value system
- Separation/loss of a valued object or situation (e.g., job, finances, property)
- Threat of loss of control of a life situation
- Unfavorable prognosis

Characteristics/Assessment Findings

- *Expresses concern with meaning of life/ death or belief systems
- Anger toward God
- Questions meaning of suffering
- Verbalizes inner conflict about beliefs
- Verbalizes concern about relationship with deity
- Questions meaning of own existence
- Inability to participate in usual religious practices
- Seeks spiritual assistance
- Questions moral/ethical implications of therapeutic regimen
- Gallows humor
- Displacement of anger toward religious representatives
- Describes nightmares/sleep disturbances
- Alteration in behavior/mood evidenced by anger, crying, withdrawal, preoccupation, anxiety, hostility, apathy, etc.
- Demonstrated interest in spiritual matters
- Expresses feelings of not being wanted/loved or valued; of unworthiness, loneliness; being cut off from source of strength, faith, hope, peace
- Questions subsequent influence of supreme being on current illness/situation
- Expresses feelings of being punished by God or supreme being for some perceived wrongdoing
- Unable to forgive oneself for perceived wrongdoing
- Lack of reconciliation with God or supreme being
- Loss or separation from religious or spiritual practices, either short- or long-term
- Expressed need for religious representative (e.g., rabbi, priest, minister, pastoral care), articles, literature, etc.
- Recognition of one's own mortality
- Searching for a spiritual source of strength

Content appearing in this typeface is additional information not included in the NANDA nursing diagnoses.

*Critical.

Expected Outcomes/Goals

The patient will

➤ express feelings about spiritual values as evidenced by
  ▷ describing personal spiritual/religious values
  ▷ discussing conflict with spiritual/religious/belief systems
  ▷ identifying source of conflict
  ▷ describing previous sources of inner strength, faith, hope, peace, joy.
➤ verbalize comfort and satisfaction from spiritual resources as evidenced by
  ▷ expressing resolution of conflict, guilt
  ▷ describing feelings of no longer being cut off from source of strength, hope, peace, forgiveness
  ▷ implementing practices or using sources of spiritual/religious strength, hope, peace, forgiveness.
➤ demonstrate maintenance of any spiritual practices desired (e.g., required foods, spiritual articles) as manifested by
  ▷ continuation of direction of spiritual development
  ▷ expressing comfort with spiritual, religious, personal, or cultural values/belief systems
  ▷ requesting dietary regimens that adhere to religious or spiritual practices/values
  ▷ instituting or reinstituting religious/spiritual practices (e.g., prayer, meditation, journaling)
  ▷ verbalizing desire for pastoral care visits, church attendance, chaplain visits, religious or spiritual articles, reading materials.

Nursing Orders with Rationale

➤ Assess and monitor for presence/absence/changes in assessment findings outlined above *in order to detect any change in status.*

➤ Assess the patient's spiritual needs:
  ▷ look at patient's environment (e.g., Bibles, religious objects, inspirational reading)
  ▷ look at patient's thought patterns, content of speech, affect
    to differentiate delusions and hallucinations from actual needs.
  ▷ look at cultural orientation and social relationships.
    Information about the patient's spiritual component is harder to obtain because it does not always lend itself to direct observation (Peterson & Nelson, 1987).

➤ Reassure patient that it is all right to verbalize religious or spiritual issues; create an atmosphere of acceptance of patient's values and level of spiritual/religious development or need.
  "Spiritual care like that of emotional care is personal availability, accessibility, compassion, listening, and dialogue: the maintenance of the human connection" (Dugan, 1987).

➤ Realize that the nurse does not need to provide answers for the patient; use the same approaches and responses (e.g., reflection, empathy, clarification) that are normally used in interactions.
  What is often needed is just someone who cares and will be present during patients' struggle with their need to find meaning, and as they learn to forgive themselves and establish a source of love and relatedness (Peterson & Nelson, 1987).

➤ Differentiate between the concepts of "spiritual" and "religious" because a patient may have spiritual needs (e.g., lack of meaning and purpose in life, guilt, need for love) but not have religious needs (e.g., want to be baptized, or read the Bible).
  Religion is an organized set of beliefs and practices. Spirituality is a transcendental relationship between the person and a higher being, that strives for reverence, awe, and inspiration, and that gives answers about the infinite (Murray, 1990).

➤ Do not assume that a patient's stated religious affiliation means that she or he accepts or lives by all the beliefs or practices.
  Because a woman is Catholic does not mean that she will automatically feel guilt about an abortion (Peterson & Nelson, 1987).

➤ Ask what spiritual practices are significant to the patient when she or he is not ill
  to help sort out the religious preoccupation that sometimes comes with illness or an exacerbation of illness (Peterson & Nelson, 1987).

➤ Ascertain what the practices mean in light of the history of the patient (e.g., guilt and fear or feelings of warmth and comfort), and in the light of the immediate stressors the patient is under (e.g., becoming more religious as a way of coping).
  This information can give a clue to possible future hopes and spiritual integrity of the patient as a person.

➤ Determine whether a patient is exhibiting pathology or expressing a legitimate spiritual concern.
  Religious beliefs or concerns can be integrated into the illness (e.g., patients who believe themselves to be Jesus Christ, or who kill because God told them to do so) (Peterson & Nelson, 1987).

➤ Determine how the patient deals with guilt (e.g., ruminates over past behaviors); how the patient responds to criticism in the present (e.g., hostility, projection, accusation of others).
  Guilt and resentment are what result when forgiveness does not happen. The need for forgiveness is frequently observed in mentally ill patients. The inability to forgive self often leads to an inability to tolerate anything that resembles criticism (Peterson & Nelson, 1987).

➤ Ask if anything or anyone contributes to the patient's sense of dignity and worth.
  A source of love and relatedness is a major issue for many mentally ill patients. Often their social skills have been poorly developed, or have deteriorated during illness, or they have difficulty establishing or maintaining relationships with others (Peterson & Nelson, 1987).

➤ Recognized that "Why did this happen to me?" questions reflect a distressed value system; help patient acknowledge that what they believed about God, life, etc., seems to be in question. "Why me?" questions indicate that the patient's beliefs about life do not provide an adequate explanation for the current situation (Hill & Smith, 1990).

➤ Encourage the expression of anger, disappointment, and fear that accompanies feeling let down or betrayed by God, life, etc.
  Releasing painful emotions allows people to think more clearly about what they believe.

➤ Discuss with the patient what gives meaning and purpose to life; what has been meaningful in the past? when did she or he recognize a sense of meaningless?
  Mentally ill patients often struggle with finding a source of meaning and purpose in their lives. Direct questions may not elicit much information unless the patient is able to think abstractly (Peterson & Nelson, 1987).

➤ Help patient clarify personal values and beliefs by giving feedback, clarifying, and lending perspective.
  Clarification, support, understanding, openness, and nonjudgmental acceptance is an inherent component of spiritual care (Dickinson, 1975).

➤ Provide an environment of acceptance; ensure privacy and time for prayer, meditation, reading, journal writing as desired.
  Spirituality is a significant component of each person and is shared by all human beings (Potter & Perry, 1988). How individuals actualize this dimension varies with each person.

➤ Pray with patient if requested; refer another source if unable to comply with request.
  Praying with patients, for nurses who are comfortable with this, can provide a sense of connectedness or community (Hover, 1986) at a time when the patient may feel isolated and alone.

➤ Discuss moral/ethical questions with patient and family; include specialist in any decisions (e.g., ethicist, clergy, lawyer); use resources (e.g., friends, family, clergy) as needed
  to provide spiritual support (Hill & Smith, 1990).

➤ Provide opportunities where patient can divert energies to others outside of self.
  A crisis of health, grief, or loss may shake the individual's fundamental view of life, self-worth, goals, meaning, and suffering (Hill & Smith, 1990). For some people, crisis can provide an opportunity for spiritual growth. Being of service to others can provide one method of spiritual growth and development and serve as a way to divert energy outside of oneself (Hall, 1986; Hill & Smith, 1990).

➤ Suggest journal writings to express daily thoughts and reflections.
  Journaling can provide a way to explore and express inner feelings, thoughts, unconscious messages or to explore deeper meaning in life (Hill & Smith, 1990).

➤ Provide touch or attendance
  to promote trust/security and to provide a sense of connection and community with others.

Charting Components

➤ Conflicts between medical regimen and spiritual beliefs
➤ Conflicts or noncompliant behavior that does not seem to conform to the person's previous response to crisis, illness, pain, or loss
➤ Ethical dilemma that needs a decision
➤ Need for or request made for clergy
➤ Role of God/religion in patient's life
➤ Spiritual practice being done in the hospital
➤ Strength of belief system to cope with illness

V. Choosing

A. COPING

1. Ineffective Individual Coping

Definition

Impairment of adaptive behaviors and problem-solving abilities of a person in meeting life's demands and roles

Related to

- Situational crises
  - altered family support
  - body-image changes
  - distorted perception of the problem
  - pain, physical abilities
  - nature of disease
  - sexual dysfunction
- Maturational crises (e.g., life-style changes)
- Personal vulnerability
- Ego deficits/developmental immaturity
- Environmental stressors
- Lack of supportive environment
- Knowledge deficit
- Chronic pain or physical disability
- Dependence on chemical substances
- Excessive anxiety
- Impaired reality testing
- Impaired thought processes

Content appearing in this typeface is additional information not included in the NANDA nursing diagnoses.

Characteristics/Assessment Findings

- *Verbalization of inability to cope/ask for help
- Inability to meet role expectations
- Inability to meet basic needs
- *Inability to problem solve
- Alteration in societal participation
- Destructive behavior toward self or others
- Inappropriate use of defense mechanisms
- Change in usual communication patterns
- Verbal manipulation
- High illness rate
- High rate of accidents
- Inadequate support system
- Reported low self-esteem
- History of substance abuse
- Perceptual distortions
- Verbalized high expectation of self
- Aggressive rather than assertive behavioral style
- Immature, maladaptive behavior

Expected Outcomes/Goals

The patient will
- identify nature of stress as evidenced by
  - describing the stress and source
  - identifying various factors involved
  - expressing feelings related to stress.
- increase adaptive ways to cope with stress as evidenced by
  - acknowledging own strengths (skills, resources) to cope with problems
  - discussing alternative ways to meet demands of current situation
  - identifying changes that could be made in current life-style.

---

*Critical.

Nursing Orders with Rationale

➤ Assess and monitor for presence/absence/ changes in assessment findings outlined above *in order to detect any change in status.*

➤ Identify patient's perception and understanding of current situation; do not be judgmental or argumentative, but accept what patient shares as valid for him or her.
Distorted perceptions can raise anxiety level and render the problem unsolvable.

➤ Assess stressors and precipitating causes of current situation.
Ineffective coping often results from the cumulative effect of various stressors, one of which has precipitated the current dysfunctional coping pattern. By understanding the nature of the stressors, the nurse can work to reduce their impact on patient's life.

➤ Identify patient's ego deficits and developmental deficiencies.
Ineffective coping may result from deficits in ego functioning (e.g., reality testing, object relatedness, impulse control, thought processes, self-perception). These deficits are commonly seen in patients with borderline, substance-abuse, and obsessive-compulsive disorders and in brief psychotic reactions (Kerr, 1990).

➤ Evaluate patient's decision-making ability; teach to identify the problem, to explore alternatives and their outcomes, to select an action, and to evaluate the results:
  ▷ reinforce positive attempts.
  ▷ display empathy when patient has setbacks.
  ▷ avoid giving advice or false reassurance; state your belief in patient's ability to make adaptive choices.
Understanding the problem-solving approach will enable the patient to apply current knowledge in a variety of situations after discharge.

➤ Reinforce patient's current skills, resources, and knowledge to deal with problems; provide opportunities to patient to make decisions in daily care.
Reinforcing patient's ego competencies helps to mobilize available external/internal resources (Kerr, 1990). Making successful decisions reinforces the patient's ability to solve some of own problems.

➤ Listen therapeutically, use open-ended questions (e.g., "How have you handled this situation in the past?")
to help patient develop coping strategies based on previous experiences and personal strengths.

➤ Identify any maladaptive behavior patient may be exhibiting (e.g., blaming others, aggression, withdrawal, substance abuse); do not encourage or reinforce it.
Reinforcement of maladaptive coping inhibits the development of adaptive coping (McFarland & Wasli, 1986).

➤ Observe for destructive behavior toward self or others; protect patient and others.
Destructive behavior is a symptom of low self-esteem, feeling overwhelmed, unable to cope successfully (McFarland & Wasli, 1986).

➤ Teach use of "I" statements to state feelings and needs (e.g., "I am upset" rather than, "You make me angry.").
Effective communication facilitates better relationships and helps to get one's needs met.

➤ Provide opportunities for patient to verbalize feelings; use reflective statements to convey empathy and understanding (e.g., "It must be very difficult for you to adjust to . . . ").
Feeling understood helps the patient to express feelings and accept new situations.

➤ Help patient to set and accomplish achievable goals.
Developing a specific plan of action helps to counteract paralysis or withdrawal that had arisen because of anxiety (Carpenito, 1989).

➤ Support therapeutic contributions of other professionals on the healthcare team.
This establishes a network of people who can function as a network of support as the patient endeavors to solve his or her problems.

➤ Evaluate with patient current life-style patterns that can be modified to develop better coping.
Alterations in rest, nutrition, or biochemistry affect a person's ability to cope. A healthy life-style is necessary if a person is to have the stamina and strength to cope with existing problems. Strategies to reduce stress and enhance wellness will help patient to develop effective coping.

Charting Components

- ➤ Evidence of effective decision making
- ➤ Expressed ability to cope with current situation
- ➤ Level of anxiety, presence of denial
- ➤ Presence/absence of support systems
- ➤ Skills, resources, knowledge identified to help with coping
- ➤ Source of stress, length of time it has existed
- ➤ Specific goals set
- ➤ Usual and current coping mechanisms
- ➤ Verbalized feelings, thoughts
- ➤ Patient/family teaching, response

2. Impaired Adjustment

Definition

The state in which the individual is unable to modify own life-style/behavior in a manner consistent with a change in health status

Related to

- ➤ Disability requiring change in life-style
- ➤ Inadequate support systems
- ➤ Impaired cognition
- ➤ Sensory overload
- ➤ Assault to self-esteem
- ➤ Altered locus of control
- ➤ **Incomplete grieving** over loss of usual health status (e.g., body part, vocation, divorce, home, family member, significant other)
- ➤ Chronic progressive illness
- ➤ Maturational crisis (e.g., adolescence, aging)
- ➤ Identity disturbance
- ➤ Unstable, inadequate interpersonal relationships
- ➤ Fear of relatedness/abandonment
- ➤ Unmet dependency needs

Content appearing in this typeface is additional information not included in the NANDA nursing diagnoses.

Characteristics/Assessment Findings

Major

- ➤ Verbalization of nonacceptance of change in health status
- ➤ Nonexistent or unsuccessful ability to be involved in problem solving or goal setting
- ➤ Severe depression
- ➤ Substance dependence
- ➤ Inadequate coping strategies
- ➤ Powerlessness
- ➤ Social isolation
- ➤ Severe anxiety
- ➤ Severe regressive behaviors
- ➤ Self-destructive behaviors
- ➤ Excessive approach/avoidance conflict
- ➤ Feelings of alienation
- ➤ Excessive/inappropriate expressions of anger

Minor

- ➤ Lack of movement toward independence
- ➤ Extended period of school, disbelief, or anger regarding change in health status
- ➤ Lack of future-oriented thinking
- ➤ Negativistic behaviors
- ➤ Inappropriate expression of anger
- ➤ Moderate anxiety
- ➤ Indecisiveness, excessive ambivalence
- ➤ Inflexibility
- ➤ Unrealistic/inappropriate guilt or lack of guilt
- ➤ Feelings of entitlement
- ➤ Social withdrawal
- ➤ Regression
- ➤ Toxic shame

Expected Outcomes/Goals

The patient will

- ➤ be able to accept the change(s) in life circumstances/health status as evidenced by
  - ▷ verbalizing feelings
  - ▷ verbalizing realistic self-expectations
  - ▷ discussing positive attributes of self to caregivers
  - ▷ demonstrating interdependence by appropriately being independent or dependent
  - ▷ identifying past stressors/losses that might be influencing the current situation
  - ▷ accepting treatment for chemical dependency
  - ▷ recognizing interpersonal manipulation strategies
  - ▷ reinforcing self positively for success-oriented behaviors

▷ effectively dealing with angry feelings
▷ using problem-solving techniques.
➤ move adaptively through the grief process as manifested by
▷ engaging in appropriate social roles
▷ differentiating successful coping strategies from maladaptive coping patterns
▷ realistically discussing the loss with caregivers
▷ making plans to adapt life-style as necessary.

Nursing Orders with Rationale

➤ Assess and monitor for presence/absence/ changes in assessment findings outlined above *in order to detect any change in status.*

➤ Identify the individual's past and present coping strategies; determine if personal resources are inadequate or unavailable
This information is needed in order to plan interventions that build on existing skills and personal strengths.

➤ Look for use of maladaptive coping strategies; recognize that substance abuse may be a response to the current situation or a past pattern of coping with stress.
Substance abuse is connected with feelings of powerlessness (Smith, 1985).

➤ Ascertain family's/significant other's perception of the situation
to help determine if the family is a source of potential help or also needs intervention (Hoff, 1984).

➤ Determine the availability and quality of social support.
Patients with a chronic mental illness often have a diminished social network. Often they receive what is termed "expressed negative emotions" from their social network.

➤ Note and point out to patient factors that are contributing to their failure to adjust.
This will enable the patient to gain an intellectual understanding of the current situation.

➤ Be alert for the presence of denial; refer to nursing care plan "Ineffective Denial"; if denial is present, accept patient's behavior without supporting it; allow patient to be distracted by nonthreatening topics or activities.
Denial is the major defense mechanism employed when a person cannot deal with the harsh reality of a situation.

➤ Help patient to express anger constructively without being judgmental:
▷ involve in large motor activity when possible.
▷ teach that anger is part of the grief process.
▷ allow to cry.
▷ suggest that patient write down feelings in a journal.
▷ help to identify fears.
Anger is often a response when grieving, feeling frustrated, fearful, or powerless. Constructive release of these feelings brings relief and increases coping ability and communication with others (Haber, Hoskins, Leach, & Sideleau, 1987).

➤ Assist patient to put anger into words.
When patients express frustration in an inpatient setting, encourage verbalization to help cut down impulsiveness and acting out feelings. Guilt over destructive outbursts can be minimized.

➤ Do not directly confront demanding and angry patients with their unrealistic expectations for special treatment or privileges. Provide a calm, matter-of-fact response.
Confronting patient directly over valuation of self may leave him or her with the opposite attitude of devaluing self; patient may act out self-destructive impulses (Sederer & Thorbeck, 1986).

➤ Support manageable goals to reduce powerlessness; refer to nursing care plan "Powerlessness":
▷ recognize progress made.
▷ help patient revisit developmental milestones by asking for examples of past success and accomplishments.
▷ focus on strengths and assets, not limitations.
▷ encourage to care for self so as to minimize frustration.
Increasing the patient's sense of control helps decrease anger, hostility, and powerlessness.

➤ Give positive reinforcement for non–stick-role behaviors.
This fosters independence and enhances self-esteem, thus allowing patients to make decisions that will allow them to live as independently as possible.

➤ Do not foster excessive dependency on nursing care.
Nurses may inadvertently foster dependency in patients when their caring is expressed as parental or coercive.

➤ Enhance the patient's self-esteem; refer to nursing care plan "Situational Low Self-Esteem":
  ▷ encourage to discuss own positive attributes.
  ▷ help to identify realistic expectations for self.
  ▷ acknowledge patient's worthiness and personal value.
  ▷ help to set and complete short-term, gratifying goals.
  ▷ assist with hygiene and grooming as needed.
  ▷ positively reinforce assertive behavior.

    When a person's self-concept is threatened by illness or disability, dependency often increases and becomes problematic. Enhancing self-esteem can encourage independence.

➤ Support patient through depression:
  ▷ help patient to recognize depression as part of the grief process.
  ▷ do not try to talk patient out of sad feelings, but rather validate the patient's reality.
  ▷ encourage expression of feelings, especially those of anger, guilt, sadness; determine if patient has an attitude that may be undermining progress (e.g., feeling worthless, weak, or "bad" as if being punished).
  ▷ assess for self-destructive thoughts and behavior.
  ▷ monitor sleep patterns and nutritional status.
  ▷ encourage as much physical activity as possible.

    Depression is often the response to anger that has been turned against the self when a person feels it is unacceptable to be angry and has guilt.

➤ Determine if current depression is linked to this current situation or if past losses are contributing to the current impairment in adjustment:
  ▷ search with the patient for similarities between the past and present experience.
  ▷ help patient identify which old memories, feelings, or thoughts might have emerged, unexplained, into consciousness.
  ▷ explain that it is often necessary for past losses to be resolved before resolution in the current situation can be complete.

    Patients with unresolved grief have been unable to work through the past losses, and this may complicate the present grieving process (Horsley, 1988).

➤ Explore with the patient activities that will add meaning to his or her life.

    Chronically ill patients have a need for activities that can be undertaken despite that presence of disease. Helping a person accomplish a meaningful contribution to society is as important an activity for nursing as assuring adherence to a particular regimen of diet or medication (Larkin, 1987).

➤ Refer patient to available community resources for support in managing the chronic illness.

    The patient must know what is available for emergency assistance or ongoing emotional support. Ultimately this fosters independence and will diminish a need to return to the acute care setting. This is especially critical for the psychiatric patient who historically has an inadequate social network (Worley & Albanesa, 1989).

➤ Emphasize the importance of community support and involvement in groups that share similar issues.

    The use of groups with similar social issues makes advocacy possible and decreases feelings of isolation (Mechanic, 1986). Many cities have club houses for the long-term mentally ill. Membership in a club house removes individuals from the patient role and enables them to participate in activities that are appropriate to their level of functioning.

➤ Support the family/significant others:
  ▷ facilitate the expression of feelings by being nonjudgmental and by using therapeutic communication techniques (e.g., reflecting feelings).
  ▷ discuss the importance of maintaining usual roles and responsibilities.
  ▷ provide accurate information about the patient's treatment and progress.
  ▷ determine the state of grief that significant others may be experiencing.
  ▷ teach about the grief response.
  ▷ discourage significant others from minimizing or distracting the patient or other family members from grieving; tell them of the importance of grief work; be sensitive to feelings of shame and embarrassment that may signal the patient/family is feeling stigmatized.
  ▷ provide a referral source for further counseling as needed.

    When one member in a family becomes dysfunctional, the entire family system is threatened (Baker, 1989).

➤ Inform the family about the Alliance for the Mentally Ill.

Family members need support in working through loss of a member to mental illness. This group not only offers emotional support but access to resources that the nurse might not be aware of. They are also active in promoting better care for the mentally ill in the community.

➤ Anticipate with the patient/family specific behavioral criteria that can be used in evaluating the need for acute hospitalization.

Many psychiatric symptoms are insidious, thus making it difficult for the patient/family to know when to contact professionals. Denial may also be present, which further complicates the issue. Having a concrete list of specific symptoms that signal a pending relapse often helps families cope in decision making.

➤ Identify readiness for health teaching; refer to nursing care plan "Knowledge Deficit":
  ▷ keep teaching sessions short; be specific, repeat information often, emphasize key points, and provide written reinforcements.
  ▷ assess for the ability to generalize and apply what has been learned to own unique life situation.

➤ Individualize teaching plans and information that is given to chronically ill patients.

For the patient who is seeking information as a way of coping, the nurse needs to be sensitive to the current needs of the patient and allow the patient to prioritize information. Some patients may need to be allowed not to acquire information at a particular time (Burckhardt, 1987).

Charting Components

➤ Ability to use social support
➤ Amount of self-initiated care
➤ Availability of support systems
➤ Degree of insight into problem
➤ Feelings expressed
➤ Problem-solving ability
➤ Self-destructive thoughts/behaviors
➤ Self-reinforcement for positive behaviors
➤ Stage of grief
➤ Subjective/objective signs of anxiety, depression
➤ Use of adaptive/maladaptive coping strategies
➤ Patient/family teaching, response

Additional Nursing Orders for
THE PATIENT WITH A CHEMICAL DEPENDENCY

➤ Observe for criteria that indicate the possible presence of chemical dependency; e.g.,
  ▷ withdrawal syndromes (Vance, 1989)
  ▷ tolerance
  ▷ frequent references to drinking or using recreational drugs
  ▷ excessive use of denial, rationalization, projection
  ▷ marital/family/relationship problems
  ▷ legal problems
  ▷ employment or school difficulty
  ▷ family history of chemical dependency or other compulsive behaviors
  ▷ heavy smoking
  ▷ abnormal laboratory values (especially toxicology screen, liver function tests, stool for occult blood, chest x-ray, urinalysis, blood sugar, electrolytes)
  ▷ alcohol on breath
  ▷ presence of associated conditions (e.g., pneumonia, pancreatitis, irritable bowel, cystitis, secondary diabetes, hypoglycemia, bruising, dehydration, edema, gastritis, cardiac arrhythmias, anemia, malnutrition, hepatitis).
    Alcohol affects all systems of the body (Kinney & Leaton, 1987).

➤ Use of matter-of-fact and nonthreatening approach when conducting a health history; assess for alcohol or recreational drug use: ask patient directly, "Do you take any alcohol?" "How much alcohol do you drink per day?" "Which drugs do you take regularly?" "When was your last drink?" "Did you drink alcohol today?"
    Direct, nonthreatening, nonjudgmental questions will elicit the most accurate information.

➤ Be aware that denial is usually present; refer to nursing care plan "Ineffective Denial."

➤ If denial persists and the condition is deemed urgent, a formal intervention process can be planned.
    Formal intervention involves the patient's family members, friends, employer, and other significant persons confronting the patient in a caring way with specific documentation of the physical, psychological, and behavioral impairments related to his or her chemical use (Tweed, 1989).

➤ Speak of chemical dependency as an illness that is treatable; remain nonjudgmental and identify counterproductive behaviors matter-of-factly.
   Present reality in a manner that displays frankness without being punitive.

➤ Do not support the patient's rationalizations; provide empathy, not sympathy.
   Empathy conveys understanding regarding the underlying anxiety that results in rationalizations and denial.

➤ Consistently focus on the problem behaviors, not the label of being chemically dependent or alcoholic.
   The ability of the counselor to provide accurate feedback to the patient, giving specific descriptions of behavior—of what the patient is doing—is very valuable as the alcoholic has lost the ability for self-assessment (Kinney & Leaton, 1987).

➤ Assess for the presence of concurrent psychopathology.
   Patients may have other psychiatric conditions in addition to substance dependency (Hesselbrock, Meyer, & Keener, 1985).

➤ Discuss the concept of loss of control rather than amount of alcohol consumed.
   This approach prevents a defense response concerning the amount consumed and keeps the focus on self-diagnosis, which is essential for successful treatment.

➤ Discuss treatment options with the patient (e.g., inpatient program for chemical dependency, outpatient therapy groups, or a 12-step program such as AA).
   Individuals with a history of unsuccessful outpatient treatment, potential withdrawal problems, medical problems, few social supports, family needs, or who have expressed ambivalence are candidates for inpatient treatment (Kinney & Leaton, 1987).

➤ Refer patient to a program that uses the therapeutic community during inpatient treatment.
   A therapeutic milieu is a group treatment environment that is supervised and provides a model of the everyday world by maximizing opportunities for patients to benefit from their social and physical surroundings (Wrisley Jack, 1989).

➤ Foster problem solving through group discussion and consensus rather than by authority figures *to encourage patients to participate in their own treatment. Power is shared by the group rather than held by professionals, as in the traditional medical model.*

➤ Provide education on substance dependency and abuse.
   Knowledge of the psychological and physical aspects of chemical dependency is a necessary component in the recovery process. It helps patients deal with misconceptions involving willpower and guilt.

➤ Involve the family in treatment.
   The systems approach is used in chemical dependency because treating only the identified patient has proven to be ineffective.

➤ Present on admission the unit rules concerning use of drugs and alcohol.
   Program rules vary, but usually a patient is given two warnings before being discharged.

➤ Involve the patient group when patient neglects unit rules or responsibilities; discuss infractions and limit testing during community meetings.
   The group will impose negative consequences when the patient does not fulfill responsibilities. Thus, everyone on the unit can learn directly or indirectly that inappropriate behavior invokes real-life restrictions.

➤ Do not try to please patients when they have unreasonable requests or placate them when they exhibit aggressiveness; rather, help them see that you have both positive as well as negative aspects to your personality.
   Splitting as a defense blocks patients from being able to integrate the negative and positive characteristics of people they care about. The nurse helps patients learn that the same person can nurture as well as frustrate.

➤ When dysfunctional anger is displayed toward the nurse, ask the patient who treated him or her with hostility in the past.
   This causes the patient to reflect on own feelings and behavior and to see that there is a historical reason for the rage. Understanding that intense anger is not caused by the current treatment relationship helps the patient accept responsibility for own behavior.

➤ Provide a structured schedule for the patient.
   The ability to test reality improves in response to external structure even though it may be resisted and may anger the patient initially.

➤ Assess for the presence of shame.
Shame is evoked by danger of unexpected exposure, humiliation, and rejection when a person feels she or he has fallen short of the ideal (Campbell, 1984).

➤ Help patient to differentiate between shame and guilt.
Shame concerns the core of who we are; guilt is remorse about something we did. Identifying one's own intergenerational shame-bound family system helps to break down the denial.

➤ Assess for codependency (e.g., rescuing, inability to define own needs, lack of self-nurturing, denial).
Codependency is a specific condition that is characterized by preoccupation and extreme dependence (emotional, social, sometimes physical) on a person or object. Eventually, this dependence on another person becomes a pathological condition that affects the codependent in all other relationships (Wegscheider-Cruse, 1987).

➤ Provide patient with a questionnaire that addresses codependency.
Specific behaviors are associated with codependency, and individuals will be able to assess their own issues effectively (Hall & Wray, 1989).

➤ Inform patients that many individuals who are chemically dependent are also codependent.
Once the individual is chemically free, other disturbing issues that involve problematic relationships and lack of self-nurturing may cause the recovering individual much distress. Often untreated codependency is present, which needs to be addressed (Zerwekh & Michaels, 1989).

➤ Set realistic goals for the patient regarding self-destructive life-styles and relationships.
Emotional pain may be the only way the patients feels connected to others because of early traumatic relationships within the family (Sederer & Thorbeck, 1986).

➤ Refer to a support group for follow-up.
The concept of powerlessness is an integral part of the philosophy of successful self-help groups such as Alcoholics Anonymous and Al-Anon. Other 12-step programs (e.g., Cocaine Anonymous, Narcotics Anonymous, CODA [CoDependence Anonymous], ACA [Adult Children of Alcoholics]) are also available as resources once the individual has sufficient recovery from the chemical dependency to begin to explore their past and work through own grief over a lost childhood.

➤ Refer to primary care provider for follow-up.
Antihypertensives, hormones, and other routine medications may need to be adjusted once abstinence has occurred (Talashek, Gerace, Miller, & Lindsey, 1995).

➤ Refer to primary care provider for the possible use of naltrexone.
Naltrexone is a long-acting opioid antagonist that has proven to be useful in relapse prevention for alcoholics (O'Brien, 1995).

Additional Charting Components

➤ Aggressiveness, shame, guilt
➤ Attendance/participation in community groups
➤ Codependency
➤ Community referrals
➤ Denial
➤ Environmental supports
➤ Family involvement, response
➤ Indicators of substance use/abuse/dependence
➤ Limit testing, infractions

Additional Nursing Orders for
THE PATIENT WITH DUAL DIAGNOSIS

➤ Assess for the presence of a mental illness or a personality disorder in all patients with a substance-abuse or dependency problem.
A dual diagnosis refers to the presence of at least one psychiatric disorder in addition to a substance-abuse or dependency problem. Substance-abuse issues are often present in persons with personality disorders, particularly those with antisocial traits. About 70% of those diagnosed with antisocial personality disorder are chemically dependent (Walker, 1992).

➤ Assess whether the mental illness symptoms are a result of intoxication or withdrawal or the effects of psychoactive substance abuse.
The use of amphetamines can produce a psychotic episode. Treatment for substance abuse would alleviate the psychotic symptoms (Wilson & Kneisl, 1996).

➤ Assess whether the patient with a major psychiatric disorder is using psychoactive substances to cope with symptoms or to get relief from psychotropic side effects.

Individuals with a psychiatric disorder are at a higher risk for having a substance-abuse disorder. The risk is twice as high for those suffering from depression, bipolar disorder, or an anxiety disorder. Self-medication with alcohol and drugs can help schizophrenic patients feel less anxious and decrease the intensity of hallucinations. Treatment for the psychiatric illness would relieve both problems (Johnson, 1993).

➤ Determine whether abstinence from a substance should be the focus of treatment or a prerequisite for treatment.

For a patient with an antisocial personality, abstinence from alcohol and drugs may be required prior to beginning treatment, while a patient with schizophrenia may be first treated for the psychiatric symptoms (Wilson & Kneisl, 1996).

➤ Assess how the symptoms or treatment of mental illness will interfere with the patient participating in program activities designed to help the substance-abuser.

Patients with religious delusions, preoccupations, and distortions find it difficult to work in a 12-step recovery program such as Alcoholics Anonymous. A substance-abuse program may discourage the use of antianxiety medications (Clement, 1993).

➤ Be aware of patients with dual diagnosis in chemical dependency groups. Use supportive gentle confrontation techniques rather than intense confrontation.

Patients may have changes in mental status or exacerbation of mental illness symptoms caused by withdrawal from substances (Keltner, Schwecke, & Bostrom, 1995).

➤ Teach patient personal signs of relapse and relapse prevention for mental illness and alcohol/drugs.

Patients need education about their mental illness, and relapse prevention strategies based on their individual needs (Keltner, Schwecke, & Bostrom, 1995).

➤ Teach patients about medication side-effect management and potential problems that may result when using alcohol or other substances with medication.

Alcohol is a CNS depressant and exacerbates the presence of clinical depression.

➤ Assess for continued signs of depression, anxiety, or insomnia.

After the acute withdrawal phase, patients with these feelings are at risk for relapse (Toro, Thom, Beam, & Horst, 1996).

➤ Refer patients to Double Trouble outpatient groups that focus specifically on the issue of dual diagnosis.

The unique problems encountered by persons with mental illness and substance abuse/dependency problems are more easily managed in this type of group.

Additional Charting Components

➤ Presence of a personality disorder
➤ Personality traits that interfere with recovery
➤ Symptoms of mental illness that interfere with recovery
➤ Response to antipsychotic and antidepressant medications
➤ Compliance with prescribed medications
➤ Use of drugs or alcohol to self-medicate
➤ Teaching done and client response
➤ Referrals to community resources

3. Ineffective Denial

Definition

A conscious or unconscious attempt to disavow the knowledge or meaning of an event to reduce anxiety/fear to the detriment of health

Related to

➤ Threat to self-esteem
➤ Defense against ego disintegration
➤ Overwhelming traumatic event
➤ Loss/bereavement
➤ Substance use/abuse
➤ Threat to biological integrity

Content appearing in this typeface is additional information not included in the NANDA nursing diagnoses.

Characteristics/Assessment Findings

Major
➤ Delays seeking or refuses to obtain health care to the detriment of health
➤ Does not perceive personal relevance of symptoms or dangers
➤ Ignores concerns expressed by family members and significant others
➤ Avoids discussing problem area
➤ Offers opinion that no problem exists

Minor
➤ Uses home remedies (self-treatment) to relieve symptoms
➤ Does not admit fear of death or invalidism
➤ Minimizes symptoms
➤ Displaces source of symptoms to other organs
➤ Unable to admit impact of disease on life pattern
➤ Makes dismissive gestures or comments when speaking of distressing events
➤ Displaces fear of impact of the condition
➤ Displays inappropriate affect

Expected Outcomes/Goals

The patient will accept the reality of the information/situation as evidenced by
➤ exploring the impact of the information/situation on own life
➤ discussing the situation, illness, problem
➤ displaying appropriate affect
➤ actively participating in decision making
➤ making statements that imply acknowledgment
➤ asking for appropriate assistance
➤ using appropriate coping strategies
➤ verbalizing feelings (e.g., regret, remorse, anxiety, depression, anger)
➤ demonstrating assertive behavior.

Nursing Orders with Rationale

➤ Assess and monitor for presence/absence/changes in assessment findings outlined above *in order to detect any change in status.*

➤ Assess the type and nature of the treat to the individual's self-image (e.g., awareness of a discrepancy between the patient's own view of self [ego ideal] and reality).
Each person's ego ideal is unique. In order to understand the nature of the threat, the nurse must understand the individual's particular ego ideal (Kerr, 1980).

➤ Provide empathic understanding of the underlying threat while avoiding inappropriate assurance (e.g., *Patient:* "I am so angry with my husband." *Inappropriate intervention:* "But anger is a natural feeling. You are being too hard on yourself. You shouldn't feel so guilty about being angry." *Empathic intervention:* "Could you tell me what that is like for you—to be angry with him?").
Inappropriate reassurance may cause the patient to retreat once again into isolation and secrecy. Empathic intervention acknowledges the patient's true dilemma, which allows the patient to explore alternative, more constructive ways to deal with the feelings of anger.

➤ Model appropriate superego evaluation of the situation/problem in a nonpersuasive way, even without the expectation of further discussion (e.g., "Gee, if that had been me, I think I would have felt angry," or "That seems like a situation that would make many people angry.").
When these kinds of interventions are offered in a consistent manner, the patient may come to alter rigid superego evaluations that make the denial necessary.

➤ Explore with patient practical problem-solving options to resolve the problem or situation.
A problem is often denied because the individual sees no way to solve or resolve it. By helping the patient to see various options, denial becomes less needed.

➤ Be aware that it will be the cumulative effect of interventions, and not one single intervention that will penetrate the defense of denial.
If the initial response to an intervention is automatic denial (e.g., "Of course I'm not angry with my husband."), the nurse may retreat for the moment. But over a period of time, with repeated interventions, the patient may become trusting enough to view the possibility with more objectivity.

Content appearing in this typeface is additional information not included in the NANDA nursing diagnoses.

➤ Share with patient your observations as a way to decrease resistance (e.g., "I noticed that when you talk about your husband you get a certain look on your face. I may be wrong about this, but it looks to me like a feeling of irritation. Were you aware of feeling that just now as we were talking?").

Sharing your observations is respectful of patients' autonomy. They are free both to consider the possibility are to reject it.

➤ Avoid collusion in the patient's denial; reflect back to the serious consequence of the denial.

Borderline patients, in particular, need more than empathy; they need reality as well.

➤ Assist the patient to gain a sense of control; refer to nursing care plan "Powerlessness."

As the patient discovers ways in which she or he can take control, the need for denial diminishes.

➤ Refer family, friends, significant others to appropriate community support systems (e.g., Al-Anon, grief groups).

A group can offer additional support in dealing with issues related to interaction with patient.

➤ Facilitate the grief process of family members/significant others (refer to nursing care plans "Anticipatory Grieving" and "Dysfunctional Grieving"):
  ▷ explain the phases of the grief response.
  ▷ assure family that grief is time limited.
  ▷ accept the expression of feelings by old family members.
  ▷ encourage family to explore their own losses.
  ▷ discuss meaning of the loss to them.
  ▷ help to express feelings of guilt.
  ▷ support the family in maintaining social outlets and activities that have been important.
  ▷ discuss realistic responsibilities for them to assume without enabling the patient to continue being self-destructive.

This information will help them to understand that their responses are not unique but are expected responses from anyone in a similar situation.

➤ Assist the patient to perceive the detrimental effects that the denial has had in his or her life:
  ▷ point out specific consequences of denial.
  ▷ discuss how the problem/issue has impacted family members and the patient's relationship with them.

Content appearing in this typeface is additional information not included in the NANDA nursing diagnoses.

  ▷ point out patient's apparent lack of concern for self (e.g., *Nurse:* "It seems to me sometimes that I feel greater concern about the impact this is having on your life than you do yourself.").

Examining the consequences of the denial provides insight into how it negatively impacts the patient's life.

Charting Components

➤ Anxiety level
➤ Appropriate/inappropriate affect
➤ Asking questions, asking for assistance
➤ Behaviors indicative of grieving
➤ Degree of compliance with treatment plan
➤ Discussion of situation/illness
➤ Feelings expressed
➤ Participation in decision making
➤ Patient's perception of the problem
➤ Use of destructive habits (e.g., smoking, overeating, excessive alcohol intake)
➤ Verbalization of acceptance
➤ Verbal reports of symptoms
➤ Patient/family teaching, response

4. Ineffective Family Coping: Disabling

Definition

Behavior of significant person (family member or other primary person) that disables his or her own capacities and the patient's capacities effectively to address tasks essential to either person's adaptation to the health challenge

Related to

➤ Significant person with chronically unexpressed feelings of guilt, anxiety, hostility, despair, etc.
➤ Dissonant discrepancy of coping styles for dealing with adaptive tasks by the significant person/patient or among significant people
➤ Highly ambivalent family relationships
➤ Arbitrary handling of family's resistance to treatment, which tends to solidify defensiveness as it fails to deal adequately with underlying anxiety
➤ Unsatisfying marital relationship
➤ Coalitions within the family unit that detract from total group communication
➤ Low self-esteem, both individually and collectively
➤ Inability to tolerate differentness (separateness) among members

➤ Dysfunctional role assignments
➤ Lack of trust among members

Characteristics/Assessment Findings

➤ Neglectful care of the patient in regard to basic human needs or illness treatment
➤ Distortion of reality regarding the patient's health problem, including extreme denial about its existence or severity
➤ Intolerance
➤ Rejection
➤ Abandonment
➤ Desertion
➤ Carrying on usual routines, disregarding patient's needs
➤ Psychosomaticism
➤ Taking on illness signs of patient
➤ Decisions and actions by family that are detrimental to economic or social well-being
➤ Agitation, depression, aggression, hostility
➤ Impaired restructuring of a meaningful life for self, impaired individualization, prolonged overconcern for patient
➤ Neglectful relationships with other family members
➤ Patient's development of helpless, inactive dependence
➤ Sexual dysfunction (e.g., lack of interest, complaints about adequacy of partner, promiscuity, infidelity)
➤ Inappropriate role assignments (e.g., parent confides in a child more than mate, incest)
➤ Child assumes adult role in family (e.g., does majority of cooking, cleaning, housework, caring for siblings in response to failure of parent to do so)
➤ Significant reduction or increase in academic achievement of child or professional achievement of an adult to the exclusion of other tasks
➤ Decreased peer interaction or other outside interests
➤ Excessive compliance by one or more members to rules of family/society
➤ Excessive noncompliance by one or more members to rules of family/society (e.g., numerous traffic citations)
➤ Acting-out behaviors by a member that require family attention and energy be focused on that member (e.g., substance abuse, running away, stealing, failure to maintain employment, failure to complete assigned family-related tasks)

➤ Disturbance in mood/affect of one or more members (e.g., depression, excessive or inadequate amounts of sleep, overeating, pervasive feelings of sadness)
➤ Children demonstrate indiscriminate attachment to or fear of strangers
➤ Lack of outside social relationships, support for individual members and for family unit
➤ Unresolved feelings of disappointment, abandonment, anger, depression by spouses toward one or more of their parents
➤ Communication patterns that employ bribery, threats, other subtle forms of coercion
➤ Focus of family is on the illness (frequently psychosomatic in nature) of a specific family member. Attempts to reframe the issue from the one member to the family are met with resistance.

Expected Outcomes/Goals

The family will
➤ assume and maintain role assignments as evidenced by
  ▷ parents maintaining a balance of shared authority and power for decision making
  ▷ parents mutually using each other (rather than children) as primary support systems
  ▷ assigning family tasks appropriate to age, developmental level, and capability of members (e.g., young children are not expected to prepare their own meals).
➤ maintain a balance of time and energy spent among various developmental tasks as evidenced by
  ▷ spending the typical number of hours per week pursuing career or academic goals
  ▷ spending time each week pursuing desired hobbies/activities
  ▷ allowing and tolerating without anxiety some unstructured time.
➤ maintain social relationships with individuals and other families as evidenced by involvement in community groups, extended family members, with friends.

Content appearing in this typeface is additional information not included in the NANDA nursing diagnoses.

➤ collaboratively problem solve around issues of excessive dysfunction demonstrated by one or more family members as evidenced by
  ▷ ensuring that one member enables continued deviance by any other member (e.g., the family decides not to give money to a substance abuser, a mother does not encourage a child to remain home from school).
➤ provide emotional/physical safety to all members as evidenced by
  ▷ verbalizing knowledge of assessment, prevention, and management of assaultive behavior
  ▷ demonstrating techniques to counteract assaultive behavior
  ▷ verbalizing interventions specific to the identified patient's diagnosis (e.g., borderline, separation-anxiety disorder).
➤ attain and maintain an individual and collective euthymic mood state as evidenced by
  ▷ normal range of mood and affect related to the salient issue
  ▷ normal patterns of eating, sleeping, work, and relaxation within and among members.

Nursing Orders with Rationale

➤ Assess and monitor for presence/absence/changes in assessment findings outlined above *in order to detect any change in status.*

➤ Assess for the possibility of domestic violence (e.g., verbal attacks, forced sexual activity, spouse battering, child abuse).
  Domestic violence is one expression of a dysfunctional family system (Carpenito, 1989).

➤ Report any suspicion of child abuse to child protective services or police.
  It is a legal requirement in most states that suspected or known child abuse be reported within 36 hours.

➤ Create a supportive professional and private environment that facilitates processing of mood and affect.
  A protective environment will encourage honest expression of feelings; significant issues can be processed and new methods of interaction tried (Satir, 1983).

➤ Instruct family about the specific illness of the identified patient including etiology, course, treatment, and prognosis.
  Education will reduce a sense of shame and guilt and decrease resistance to change (Nunnally, Chilman, & Cox, 1988).

➤ Teach principles of prevention, assessment, and management of problematic social/psychological or physical behaviors that are specific to the disorder and to the patient (e.g., reinforce reality when a schizophrenic becomes delusional, do not give a clearly diagnosed drug addict money).
  This knowledge will help the family to feel more competent to respond to patient's problematic behaviors; setting limits on problematic areas will increase patient's sense of safety (Nunnally et al., 1988).

➤ Help family members understand that the patient also is experiencing feelings related to his or her illness, change in role, and hospitalization.
  Understanding the process that the identified patient is undergoing will build empathy among family members and facilitate communication (Satir, 1983).

➤ Provide an opportunity for family members to talk individually about any abuse and their feelings.
  There may be fear for safety or guilt about revealing the abuse, and myths that it will stop in time.

➤ Provide a list of community agencies available to victim and abuser (e.g., hotlines, legal aid, shelters, counseling).
  Frequently, families are isolated and lack knowledge of the severity of the problem, community resources available, and legal rights (Carpenito, 1989).

➤ Help to identify nonstressful therapeutic ways to spend time with the patient; provide highly structured passes initially to a patient who argues a great deal.
  Such structure will increase opportunities for positive experiences.

➤ Clarify misconceptions regarding the relationship among all aspects of the illness and the family belief system (e.g., a sexually provocative adolescent does not have the devil operating within her).
  Clarification will increase family responsiveness to intervention and willingness to participate in treatment (McGoldrick, Pearce, & Giordano, 1982).

➤ Teach the importance of achieving a balance between work and leisure time; assign members the task of documenting how each spends his or her time.
  Assigning a specific task will provide concrete evidence of excesses or insufficiencies of time devoted to specific areas, which can serve as a motivator for change.

➤ Assist in the appropriate redistribution of role assignment (e.g., intervene to correct children who answer questions posed to parents, encourage adults to make decisions jointly).
> *Reviewing tasks with the family and making appropriate role assignments will foster appropriate communication and interaction between members (Minuchin & Fishman, 1981).*

➤ Assist family to identify (both individually and collectively) people, groups, activities that are external to the family.
> *Involvement outside the family allows what may be a closed system to receive input from sources other than itself.*

➤ Interrupt efforts made by members to speak for or to answer questions for each other; allow individuals within the family to struggle to find their own words to express themselves; acknowledge how difficult this is for someone who is used to having others think and feel for him or her.
> *Individual efforts will lead to the establishment of an individual sense of self (Minuchin & Fishman, 1981).*

➤ Illuminate areas where patient and family continue to function effectively; point out when they have attained a goal or resolved a problem.
> *This positive reinforcement will promote a sense of competence within and among members.*

➤ Provide names of support groups that are specific to the diagnosis (e.g., Al-Anon).
> *Support groups provide emotional support and aid the family in opening their system to others. In addition, having another source of input to the family will facilitate the transition back to the community.*

Charting Components

➤ Interventions to counter acting out by a family member
➤ Involvement in community groups, activities, people outside family
➤ Ratio of time spent on work, leisure, unstructured time
➤ Role and task assignments of family members: appropriateness regarding developmental age, capability
➤ Family teaching, response

5. Ineffective Family Coping: Compromised

Definition

A usually supportive primary person (e.g., family member or close friend) is providing insufficient, ineffective, or compromised support, comfort, assistance, or encouragement that may be needed by the patient to manage or master adaptive tasks related to his or her health challenge

Related to

➤ Inadequate or incorrect information or understanding by a primary person
➤ Temporary preoccupation by a significant person who is trying to manage emotional conflicts and personal suffering and is unable to perceive or act effectively in regard to patient's needs
➤ Temporary family disorganization and role changes
➤ Other situational or developmental crises or situations the significant person may be facing
➤ Little support provided by patient, in turn, for primary person
➤ Prolonged disease or disability progression that exhausts supportive capacity of significant people
➤ Stressful contact of one member or the whole family with extrafamilial forces
➤ Situational stressors within the family
➤ Time of onset
➤ Family-belief system
➤ Affective responses of members
➤ Interface with extended family and other larger systems
➤ Structure of the family before and after onset of the illness

---

Content appearing in this typeface is additional information not included in the NANDA nursing diagnoses.

Characteristics/Assessment Findings

Subjective

➤ Patient expresses or confirms a concern or complaint about significant other's response to patient's health problem

➤ Significant person describes preoccupation with personal reaction (e.g., fear, anticipatory grief, guilt, anxiety) to patient's illness, disability, or to other situational or developmental crises

➤ Significant person describes or confirms an inadequate understanding or knowledge base, which interferes with effective assistive or supportive behaviors

Objective

➤ Significant person attempts assistive or supportive behaviors with less than satisfactory results

➤ Significant person withdraws or enters into limited or temporary personal communication with the patient at the time of need

➤ Significant person displays protective behavior disproportionate (too little or too much) to the patient's abilities or need for autonomy

Other Possible Characteristics

➤ Family verbalizes a number of previously performed functions that are no longer being done (e.g., cooking, child care, employment); family or member complain of being unable to meet financial obligations

➤ Family belief system interferes with adherence to prescribed treatment regimen (e.g., meds)

➤ Inability to make decisions concerning a specific family member or other issues pertaining to the family as a whole

➤ Nuclear family verbalizes fear of response of extended family and nonfamily members

➤ Members of family other than the identified patient exhibit disturbance in appetite, mood, affect

➤ Identified patient exhibits behavioral problems (e.g., refusal to comply with medications, assaultiveness, verbal abusiveness)

➤ Family verbalizes feelings of guilt related to the identified patient.

Content appearing in this typeface is additional information not included in the NANDA nursing diagnoses.

Expected Outcomes/Goals

The family will

➤ reestablish equilibrium within the family as evidenced by
  ▷ seeking help to solve problems
  ▷ implementing effective coping mechanisms
  ▷ correcting distorted perceptions.
➤ increase contact with patient as evidenced by
  ▷ visiting patient regularly
  ▷ telephoning patient
  ▷ taking patient out on pass as permitted.
➤ establish an organization and structure that enables necessary roles and functions to be carried out as evidenced by assigning economic, household, child care, and other tasks to appropriate members.
➤ make decisions about treatment and care of ill family member as evidenced by authorizing or consenting to prescribed medications and treatment.
➤ discuss impact of crisis on family and individuals as evidenced by verbalizing feelings of guilt, shame, and loss.
➤ maximize optimal level of biopsychosocial function of ill member as evidenced by
  ▷ fostering patient independence
  ▷ encouraging patient to comply with treatment recommendations
  ▷ assigning a realistic family role to patient.
➤ act to ensure maintenance of its newly adaptive adjustment to ill family member as evidenced by
  ▷ openly discussing feelings about the patient and newly established roles, relationships, tasks
  ▷ obtaining assistance of relevant resources to problem solve around issues of economics and care of the patient
  ▷ planning vacations or determining other sources of respite care for the ill family member.

Nursing Orders with Rationales

➤ Assess and monitor for presence/absence/ changes in assessment findings outlined above *in order to detect any change in status.*

➤ Identify underlying situation that may contribute to inability of family to provide needed assistance to patient.
    The family crisis may be intensified by long-term situations that need attention.

➤ Meet with family before and after each visit with patient.
    Ensuring a protective environment will encourage honest expression of feelings and ultimately assist to normalize mood and affect.

➤ Identify the role of patient in family and how his or her illness has changed the family organization.
   Mental illness often results in the patient withdrawing or acting in unfamiliar ways that disrupt a heretofore functioning family.

➤ Assess information available to and understood by the family
   in order to develop a teaching plan regarding patient's condition, prognosis, treatment.

➤ Teach the family specific interventions to use in response to behavioral or social problems presented by the changes in the patient; refer to nursing care plan "Ineffective Individual Coping" for more interventions.
   A repertoire of successful adaptive strategies will help the family regain a sense of competence and self-worth and increase bonds between members.

➤ Instruct the family about patient's illness, including etiology, onset course, and prognosis.
   Education will reduce the sense of guilt, stigma, and shame the family experiences. It will also enable anticipatory problem solving as the illness continues (Nunnally, Chilman, & Cox, 1988).

➤ Teach principles of prevention, assessment, and management of problematic social, psychological, or physical behaviors that are specific to the patient.
   Knowledge of these principles will decrease the feelings of danger and threat to security that the family might be experiencing in response to the patient's illness. A decrease in these negative feelings will lead to increased patient contact (Nunnally et al., 1988).

➤ Help family members understand that the patient also is experiencing feelings related to his or her illness, changes in role, hospitalization, and recovery.
   Understanding the process that the ill member must go through will enable the family to be more sympathetic and empathic to the ill member and to continue to view him or her as an individual and not as a disease (Satir, 1983).

➤ Help family to identify and explore private and community resources.
   Using these resources will decrease the burden the family is experiencing in response to the illness.

➤ Clarify misconceptions regarding relationships among all aspects of the illness and the family-belief system.
   Clarification will decrease resistance to prescribed treatment and alternatives. It will also enable the family to act as an advocate for its ill member (McGoldrick, Pearce, & Giordano, 1982).

➤ Assist the family to identify nonstressful ways to spend time with the patient.
   Therapeutic interactions that are consistent with the needs of the family and patient will increase cohesion and support, and will ensure the maintenance of an adaptive role for the ill member within the family system (Nunnally et al., 1988).

➤ Identify and share with the family areas where both the recovering member and the family continue to function effectively.
   This identification can promote a sense of competence and mastery of the illness.

➤ Encourage the family to identify and use respite care.
   Planned respite from care will assist in avoiding burnout and maintaining participation in the care of the recovering member.

➤ Collaborate with family in decision making around planning treatment of recovering member.
   Participation in decision making increases the sense of competency and responsibility.

➤ Recommend participation in care based on assessment of family adaptation to the recovery.
   Appropriate levels of participation will foster commitment without engendering feelings of inadequacy or resentment.

➤ Keep family informed regarding patient status.
   Knowledge will alleviate feelings of helplessness and increase sense of competence to make decisions around patient care.

➤ Assist family to evaluate role assignments and to adjust them to ensure appropriate distribution of responsibility.
   Appropriate role assignment will help to maintain a healthy equilibrium and reintegration of the recovering member into the family (Minuchin & Fishman, 1981).

➤ Give family a list of problematic behaviors that may signal a pending relapse or a need for a medication change.
   A concrete list of problematic behaviors enables the family to make an objective assessment.

Charting Components

➤ Authorizing/consenting to patient treatment
➤ Contacting/using community resources
➤ Discussion of family roles, tasks, relationships
➤ Expression of feelings (e.g., guilt, shame, embarrassment, loss)
➤ Family contacts with patient: types, frequency
➤ Past and current methods of assigning family roles and functions
➤ Plans for respite care
➤ Supporting/encouraging patient in treatment program

6. Family Coping: Potential for Growth

Definition

Effective managing of adaptive tasks by family member involved with the patient's health challenge, who now is exhibiting desire and readiness for enhanced health and growth in regard to self and in relation to the patient

Related to

➤ Needs sufficiently gratified and adaptive tasks effectively addressed to enable goals of self-actualization to surface
➤ Reestablishment of roles and tasks of individual family members to allow an equilibrium between members, including the recovering patient, to recur

Characteristics/Assessment Findings

➤ Family member attempting to describe growth impact of crisis on own values, priorities, goals, relationships
➤ Family member moving in direction of health promotion and life-style enrichment that supports/monitors maturational processes and audits/negotiates treatment programs; generally chooses experiences that optimize wellness
➤ Individual expressing interest in making contact on one-to-one or mutual-aid group basis with another person who has experienced a similar situation

Expected Outcomes/Goals

The family will
➤ express willingness to undertake tasks leading to growth and change as evidenced by
  ▷ verbalizing need to change self and family
  ▷ verbalizing need for commitment to change.
➤ express willingness to look at own role in the growth of the family as evidenced by
  ▷ identifying areas within self that need to be changed
  ▷ identifying ways they can contribute to the family making changes.
➤ express feelings of self-confidence regarding ability to make changes as evidenced by
  ▷ verbalizing satisfaction with progress
  ▷ statements of hope for the future
  ▷ excitement regarding new possibilities.

Nursing Orders with Rationale

➤ Assess and monitor for presence/absence/changes in assessment findings outlined above *in order to detect any change in status.*

➤ Assess the family situation and adaptive skills being used by each family member *to build on the strengths already existing in the family.*

➤ Determine what stage of growth the family is in and discuss with family what the next step might be. *Families have a unique developmental process much like an individual, and go through several stages before the family is functioning at its highest potential (Bomar, 1989).*

➤ Assess the psychosocial characteristics of each family member (e.g., life stage, value orientation, previous experience with transitions). *Information about each person provides a means for identifying the degree of stress and potential family strengths (Bomar, 1989).*

Content appearing in this typeface is additional information not included in the NANDA nursing diagnoses.

➤ Explore concerns with family regarding past events that have disabled or compromised family functioning.

Moving forward in growth requires that the family understand why disruptive event occurred, how it happened, and how the family can best cope with the effects of having a family member with a mental illness (Bomar, 1989).

➤ Assess communication patterns of the family; discuss importance of open communication and of not keeping secrets.

Open and honest communication facilitates understanding, empathy, and successful interactions among family members.

➤ Teach family communication skills (e.g., "I" messages, active listening, problem-solving techniques).

Effective communication skills enhance respect for support for each family member (Carpenito, 1989).

➤ Promote wellness by providing examples of role models with whom the family may identify.

Families may need a realistic example of how a high functioning family interacts and lives up to its fullest potential (Doenges & Moorhouse, 1985).

➤ Identify community support groups (e.g., churches, recovery groups, social clubs) that cater to families and encourage family development.

Community activities enhance shared leisure time and foster a sense of family togetherness (Bomar, 1989).

➤ Work with the family to help them develop a sense of shared responsibility and respect for each member's contribution to the family.

Respect and responsibility within a family promote a feeling of being valued and of belongingness (Doenges & Moorhouse, 1985).

➤ Teach the importance of developing and following family rituals and traditions (e.g., holidays, vacations, prayer).

Rituals help to solidify a strong sense of family and a feeling of uniqueness about traditions that are passed down from grandparents to parents to children (Bomar, 1989).

➤ Emphasize the importance of humor and play *to keep a perspective and balance between family members.*

➤ Encourage family members to discuss ways they can respect the privacy of others *to ensure that each family member has both alone time and time with the family (Carpenito, 1989).*

➤ Assist family members to learn new, effective ways of dealing with feelings; encourage expression of feelings rather than acting out or withdrawing.

Verbal expression of feelings decreases tension, opens up communication, and facilitates understanding and empathy.

Charting Components

➤ Communication patterns
➤ Data about each family member regarding role, developmental stage, concerns, needs, goals
➤ Developmental stage of family
➤ Discussion of family roles, tasks, relationships
➤ Expression of feelings
➤ Family activities
➤ Impact of crisis on family/individual members
➤ Statements about progress, hope for the future
➤ Willingness of each member to make changes
➤ Family teaching, response

B. PARTICIPATION

1. Noncompliance

Definition

A person's informed decision not to adhere to a therapeutic recommendation

Related to

- Patient value system
  - health beliefs
  - cultural influences
  - spiritual values
- Patient-provider relationship
- Nontherapeutic environment
- Side effects of therapy
- Extensive therapy
- Knowledge deficit
- Complex, prolonged, or undersupervised therapy
- Anxiety
- Lack of support by significant others
- Denial of condition
- Sensory overload
- Alteration in thought processes (organic/functional)
- Past negative experiences with healthcare providers

Characteristics/Assessment Findings

- *Behavior indicative of failure to adhere (by direct observation or by statements of patient or significant others)
- Objective tests (e.g., physiological measures, detection of markers)
- Evidence of development of complications
- Evidence of exacerbation of symptoms
- Failure to keep appointments
- Failure to progress
- Progression of disease process
- Ineffective individual coping patterns
- Increased objective signs of anxiety
- Verbalization of fear
- Low self-esteem
- Verbalization of hopelessness
- Spiritual distress
- Missed group sessions
- Verbal refusal to take medications
- Return to previous self-destructive life-style

Expected Outcomes/Goals

The patient will adhere to the treatment plan in an informed, responsible manner as evidenced by

- demonstrating problem-solving ability by verbalizing correct information about condition, benefits of treatment, risks of treatment, treatment options.
- participating in decision making concerning treatment plan.
- verbalizing potential obstacles that might interfere with compliance (e.g., conflicting values, beliefs, socioeconomic influences).
- discussing the impact of illness on life-style.
- establishing a trusting, supportive, and therapeutic relationship with caregivers.

Content appearing in this typeface is additional information not included in the NANDA nursing diagnoses.

---

*Critical.

Nursing Orders with Rationale

➤ Assess and monitor for presence/absence/ changes in assessment findings outlined above *in order to detect any change in status.*

➤ Practice introspection and clarification of own attitudes, beliefs, and values that might influence perception of the patient, the illness, and the treatment decisions.

The nursing diagnosis of noncompliance is highly subjective and requires the nurse to have self-awareness. Judgment needs to be based on objective data, scientific knowledge, and contributing factors rather than on personal beliefs.

➤ Establish a trusting, therapeutic relationship with patient/significant others:

▷ be punctual and keep appointments; inform patient of a change in your schedule well ahead of time.

▷ use therapeutic communication techniques (e.g., reflecting feelings, minimal encouraging, active listening); restate the content, feelings, and meaning of the message; use open-ended statements (e.g., "Tell me about . . . ").

▷ communicate a commitment to engage in cooperative problem solving by being nonjudgmental.

▷ use silence to allow the patient time to gather thoughts, state opinions and feelings.

▷ be honest and use language appropriate to the patient's experience, age, educational background; avoid contradictory messages and ones in which the verbal and nonverbal cues are incongruent.

There is evidence that expressing warmth, accurate understanding, and cooperative intentions increases trust in a relationship and facilitates change (Kanfer, Goldstein, & Goldstein, 1980).

➤ Assess the possible contributing factors leading to noncompliance.

A patient who is noncompliant is expressing a need; the behavior has meaning and helps patients meet their needs (Miller, 1983).

➤ Remove communication barriers:

▷ use interpreters whenever necessary.

▷ explain treatment using nontechnical language.

▷ provide written material for the patient to review and take home.

▷ provide privacy and uninterrupted time.

▷ schedule enough time for questions and discussion.

▷ when possible, assign patient to same caregiver.

▷ schedule team conferences to facilitate communication among the different disciplines.

Accurate needs assessment can only occur when communication is enhanced and information easily exchanged (Moree, 1985).

➤ Promote a method of scheduling appointments in a comfortable environment that enhances the patient's perception of the healthcare delivery system:

▷ schedule individual appointments rather than on a first-come, first-served basis.

▷ schedule appointments so that waiting is minimized.

▷ collaborate with other departments so that appointments involving other disciplines can be coordinated.

Patients who have positive experiences with the healthcare delivery system are more likely to comply with treatment as they perceive the facility to be cooperative and invested in their welfare.

➤ Facilitate expression of feelings by using interpersonal communication techniques (e.g., broad openings/lead-in phrases, active listening, allowing for silence, reflecting back feelings, making observations for clarity/confirming nonverbal behaviors).

When patients feel free to express both the positive and negative feelings they have in regard to their treatment the nurse can better assess the psychosocial barriers that might block compliance.

➤ Provide positive reinforcement for the expression of feelings.

Low self-esteem is often associated with noncompliant behavior; positive reinforcement enhances the patient's self-esteem.

➤ Help patient to reduce anxiety to mild level; refer to nursing care plan "Anxiety."

Problem solving is enhanced during mild anxiety but when anxiety is moderate or severe, the patient cannot accurately perceived information or focus attention productively (Haber, Hoskins, Leach, & Sideleau, 1987).

➤ Assess the patient's perception of the illness/condition; promote a realistic perception by giving accurate information; refer to nursing diagnosis "Ineffective Denial."

When denial is present, the patient may not be able to perceive the illness or disability accurately and thus may not be compliant to treatment because of the necessity of maintaining his or her defensive system.

➤ Help patients to work through angry feelings.
When anger is not openly expressed, it will be expressed indirectly through maladaptive behaviors such as procrastination, negativism, development of physical symptoms, noncompliance.

➤ Assist patient to gain a sense of control:
  ▷ provide individualized care to counteract the many impersonal aspects of the setting.
  ▷ have patients participate in planning care, emphasizing the importance of their involvement.
  ▷ enlist patient's support in recording and reporting side effects of treatments/medications promptly to caregiver.
  ▷ work with patient to set realistic expectations of treatment.
  ▷ encourage to participate in decision making.
  ▷ develop with patient a method of monitoring progress.
  Powerlessness results when individuals feel they have no control over outcomes. When a person regains a sense of control in own life, that person is more likely to be compliant with the program.

➤ Attempt to contact patient if appointment is missed.
Assess why the patient has missed the appointment to determine if the patient is feeling a loss of control or motivation.

➤ Make a compliance contract with patient; review it periodically and stress importance of follow-up care.
Often patients will be compliant initially, but as time lapses and the condition becomes chronic, compliance tends to decrease (Miller, 1983).

➤ Reduce the complexity of the treatment program as much as possible:
  ▷ prioritize treatments so they need not all be initiated at once.
  ▷ schedule medications twice a day instead of four times a day, if possible.
  ▷ provide family information about medications, treatments, schedules.
  ▷ have patient write down a schedule that is realistic for his or her life-style.
  ▷ discuss time management.
  Compliance decreases with the complexity of treatment (Miller, 1983).

➤ Refer to a support group as needed.
Often a support group can offer creative possibilities for complex treatment regimens because of direct personal experience.

➤ Identify patient's personal habits that may need to be changed; educate on health risks if such habits continue; express empathy and be nonjudgmental.
Compliance is hardest to achieve when personal habits such as smoking, drinking, or overeating must be broken.

➤ Provide the family with information about diagnosis, medications, treatments; assess degree of family support and involvement; assess attitudes about health and determine sociocultural variations; refer family to support group if indicated.
Patients who receive positive social support from families are less likely to be noncompliant.

➤ Use rehearsal, practice, role playing, or other teaching aids to reduce confusion when demonstrating a procedure or treatment; observe the patient's technique(s).
Lack of supervision is a major variable in noncompliance.

➤ Assess financial resources and refer to social services as necessary.
Inability to afford healthcare is a major contributing factor in noncompliance (Moree, 1985).

Charting Components

➤ Anxiety level
➤ Behavior that demonstrates compliance (e.g., adhering to treatment plan, discussing impact of illness on life-style)
➤ Behavior that demonstrates noncompliance (e.g., refusing treatment, medications; verbal quotes of noncompliance)
➤ Objective and subjective evidence of noncompliance
➤ Participation in decision making regarding treatment plan
➤ Patient/family teaching, response

Additional Nursing Orders for THE PATIENT WHO REFUSES TO TAKE MEDICATION

➤ Provide accurate information about the medication regimen:
  ▷ provide information about side effects of medications.
  ▷ present a clear understanding of the drug's positive effect.
  ▷ explain how the medication works, why it helps.

▷ teach what to do about missed doses.

▷ provide resources to call for information if in doubt about continuing the drug.

▷ emphasize the importance of continuing the full course of treatment.

▷ identify the present medication therapy including over-the-counter medications to detect possible drug interactions.

▷ explain lab tests and other indicators that will enable caregivers to assess progress.

▷ discuss controversies over treatment, explain when and why there might be differing medical opinions.

Individuals who perceive a relationship between their actions and outcomes desire a great deal of information about their illness and treatment in order to control their disease. Others who do not necessarily rely on internal cues will comply more with the prescribed regimen when the information is presented accurately by a professional they believe to be an authority (Miller, 1983).

➤ Inform patient that antidepressant medication, lithium, and the neuroleptics (major tranquilizers) are restorative medications; they will not cure the illness, but will help stabilize the body's chemistry.

Patients often feel that psychotropic medication will cure their mental illness; they become disillusioned when it does not and discontinue taking it. Informing patients that the intent is not to cure but to stabilize their mood and behavior will enhance compliance. Telling patients that these medications are not addictive decreases anxiety over prolonged use of the medication.

➤ Approach the suspicious patient with the expectation that medication will be taken, even if refused previously; say, "Here is your medication, Mrs. Taylor"; if the patient hesitates, say, "Put it in your mouth and swallow it."

A hesitant approach may arouse the patient's suspicion about medication (Davies & Janosik, 1991). Decreasing ambivalent situations by limiting choices and giving concrete suggestions can help the patient with schizophrenic negativism by reducing anxiety.

➤ Offer the same form of medication each time (e.g., if liquid concentrate is given, always mix the same flavor; if 150 mg Thorazine are ordered, always give 3 × 50 mg tablets or 1 × 100 mg and 1 × 50 mg); be consistent.

Consistency prevents confusion and saves time and discussion (Davies & Janosik, 1991).

➤ Do not try to trick a patient by putting medication in food or drink.

Discovery of this by the patient destroys any trust established and gives his or her suspicions a basis of objective reality. The patient may stop eating or drinking (Beck, Rawlins, & Williams, 1988). In most states, taking psychotropic medication requires a signed consent from the patient.

➤ Give injections quickly and with as few restraints as possible
to protect the safety and dignity of the patient.

➤ Decrease patient hyperactivity by providing a quiet, nonstimulating environment.
Refusal of medication has been associated with elevated mood; reducing stimuli helps stabilize mood.

➤ Collaborate with physician when patient refuses medication; check hospital policy and state laws.
Most states make provisions for administering medication on an emergency basis. Courts have agreed that the right to treatment is a fundamental right, as is the right to refuse medication under certain circumstances. These rights extend to involuntary patients (Oriol & Oriol, 1986).

➤ Determine whether a different medication, a lesser dosage, or a different kind of therapy might be acceptable to the patient.
Under the concept of least restrictive treatment, the patient retains the right to refuse medication if there is an equally effective therapy available. Offering a less potent medication or decreasing the dosage could be viewed as less restrictive (Oriol & Oriol, 1986).

Additional Charting Components

➤ Form of medication given
➤ Interventions that convinced patient to take medication
➤ Patient's understanding of role of medication in treatment

C. JUDGMENT

1. Decisional Conflict (Specify)

Definition

The state of uncertainty about course of action to be taken when choice among competing actions involves risk, loss, or challenge to personal life values

Related to

➤ Unclear personal values/beliefs
➤ Perceived threat to value system (incompatible personal values)
➤ Lack of experience or interference in decision making
➤ Lack of relevant information
➤ Support system deficit
➤ Multiple or divergent sources of information
➤ Ambivalence
➤ Fear of making a mistake
➤ Feelings of dependency
➤ Need to please others
➤ Difficulty in processing complex messages
➤ Bombardment by thoughts and feelings, environmental stimuli
➤ Anxiety
➤ Impairment in ability to communicate

Characteristics/Assessment Findings

Major
➤ Verbalization of uncertainty about choices
➤ Verbalization of undesired consequences of alternative actions being considered
➤ Vacillation between alternative choices
➤ Delayed decision making

Minor
➤ Verbalization of feeling of distress while attempting to make a decision
➤ Self-focusing (e.g., statements focus on risks to self or caring for self)
➤ Physical signs of distress or tension (e.g., increased heart rate/muscle tension, restlessness)
➤ Questioning personal values and beliefs while attempting a decision

Expected Outcomes/Goals

The patient will
➤ identify strategies to decrease/resolve conflict as evidenced by
  ▷ statements of a plan for decision making
  ▷ statements of peace with decisions.
➤ tolerate feelings of ambivalence as evidenced by decrease in ritualistic behavior, negativism, and overcompliance.

Nursing Orders with Rationale

➤ Assess and monitor for presence/absence/ changes in assessment findings outlined above *in order to detect any change in status.*

➤ Assess values, goals, decision-making skills, level of distress, adequacy of knowledge, and supports. *Assessment data are need to identify a baseline for ongoing evaluation of progress and to prioritize interventions.*

➤ Employ therapeutic communication:
  ▷ use active listening (e.g., focus attention on patient, be sensitive to meaning of words and emotional context, give feedback, demonstrate understanding).
  This will encourage patient to express self, to explore the conflict, and to come to own conclusions (Helms, 1985).

  ▷ use presence (i.e., be physically available to patient; give attention to needs; use empathy, touch, reassurance)
  to develop a caring, supporting relationship with the patient (Gardner, 1985).

➤ Assist with gathering new information (refer to nursing care plan "Knowledge Deficit"):
  ▷ provide relevant information about alternatives (e.g., books, tapes, pamphlets, demonstrations) and risks/benefits.
  ▷ assist to evaluate discrepancies in information.
  ▷ refer to appropriate healthcare team professionals.

Content appearing in this typeface is additional information not included in the NANDA nursing diagnoses.

▷ assist with reexamination of alternatives with incorporation of new information.
  Providing adequate, relevant information will decrease confusion, leading to informed decision making.

➤ Assist with values clarification to identify and clarify most important personal life principles or values:
  ▷ use a clarifying response
    to assist patient to reflect on situation, to review goals/values, and to identify important goals/values (Wilberding, 1985).

  ▷ use values-clarification exercises (e.g., rank order values or alternatives); help to list, prioritize, choose, and explain values; search for alternatives/consequences (list alternatives, identify consequences, identify willingness to try each alternative)
    to help patient increase awareness of own values and priorities (Wilberding, 1985).

➤ Help to develop decision-making skills
  to increase/develop problem-solving skills and to provide an environment for quality decision making (Tauer, 1983).

  ▷ help to set goals incorporating important values
    to assist patient to begin a plan that will integrate personal values (Tauer, 1983; Wilberding, 1985).

  ▷ provide information regarding alternatives
    to give opportunity for informed decision making.

  ▷ discuss consequences, risks, benefits of each alternative (e.g., write lists, make balance sheet)
    to assist in weighing each alternative.

  ▷ assist to identify course of action (solutions) acceptable to patient
    to ensure that decision has high value to patient (Wilberding, 1985).

  ▷ provide an atmosphere that permits free choice among alternatives
    to ensure that patient is acting on personal values (Wilberding, 1985).

  ▷ assist to test choice(s) (e.g., rehearse, role play)
    to practice action plan and gain confidence, to develop a contingency plan in the event the first choice may not be feasible.

➤ Assist to reduce stress:
  It is important to decrease distress while making decisions (Scandrett & Uecker, 1985).

  ▷ review and identify effective stress-reduction strategies
    to use previously successful techniques.

  ▷ provide opportunity for use of effective stress-reduction techniques
    to facilitate practice of effective techniques to increase success in different environment (Snyder, 1985).

  ▷ teach/review preferred relaxation techniques (e.g., rhythmic breathing, relaxation response, progressive relaxation, guided imagery, exercise)
    to provide new information to support stress-reduction skills (Scandrett & Uecker, 1985).

Charting Components

➤ Decisions made by patient
➤ Physical signs of distress or tension (e.g., increased heart rate, increased muscle tension, restlessness)
➤ Referrals made
➤ Statements regarding
  ▷ adequacy of information or resources
  ▷ description of decision-making process
  ▷ feelings of distress
  ▷ outcomes of decisions
  ▷ personal goals, values, beliefs, desires
  ▷ plan for decision making
  ▷ risks/consequences of alternative actions
➤ Patient/family teaching, response

Additional Nursing Orders for
THE PATIENT WITH AMBIVALENCE

➤ Minimize the need for the schizophrenic patient to make choices; offer only two choices when anxiety level is lower.
  Ambivalence results in difficulty with decision making. Schizophrenics may debate endlessly about the alternatives in a situation that requires making a choice (Stuart & Sundeen, 1987).

➤ Limit choices to simple ones for the depressed person; if the patient is unable to choose, make the decision for him or her.
  This will prevent the patient from being overwhelmed.

➤ Listen with empathy to the feelings of an obsessive-compulsive person who has paralyzing doubt in the face of choices.

These patients often consciously experience both love and hate toward their objects. The opposing emotions may be seen in the doing-undoing patterns of behavior and the inability to make a decision (Kaplan & Sadock, 1985).

➤ Be aware that the highly suspicious individual may continually alternate between choices, expressing a wish to do first one thing and then another.

The constant indecision of the ambivalent person most likely indicates that a conscious or unconscious motivation to accomplish a task is not present (Beck, Rawlins, & Williams, 1988).

➤ Watch for overcompliance in patients who attempt to deny responsibility for any action by doing only what another exactly instructs should be done.

Ambivalent feelings can seriously disrupt the individual's ability to function and may produce overcompliance, negativism, and compulsive rituals (Beck et al., 1988).

➤ Teach the patient steps that will facilitate problem solving as decision-making ability grows:

▷ clearly define the problem using behavioral terms.

▷ think of possible solutions and write down several options.

▷ have patient think about what advice she or he would give someone else with the same problem.

▷ have patient choose preferred option and try it.

▷ remind patient that no decision is a decision not to make a decision; point out the consequences of not deciding.

▷ evaluate the option chosen, discuss outcome with patient.

Decision making entails responsibility for the outcome of the decision. Helping the patient assess all the facets of a decision, then giving support for the choice made, strengthens the idea that she or he can make a good decision (Dreyfus, 1988).

Additional Charting Components

➤ Ability to choose between two things offered
➤ Compulsive ritualistic behavior employed
➤ Decisions made and acted on
➤ Degree of interference in functioning
➤ Overcompliance as a way to decrease responsibility for decisions
➤ Reaction to simple choices offered

VI. Moving

A. REST

1. Sleep-Pattern Disturbance

Definition

Disrupton of sleep time causes discomfort or interferes with desired life-style

Related to

- ► Sensory alterations: internal (e.g., illness, psychological stress)
  - ▷ psychiatric disorders (e.g., depression, personality disorders, functional psychosis, anxiety, alcohol withdrawal, PTSD)
  - ▷ serious illness (e.g., pain, discomfort, coughing, hospital noise)
  - ▷ sleep-related medical problems (e.g., sleep apnea, restless leg syndrome, narcolepsy, epileptic seizures, bruxism, head banging, painful erections, cluster headaches, abnormal swallowing, asthma, cardiovascular symptoms, gastroesophageal reflux)
  - ▷ need to urinate frequently
  - ▷ fear
  - ▷ sleepwalking
  - ▷ sleep terror (e.g., nightmares, "night frights")
  - ▷ bed wetting
  - ▷ pregnancy
- ► Sensory alterations: external (e.g., environmental changes, social cues)
  - ▷ changes in sleep-wake cycle (e.g., time-zone change, jet lag, work shift change)

- ▷ medications that disrupt REM sleep (e.g., tranquilizers, sedatives, hypnotics, antidepressants, steroids, amphetamines, barbiturates, MAO inhibitors)
- ▷ life-style disruptions (e.g., situational stress, environmental change, minor illness, interruptions in sleep)
- ▷ use of drugs and alcohol (excessive or chronic use, withdrawal from drugs or alcohol)
- ▷ bad sleep habits (e.g., bedroom not restful, irregular sleep habits, too little or too much food, eating in bed, no bedtime rituals)
- ▷ lack of exercise

Characteristics/Assessment Findings

- ► *Verbal complaints of difficulty falling asleep
- ► *Awakening earlier or later than desired
- ► *Interrupted sleep
- ► *Verbal complaints of not feeling well rested
- ► Changes in behavior and performance (e.g., increasing irritability, restlessness, disorientation, lethargy, listlessness)
- ► Physical signs (e.g., mild fleeting nystagmus, slight hand tremor, ptosis of eyelid, expressionless face, dark circles under eyes, frequent yawning, changes in posture)
- ► Thick speech with mispronunciation and incorrect words
- ► Dozing during the day
- ► Lack of energy, fatigue
- ► Loss of train of thought
- ► Moodiness, agitation
- ► Subjective report or objective observation of little or no sleep for 36 hours or more
- ► Conditioned arousal at bedtime
- ► Anticipatory anxiety about the prospect of sleepless nights, days of fatigue
- ► Excessive amount of time spent in bed to compensate for lost sleep

---

*Critical.

Content appearing in this typeface is additional information not included in the NANDA nursing diagnoses.

Expected Outcomes/Goals

The patient will
➤ remain free from signs of sleep deprivation as evidenced by
  ▷ absence of dozing, dark circles under eyes, or yawning
  ▷ improved mood
  ▷ oriented to time
  ▷ increased energy.
➤ verbalize satisfaction with sleep-rest pattern as evidenced by phrases such as, "I slept well," or "I feel rested."

Nursing Orders with Rationale

➤ Assess and monitor for presence/absence/ changes in assessment findings outlined above *in order to detect any change in status.*

➤ Assess the problem of insomnia thoroughly. *Adequate assessment can identify medical problems that may disrupt the sleep pattern (i.e., nocturnal dyspnea, pain) (Gournay, 1988).*

➤ Ask about use of drugs; discourage patient reliance on benzodiazepine hypnotic agents. *Habituation and tolerance to these drugs represent the third most common cause of insomnia (Doghramji, 1989).*

➤ Have patient keep a sleep/rest diary and record in it sleep patterns, medications, timing of meals, and naps. *A sleep/rest-pattern diary illustrates the patient's actual sleep pattern so that any disruptive behaviors can be identified and modified (Gournay, 1988).*

➤ Refer persistent insomniacs and sleep-wake complaints to a sleep-disorder center for evaluation when psychotherapy, behavioral therapy, and medications are ineffective. *Polysomnographic findings provide a more accurate diagnosis of the underlying problem (Doghramji, 1989).*

➤ Instruct patient to establish a regular wake-up time; gently, but firmly, awaken patient at same time every day if patient does not get up. *Patients who do not want to face a new day often have difficulty getting out of bed in the morning. A regular wake-up time strengthens the circadian cycle (Cole & Rogers, 1984).*

➤ Encourage patient to sleep as much as needed to feel alert during the day, but not more. *Curtailing the time in bed seems to solidify sleep; excessive time spent in bed seems to fragment sleep (Doghramji, 1989).*

➤ Eliminate or reduce sleep interruptions (e.g., unplug telephone, close door, pull curtains). *Sleep interruptions from noise or changes in the environment will disrupt sleep (Gournay, 1988).*

➤ Eliminate factors that exacerbate sleep disruption (e.g., noisy room, irregular sleep habits, excessive use of drugs or alcohol); avoid unnecessary procedures during the night. *Life-style changes and stress can exacerbate sleep-pattern disturbance (McNeil, Padrick, & Wellman, 1986).*

➤ Offer a small bedtime snack to prevent nocturnal hunger. *A light snack may improve sleep by preventing nocturnal hunger. A large meal and excessive fluids close to bedtime can have the opposite effect.*

➤ Establish a bedtime ritual with pillows, quiet activity, baths, massage, and a glass of warm milk. *A bedtime ceremony or ritual stimulates sleepiness (Geach, 1987).*

➤ Instruct to eliminate or reduce caffeine, nicotine, alcohol intake. *Intake of stimulants can prevent sleepiness or disrupt sleep. Alcohol intake is disruptive to sleep (Hopson, 1986).*

➤ Teach patient to use bed for sleep only, arising if unable to sleep. *When bed is associated with successful sleep only, sleeping is enhanced (Speilman, Saskin, & Thorpy, 1987).*

➤ Tell patient to avoid catnaps to catch up on sleep. *Catnaps reduce sleepiness and further disrupt a sleep-pattern disturbance (Hopson, 1986).*

➤ Encourage daily exercise that is not too close to bedtime. *A steady exercise program deepens sleep (Speilman, Caruso, & Glovinsky, 1987).*

➤ Schedule intake of diuretic medications so large-volume urination occurs in the daytime. *Diuretic medications should be scheduled so that peak effect or urination occurs during nonsleep time (Speilman, Caruso, & Glovinsky, 1987).*

➤ Teach to use relaxation techniques (e.g., deep breathing, soft music, guided imagery) and biofeedback; encourage regular use of an audiotape made specifically to induce sleep.

> *Relaxation techniques can induce sleepiness (Gournay, 1988).*

➤ Use behavioral and cognitive techniques to reestablish a connection between being in bed and sleeping.

> *Patients are conditioned to wakefulness at bedtime and can be reprogrammed to associate bedtime and their bed with sleepiness (Speilman, Saskin, & Thorpy, 1987).*

➤ Institute sleep-restriction therapy:
  ▷ have patient complete sleep log for two weeks.
  ▷ review log to determine time spent in bed compared to time asleep.
  ▷ prescribe time in bed equivalent to patient's mean daily total sleep time.
  ▷ have patient report regularly the estimated time spent asleep.
  ▷ calculate the subjective sleep efficiency (ratio of total time spent asleep to the time spent in bed).
  ▷ adjust the time spent in bed to keep sleep efficiency between 85% and 90%.

> *The sleep pattern of many insomniacs is highly fragmented due to nocturnal awakening and daytime naps. Patients have reported significant and lasting improvement after eight weeks of sleep-restriction therapy (Speilman, Saskin, & Thorpy, 1987).*

➤ Institute stimulus-control therapy; have patient
  ▷ get up at the same time each morning.
  ▷ go to bed only when sleepy.
  ▷ do nothing else in the bedroom that competes with sleep (except sexual activity).
  ▷ if unable to sleep after 10 minutes or if awake during the night, leave the bedroom and do something distracting.
  ▷ return to bed when sleepy.

> *Stimulus-control therapy is a reprogramming method of relearning healthy sleep habits and unlearning the idea that going to bed always leads to insomnia (Gournay, 1988).*

➤ Institute progressive muscular relaxation:
  ▷ do the relaxation exercise in a quiet, darkened room.
  ▷ position patient comfortably on a couch/chair.
  ▷ instruct to take deep breaths and give advice on adequate diaphragmatic breathing.
  ▷ ask patient to tense and relax various muscle groups; start at the toes and work upward.
  ▷ ask patient to visualize a relaxing scene such as a sunny beach, pretty flower garden.

> *Progressive muscular relaxation teaches the patient to become more sensitive to the signs of muscular tension and learn how to achieve a more relaxed state (Gournay, 1988).*

➤ Refer for biofeedback training.

> *The use of physiological monitoring apparatus trains patients to recognize physical tension and helps them relax (Gournay, 1988).*

➤ Evaluate patients with Alzheimer's disease and dementia sleep pattern for obstructive sleep apnea.

> *Patients with Alzheimer's disease are especially vulnerable to developing obstructive sleep apnea and may have up to eight times the frequency of apnea of normal older persons. Effective treatment of apnea may alleviate some of the cognitive impairments (Hoch, Reynolds, & Kupfer, 1987).*

➤ Ensure that depressed patients take their antidepressant medication.

> *Polysomnography has revealed characteristic alterations in the sleep pattern of depressed people. Many antidepressants suppress the propensity for REM sleep, thus reversing the abnormalities in the REM latency and duration of the first REM period (Doghramji, 1989).*

➤ Consider sleep manipulations with severe depression when more conventional treatment modalities are ineffective:
  ▷ deprive REM sleep by awakening patient every 90 minutes.
  ▷ deprive from total sleep by keeping up for 24 to 36 hours.
  ▷ deprive from partial sleep by restricting sleep from 10 P.M. to 2 A.M.

> *Manipulation of sleep can lift the severest depression within days. Studies have shown that REM deprivation applied for a few weeks has lasting antidepressant effects. Other sleep deprivations have more transient effects (Doghramji, 1989).*

➤ Monitor closely sleep patterns in depressed and bipolar patients to avert the transition into mania. *Studies show that stressful emotional experiences (e.g., job, losses, medications) can result in sleep loss and precipitate mania (Wehr, Sack, & Rosenthal, 1987).*

Charting Components

➤ Bed-time ritual
➤ Effectiveness of treatments/therapies initiated
➤ Effects/side effects of medications
➤ Environmental change(s)
➤ Etiology of sleep disturbance, if known
➤ Hours of sleep
➤ Physical appearance, behavior indicating sleep loss
➤ Situational stress (e.g., pain, coughing)
➤ Sleep interruptions
➤ Sleep/rest pattern
➤ Subjective report of sleep disturbance, improved sleep
➤ Patient/family teaching, response

B. RECREATION

1. Diversional Activity Deficit

Definition

The state in which an individual experiences a decreased stimulation from or interest/engagement in recreational or leisure activities

Related to

- Environmental lack of diversional activity (as in long-term hospitalization, frequent lengthy treatments)
- Change in living environment
- Decreased economic resources
- Immobility or inactivity
- Lack of membership or reference group outside work
- Lack of skills to perform an activity
- Loss of ability to perform usual or favorite activities
- Loss of significant others
- Overachievement orientation to work/education
- Recent retirement
- Skeletal-muscular impairments (e.g., rheumatoid arthritis, neuromuscular impairment, multiple sclerosis)
- Social isolation

Characteristics/Assessment Findings

- Patient's statement regarding boredom, wish for something to do, to read, etc.
- Inability to undertake usual hobbies in hospital
- Avoidance of retirement planning
- Depression
- Increased somatic complaints
- Insomnia, frequent daytime napping
- Lack of interest in self and others
- Lack of participation in care
- Overinvolvement in occupation or profession
- Problems in parent-child relationship
- Passiveness
- Poor muscle tone
- Restlessness

Content appearing in this typeface is additional information not included in the NANDA nursing diagnoses.

Expected Outcomes/Goals

The patient will
- identify strengths and limitations regarding involvement in diversional activities as evidenced by
  - setting realistic goals
  - seeking out realistic opportunities
  - adapting diversional activities to changing health status.
- engage in diversional activities within personal limitations as evidenced by verbalizing satisfaction with selected activities.
- identify available diversional activities as evidenced by listing community services and agencies that can be used for hobbies or recreational activities.

Nursing Orders with Rationale

- Assess and monitor for presence/absence/changes in assessment findings outlined above
  in order to detect any change in status.

- Observe patient's activity level; compare to usual daily routine
  to determine signs of boredom.

- Vary daily routine when possible (e.g., take shower in afternoon); involve patient when scheduling daily activities
  to promote a sense of control (Doenges & Moorhouse, 1985).

- Consider using a volunteer to spend time helping the patient with an activity
  to provide opportunity for self-expression and socialization (Gettrust, Ryan, & Engleman, 1985).

- Assist patient to recognize need for diversional activity by discussing benefits of involvement in such activities.
  Being aware that one is bored allows one to redirect activities to increase stimulation (Carpenito, 1989; Gettrust et al., 1985).

- Help patient to recognize feelings of boredom/restlessness by using empathy, reflection, clarification (e.g., "I notice you seem to be more restless when you have nothing of interest to do.")
  to provide a starting point for directing activities (Gettrust et al., 1985).

➤ Work with patient to identify activities that are seen as valuable and important; review past interests, hobbies; suggest new ones (e.g., reading, games, learning a new skill, music, social events)

  to support motivation toward accomplishing an activity that fosters a positive image (Gettrust et al., 1985).

➤ Encourage involvement in new interests; bring in announcements for events, book reviews, articles on various topics.

  New interests prevent boredom (Doenges & Moorhouse, 1985).

➤ Encourage activities that provide opportunity for patient to socialize (e.g., use day room with other patients/personnel).

  Patient will have an opportunity to establish relationships with others who have common goals or interests (Gettrust et al., 1985).

➤ Work with patient daily to plan an activity

  to provide something for patient to look forward to. Satisfaction with use of time positively gives a feeling of well-being and provides the patient an opportunity to have some control over the day (Gettrust et al., 1985).

➤ Spend time discussing topics of interest with patient.

  New interests prevent boredom (Gettrust et al., 1985).

➤ Increase stimuli in the patient's environment (e.g., radio, TV, pictures, telephone, books, visitors)

  to vary monotonous environment and to stimulate interest (Carpenito, 1989; Doenges & Moorhouse, 1985; Gettrust et al., 1985).

➤ Encourage family/significant other to bring in hobbies from home

  to provide patient the opportunity to continue with desirable activities (Carpenito, 1989).

➤ Provide positive feedback for patient's effort to participate in any activity.

  Behavior that is reinforced tends to be repeated (Gettrust et al., 1985).

➤ Refer to community resources (e.g., mobile library, senior citizen's group, city/county recreational department, vocational schools, day treatment, community mental health center, club house for the long-term mentally ill).

  This increases a person's options in selecting activities (Thompson, McFarland, Hirsch, Tucker, & Bowers, 1989).

Charting Components

➤ Complaints of boredom; restlessness, agitation
➤ Daily activities
➤ Diversional activities identified, selected, pursued; patient response
➤ Frequency of napping
➤ Goals set by patient; outcomes
➤ Insight into activity deficit
➤ Interaction with other patients/family/staff
➤ Interest in community referrals
➤ Mood (e.g., cheerful, depressed)
➤ Somatic complaints

C. SELF-CARE DEFICIT

1. Self-Care Deficit

Definition

A state in which an individual experiences an impaired ability or an unwillingness to complete bathing/hygiene, dressing/grooming, feeding, or toileting activities for self

Related to

- Decreased strength and endurance
- Pain, discomfort
- Perceptual or cognitive impairment
- Neuromuscular/musculoskeletal impairment
- Depression
- Severe anxiety
- Psychosis, catatonic state
- Delirium, confusion
- Altered thought processes
- Psychomotor retardation
- Hyperactivity
- Delusions
- Sensory/perceptual alterations
- Apathy, lack of motivation
- Tremors, spasticity, flaccidity
- Conversion symptoms
- Debilitated state
- Distractibility
- Inability to make decisions
- Inability to perform ADL associated with overwhelming feelings
- Physical/mental deficit
- Ritualistic behaviors

Content appearing in this typeface is additional information not included in the NANDA nursing diagnoses.

Characteristics/Assessment Findings

- Feeding self-care deficit
  - inability to bring food from receptacle to mouth
  - sloppy eating manners, spitting up food
  - eating with hands rather than utensils
  - refusing to eat
- Bathing/hygiene self-care deficit
  - inability to wash body or body parts
  - inability to regulate temperature or flow
  - body odor; unshaven, greasy hair
  - halitosis
- Dressing/grooming self-care deficit
  - impaired ability to put on or take of necessary items of clothing
  - inability to maintain appearance at a satisfactory level
  - slovenly or inappropriately dressed
  - dirty, wrinkled clothes
- Toileting self-care deficit
  - inability to get to toilet or commode
  - inability to manipulate clothing for toileting
  - inability to carry out proper toilet hygiene
  - inability to flush toilet/empty commode
  - urinating on self

Expected Outcomes/Goals

The patient will
- meet basic needs as evidenced by
  - accepting help with ADL
  - ingesting adequate diet and fluids
  - establishing adequate elimination
  - achieving adequate sleep/rest.
- independently perform ADL as evidenced by
  - bathing daily
  - brushing teeth
  - combing and brushing hair
  - dressing in appropriate, clean clothing
  - performing proper toileting hygiene.
- meet self-care needs in a socially acceptable way and without total dependence on others as evidenced by
  - clean, appropriate appearance
  - attending to hygiene regimen every morning
  - eating with socially acceptable manners
  - performing self-care activities alone or with minimal assistance.

Nursing Orders with Rationale

➤ Assess and monitor for presence/absence/ changes in assessment findings outlined above *in order to detect any change in status.*

➤ Assess level of ability to care for self, including comprehension, awareness, cognition, and affect. *Impaired cognitive functioning with poor reality orientation or depression may cause decreased ability to be aware of and meet basic self-care needs (Beck, Rawlins, & Williams, 1987).*

➤ Provide assistance with bathing, diet, grooming, toileting as needed; monitor oral hygiene; assist with clothing choice; work with the patient to establish a daily routine for bathing, shampooing, and grooming. *Decreased self-esteem, regressive behavior, negative or apathetic attitudes, contribute to lack of interest in appearance, cleanliness, and grooming (Davies & Janosik, 1991).*

➤ Protect the patient from embarrassment over inability to eat properly, incontinence, inappropriate dress, and poor hygiene *to decrease shame over impaired functioning.*

➤ Have patient do as much self-care as possible; consider safety and keep expectations realistic given the patient's level of functioning and impairment. *Doing as much for self as possible will help patient to decrease feelings of dependency and poor self-concept (Carpenito, 1989). Realistic expectations will decrease frustration.*

➤ When patient becomes frustrated, lower your demands/expectations. *Patient needs to succeed and to increase sense of achievement before moving on to more difficult self-care needs.*

➤ Do not argue with patient who will not perform ADL; avoid judgmental or disapproving responses; try again later. *Forcing the patient to do something against his or her will promotes more negative behavior.*

➤ Do not act quickly and perform tasks for patient yourself; give patient as much time as she or he needs. *Some patients tend to follow directions slowly (e.g., demented, psychotic/catatonic). Allowing patients adequate time will increase their sense of mastery and their self-concept.*

➤ Set a realistic time frame with patient for carrying out ADL. *Providing structure decreases anxiety. Having patient participate in setting the time frame conveys respect.*

➤ Provide appropriate privacy for self-care activities *to promote self-worth and dignity (Carpenito, 1989).*

➤ Encourage patient to participate in planning for ADL and self-care; reward all efforts and accomplishments. *Participating in planning care gives patient a sense of control over daily living, helps reduce feelings of powerlessness (Carpenito, 1989), and promotes feelings of self-worth, control, and freedom.*

➤ Avoid showing rejection or belittling patient's struggles to change self-care behaviors; give positive feedback about improvement in self-care activities. *Positive reinforcement will promote improved self-concept (McFarland & Wasli, 1986).*

➤ Plan ADL with patient with ritualistic behaviors; allow to make choices and to include time for rituals; set reasonable limits on ritualistic behavior. *Interrupting ritualistic behavior can result in extreme anxiety and cause the patient to panic or decompensate (Reighley, 1988).*

➤ Adjust phobic patient's ADL routine to avoid contact with feared situation; refer to nursing care plans "Anxiety" and "Fear" for interventions on decreasing anxiety associated with phobias. *Avoidance of feared situation will help to increase compliance with self-care.*

➤ Allow patient to make simple choices in ADL (e.g., "Do you want to wear the green shirt or the brown shirt today?" rather than, "What do you want to wear?"). *Limiting choices diminishes ambivalence in the regressed patient but allows some control.*

➤ Offer to assist patient in making a chart of daily grooming and hygiene tasks to be performed in the morning and evening. *Involving the patient in a concrete task such as making a chart for the room promotes reality orientation and reinforces a grooming ritual.*

➤ Assure patient that it is acceptable to be dependent on others for a limited amount of time to provide basic needs.
  There may be a decreased level of comprehension of the need to feed, bathe, dress, or otherwise care for self in major depression (Davies & Janosik, 1991).

➤ Assess for vegetative signs that interfere with the patient's ability to perform ADL.
  The depressed patient may be unable to perform self-care activities in a manner consistent with body requirements (Reighley, 1988).

➤ Be aware that patient may lack motivation to do anything for self and may be experiencing strong feelings of dependency.
  A defense mechanism such as regression may occur as a way of dealing with depression (Davies & Janosik, 1991).

➤ Monitor food and fluid intake; record I&O if necessary; weigh weekly; monitor for urinary retention and constipation; assess need for laxatives.
  Lack of appetite and activity and slowed metabolism, which occur in a severely depressed person, can result in malnutrition, urinary retention, and constipation (Reighley, 1988). Medication can cause constipation.

➤ Avoid frequent discussion and inquiries about bowel movements
  to avoid development of ruminative thoughts about bowels.

➤ Determine favorite foods and offer small portions to depressed patients who have lost their appetite
  to increase nutritional intake.

➤ Determine favorite foods and offer small portions to depressed patients who have lost their appetite
  to increase nutritional intake.

➤ Offer fortified fluid refreshment (e.g., juice, milkshakes) or snack foods (e.g., peanuts, granola bar) for manic patients that can be consumed while standing or moving
  to increase intake of nutrients.

➤ Ensure that the manic patient has flexible opportunities to bathe, eat, groom, and sleep; encourage all attempts at self-care.
  The individual experiencing a manic episode is unable cognitively to focus on purposeful activity such as caring for body hygiene and feeding self (Reighley, 1988).

Charting Components

➤ ADL performed, daily routine
➤ Elimination patterns, toileting habits
➤ Factors interfering with self-care
➤ General appearance, grooming done
➤ Improvement in performance of self-care activities
➤ Level of frustration with ability to perform ADL
➤ Level of impairment (cognitive, affect, regression)
➤ Limitations in ADL
➤ Motivation or lack of to do ADL
➤ Nutritional status, eating habits

VII. Perceiving

A. SELF-CONCEPT

1. Body-Image Disturbance

Definition
Disruption in the way one perceives one's body image

Related to
- Biophysical factors (e.g., illness, injury, surgery, birth defect, aging, aging, obesity, pregnancy)
- Cognitive/perceptual factors (e.g., anorexia nervosa)
- Psychosocial factors (e.g., societal values placed on youth and beauty)
- Cultural or spiritual factors

Characteristics/Assessment Findings

A or B must be present to justify the diagnosis of "Body-Image Disturbance":
*A = verbal response to actual or perceived change in structure or function of the body.
*B = nonverbal response to actual or perceived change in structure or function.
The following clinical manifestations may be used to validate the presence of A or B:

Objective
- Missing body part
- Actual change in structure/function of a body part
- Not looking or touching body part
- Hiding or overexposing body part
- Trauma to nonfunctioning body part
- Change in patient's social involvement with others
- Change in ability to estimate spatial relationship of body to the environment
  - increasing dependence on others

  - self-destructive behavior (e.g., anorexia, bulimia, substance abuse, obesity)

Subjective
Verbalization of
- Change in life-style
- Fear of rejection or of reaction by others
- Focus on past strengths, functions, appearance
- Negative feelings about body or body parts
- Feelings of helplessness, hopelessness, powerlessness, vulnerability
- Preoccupation with change or loss
- Emphasis on remaining strength, heightened achievement
- Extension of body boundary to incorporate environmental objects
- Personification of body part
- Depersonalization of part or loss by impersonal pronoun
- Refusal to verify actual change
- Fear of loss of sexual attractiveness or function
- Shame, embarrassment, guilt, revulsion
- Perceived distortion of body image (e.g., seeing self as fat when body is actually very thin)

Expected Outcomes/Goals

The patient will
- demonstrate adaptation of altered body image into positive self-concept as evidenced by
  - implementing new coping patterns
  - verbalizing/demonstrating acceptance of appearance
  - improving grooming, dress, posture, and positive presentation of self.

Content appearing in this typeface is additional information not included in the NANDA nursing diagnoses.

*Critical.

➤ correct distorted body image as evidenced by
   ▷ stating a congruency between actual body size and perception of body size
   ▷ maintaining an ideal weight agreed on by staff and patient.
➤ demonstrate ability to manage self-care as evidenced by performing ADL without assistance.
➤ seek appropriate social and psychological support systems as evidenced by
   ▷ making plans to participate in/reenter a support group
   ▷ spending time with friends and family.

Nursing Orders with Rationale

➤ Assess and monitor for presence/absence/ changes in assessment findings outlined above *in order to detect any change in status.*

➤ Encourage verbalization of negative feelings by using empathy and reflective statements (e.g., "You sound angry about the prospect of having to gain 7 lb.").
   Expressing feelings can be helpful in diffusing anger and helplessness. Once verbalization about negative feelings begins, the foundations toward acceptance of change can start.

➤ Acknowledge patient's feelings of hostility, grief, fear, and dependency.
   Acknowledging feelings conveys understanding and caring, and encourages patient to ventilate.

➤ Allow patient to use denial appropriately, but do not reinforce it; discuss realistic expectations as soon as possible.
   Denial is a natural initial response to a change in body image; it becomes destructive when maintained in the face of an everpresent problem.

➤ Encourage patient to grieve for what has been lost.
   Voicing what has been lost is a first step in removing denial and in beginning the process of grief work.

➤ Encourage to assess meaning of loss of function or body part.
   The patient may feel betrayed by changes in his or her own body; one's attitudes toward own body may reflect important aspects of the self (Davies & Janosik, 1991).

➤ Encourage to touch own body and to examine self in the mirror.
   Touch is the main mode for the brain to incorporate new body boundaries into a new concept of self (Kolb, 1974).

➤ Encourage to seek information/feedback from significant others.
   Each person has a mental image of own appearance, which may or may not be real. All sources of feedback will help the patient to incorporate any changes or to accept own body as it really is.

➤ Help patient to explore and examine any self-esteem issues; refer to nursing care plan "Chronic Low Self-Esteem."
   The body represents the individual self. The more accepting one is of one's own body, the more secure the individual.

➤ Use visual aids to explore changes in body image and to confront the patient's denial (e.g., mirrors, pictures, videotapes); encourage activities in which the patient confronts the new body image (e.g., shopping for clothes, movement/exercise).
   Changes in one's body must be incorporated gradually through exploration of the alterations that have taken place. These explorations can be through body movement, visualization methods, and physical exercises until the schemata in the brain have altered its boundaries.

➤ Provide accurate information about care at patient's level of acceptance; clarify misconceptions and encourage patient to ask questions.
   Information and knowledge enable the patient to make choices about life-style changes and to incorporate new aspects of self into the self-image (Doenges, Moorhouse, & Geissler, 1989).

➤ Set limits on maladaptive behavior (e.g., induced vomiting, excessive exercising)
   to prevent self-destructive behaviors.

➤ Teach strategies for coping with emotions.
   Exploring and teaching new techniques for stress reduction facilitates adaptation to change.

➤ Help patient to discuss life-style changes that may occur with changes in function or body part.
   Exploring and implementing any necessary adaptations will help to remove denial and ease the transition to the changes.

➤ Encourage discussions about sexuality as it relates to the patient's current body image (e.g., the patient's own perception of sexual attractiveness, how the patient's significant other may respond to change); refer to nursing care plans "Altered Sexuality Patterns" and "Sexual Dysfunction" for more interventions.

The patient may feel disfigured and afraid of significant other viewing scars (Doenges et al., 1989). Talking about it provides an atmosphere of social acceptance and allows the patient to feel more comfortable about own body.

➤ Provide information about sexuality and specific alteration in body image (e.g., obesity, emaciation, aging).

Information allows the patient to deal with reality and helps to diffuse anxiety and fear (Doenges et al., 1989).

➤ Make appropriate referrals to support groups or other healthcare professionals.

Support groups provide opportunities for sharing experiences, practical problem solving, and mutual support, which can help to decrease alienation and helplessness (Doenges et al., 1989).

➤ Help the family to cope with their feelings about changes occurring in the patient.

Each person in the family system has a personal ideal and expectations of each of the others in the system. Exploration of the losses is an important step in reforming the family system around the altered person.

➤ Teach family any necessary alterations in life-style that result from a change in patient's body image.

Charting Components

➤ Behaviors indicating acceptance/denial in dealing with altered body image
➤ Level of acceptance of sexual self
➤ Level of self-care
➤ New coping mechanisms
➤ Referrals made
➤ Self-esteem
➤ Significant other's reactions to patient's condition
➤ Statements of congruence between actual and perceived body size/shape
➤ Time spent with family/friends
➤ Patient/family teaching, response

Additional Nursing Orders for THE PATIENT WITH AN EATING DISORDER

➤ Monitor eating patterns for adequate intake.

Inability to meet metabolic requirements results in loss of weight, poor health, and inability of body to grow or heal itself; all are involved in body image (Carpenito, 1989).

➤ Refer to nursing care plan "Chronic Low Self-Esteem" for interventions on how to approach the anorexic patient.

Young women who are anorexic reject their growing feminine body configuration and strive for a childlike smallness due to lack of acceptance of self (Davies & Janosik, 1991).

➤ Be aware of and discuss with patient the cultural definition of ideal body image (e.g., thinness is valued in the United States) and how this impacts negatively on some people.

The idealization of slimness can assist the anorexic girl to justify her behavior by entering modeling, theater, or dance (Stuart & Sundeen, 1987).

➤ Realize that the anorexic patient has a distorted body image, perceives self as fat even when emaciated, and will persist in the attempt to lose weight.

The patient will literally starve herself to achieve the goal of being thin; however, because of the distortion in body image, the goal is unattainable (Beck, Rawlins, & Williams, 1988).

➤ Educate the family to the concept of control; discuss the reason for power struggles between the anorexic patient and the family member who recognizes the destructiveness of the refusal to eat and tries to change it.

Control is the reason for noncompliance. When the patient surrenders to family's or staff's wishes to eat, the patient will feel a loss of self-esteem and a fear of becoming a fat, powerless, individual (Beck et al., 1988).

Additional Charting Components

➤ Amount, intensity of exercise
➤ Caloric intake, eating patterns
➤ Episodes of induced vomiting
➤ Feelings expressed about self, family
➤ Nutritional status
➤ Self-image
➤ Weight

2. Chronic Low Self-Esteem

Definition

Long-standing negative self-evaluation/feelings about self or own capabilities

Related to

➤ Excessively idealized ego ideal (e.g., unrealistic self-expectations)
➤ Lack of ego competencies
➤ Substance abuse
➤ Auditory hallucinations
➤ Intellectual impairment
➤ Avoidant and dependent patterns
➤ Lack of integrated self view (e.g., persistence of splitting as a psychological defense)
➤ Depression
➤ Shame, guilt

Characteristics/Assessment Findings

Major (Long-standing or Chronic)
➤ Self-negating verbalization
➤ Expresses feelings of shame and guilt
➤ Evaluates self as unable to deal with events
➤ Rationalizes away/rejects positive feedback and exaggerates feedback about self
➤ Hesitant to try new things/situations
➤ Expresses suicidal thoughts/impulses
  ▷ shares self-evaluation of being worthless
  ▷ demonstrates self-destructive/self-defeating behavior patterns
  ▷ uses/abuses chemicals to "mask" painful feelings of inadequacy
  ▷ exhibits symptoms of depression (e.g., insomnia, weight gain/loss, despondency, hopelessness)

Minor
➤ Frequent lack of success in work or other life events
➤ Overly conforming, dependent on others' opinions
➤ Lack of eye contact
➤ Nonassertive, passive
➤ Indecisive
➤ Excessively seeks reassurance
➤ Verbalizes feelings of helplessness
➤ Lacks self-initiative
➤ Inability to set goals

Expected Outcomes/Goals

The patient will accept self as a person having both strengths/competencies as well as certain vulnerabilities/problems as evidenced by
➤ giving an accurate, specific, and nonjudgmental description of self
➤ verbalizing a positive and integrated view of self
➤ ceasing to use chemicals to deal with dysphoria/internal feelings
➤ reporting freedom from symptoms of major depression
➤ modifying excessive and unrealistic self-expectations
➤ reporting decreased feelings of shame and guilt.

Nursing Orders with Rationale

➤ Assess and monitor for presence/absence/changes in assessment findings outlined above *in order to detect any change in status.*

➤ Refer to nursing care plans "Situational Low Self-Esteem" and "Ineffective Individual Coping" for additional interventions.

➤ Demonstrate an affirming and caring attitude. *A modification in self-esteem can occur as the patient incorporates or identifies with the respect and affirmation provided by the nurse (Kerr, 1987/1988).*

➤ Communicate concern for the patient's well-being by attention to his or her needs for adequate nutrition, exercise, rest, hygiene, and involvement in the milieu. *Attending to grooming, hygiene, and physical appearance is often not well received by a person with low self-esteem. The nurse who refuses to allow such a patient to look sloppy and unkempt can mobilize the patient's hope that there is something worthwhile about him or her (Kerr, 1987/1988).*

➤ Assist patient to express the anger that is turned against the self. *The patient may not be aware of feeling angry, resentful, or disappointed in others. The feeling remains unconscious because awareness of it would threaten the person in some way. Assisting the patient to "label" the feelings helps to decrease low self-esteem.*

Content appearing in this typeface is additional information not included in the NANDA nursing diagnoses.

➤ Help patient to take a self-concept inventory (e.g., physical appearance, relationships, performance at work/school/daily tasks of life, sexuality, personality):
  ▷ write down words/phrases that describe self in each category.
  ▷ put a "+" for strengths or a "–" for weaknesses after each item.
  ▷ revise the list of weaknesses by changing judgmental words to objective ones (e.g., "buck teeth" to "prominent front teeth").
  ▷ identify exceptions to the weaknesses (e.g., mentally lazy about current issues but an avid reader of medical information).
  ▷ rewrite list of strengths into complete sentences.
    Raising self-esteem requires a clear and accurate self-description that acknowledges strengths and describes weaknesses nonjudgmentally (McKay & Fanning, 1987).

➤ Review with the patient the types of cognitive distortions that affect self-esteem:
  ▷ *overgeneralization:* taking one fact or event and making a general rule out of it
  ▷ *filtering:* selectively paying attention to negative facts and ignoring the positive ones
  ▷ *polarized thinking:* dividing all actions, events, and feelings into black/white, either/or, always/never, success/failure with no possibility of a middle range
  ▷ *self-blame:* blaming self for everything, whether at fault or not (e.g., excessive apologizing)
  ▷ *mind reading:* assuming others don't like you, etc., without any real evidence that assumptions are correct.
    Cognitive distortions are habitual and are used to interpret reality in an unrealistic manner. They tend to reinforce a lopsided, negative, inaccurate perception of self (McKay & Fanning, 1987).

➤ Help patient identify distorted cognitions by asking, "What are you saying about yourself in this situation?" which elicits the distortion (e.g., "They will reject me." [mind reading]).
    Analysis of self-statements provides insight into how the person is contributing to the low self-esteem.

➤ Teach patient to combat cognitive distortions by using the three-column technique of analysis and rebuttal:
  ▷ *self-statement:* "They will reject me."
  ▷ *distortion:* mind reading
  ▷ *rebuttal:* "I have no way of knowing what they will think of me."
    Rebuttals must be strong, nonjudgmental, specific, and balanced to combat distorted thinking effectively (McKay & Fanning, 1987).

➤ Help patient develop compassion and forgiveness for self:
  ▷ understand what needs she or he is trying to meet.
  ▷ accept self, the situation, or other person as is.
  ▷ let go of a situation when it is over because nothing more can be done (e.g., give up ideas of retaliation, restitution).
    Compassion for self is the essence of self-esteem. The ability to forgive oneself and others fosters reasonable expectations (McKay & Fanning, 1987).

➤ Encourage patient to do visualizations that will improve self-image, self-confidence, and self-worth (e.g., relax body, clear mind, imagine positive scenes).
    Visualization raises self-esteem by replacing negative self-statements/images with conscious, positive ones. This process reprograms the mind to recognize and choose more positive actions, thoughts, and feelings.

➤ Provide physical outlets for aggressive energy.
    Activities that allow for physical sublimation of aggressive drives (e.g., tennis, running) are almost always helpful, even when the patient does not become consciously aware of the aggressive feelings that reside within (Kerr, 1987/1988).

➤ Help patient to develop appropriate problem-solving skills: assess patient's current process, point out strengths, suggest options for weak areas.
    Strengthening patient's ability to solve problems will enhance patient's self-esteem.

➤ Assess patient's ego competencies (e.g., reality testing, impulse control); support those areas where deficits exist.

A person's level of ego strength helps to determine feelings of self-worth and sense of competency in the world.

➤ Help patient to express feelings of grief, sadness, or loss by using empathic communication techniques (e.g., *Patient:* "I just don't know how I will manage with him gone. It all seems so useless." *Nurse:* "You feel scared and empty without your husband, as if everything is without meaning?")

Empathic communication conveys understanding and helps the patient verbalize feelings.

➤ Assess suicidal lethality by openly and directly querying patient, discussing any ideation or intent with patient; refer to nursing care plan "Potential for Violence: Self-Directed."

Patients may have suicidal thoughts that are never verbalized because the nurse does not ask if they are present. They will be rendered less potent to the degree patients feel understood, supported, cared about, and protected from their own impulses (Kerr, 1987/1988).

➤ Maximize the patient's participation in the therapeutic relationship:
  ▷ increase patient's participation in decisions that affect own care.
  ▷ convey to the patient that she or he is a responsible individual.

  Sharing ideas is necessary for the patient to assume ultimate responsibility for own ideas.

➤ Assess for chemical dependency. See nursing care plans "Impaired Adjustment, Additional Nursing Orders for Chemical Dependency."

Charting Components

➤ Behaviors indicative of low self-esteem
  ▷ indecisiveness
  ▷ lack of eye contact
  ▷ lack of self-care
  ▷ refusal to look in mirror
  ▷ inability to ask for help
➤ Behaviors indicative of increasing self-esteem
  ▷ attention to grooming and appearance
  ▷ smiling
  ▷ relaxed posture
  ▷ interacting with others

➤ Effectiveness of past/current coping strategies
➤ Ego competencies/deficits; support provided
➤ Feelings expressed
➤ Patient's description of self
➤ Planning, participating in ADL
➤ Statements of low/increasing self-esteem
➤ Symptoms of major depression

3. Situational Low Self-Esteem

Definition

Negative self-evaluation or feelings about self that develop in response to a loss or change in an individual who previously had a positive self-evaluation

Related to

➤ Anxiety
➤ Body-image disturbance (real or anticipated loss of body part or function)
➤ Diagnosis of chronic illness
➤ Dependency
➤ Depression
➤ Hospitalization
➤ Immobility
➤ Noncompliance
➤ Pain
➤ Powerlessness
➤ Role change
➤ Separation
➤ Trauma
➤ Loss of valued person/object

Content appearing in this typeface is additional information not included in the NANDA nursing diagnoses.

Characteristics/Assessment Findings

Major
- Episodic occurrence of negative self-appraisal in response to life events in a person with a previous positive self-evaluation
- Verbalization of negative feelings about the self (e.g., helplessness, uselessness)

Minor
- Self-negating verbalizations
- Expressions of shame/guilt
- Self-evaluation as unable to handle situations/events
- Difficulty making decisions

Other Possible Characteristics
- Anger, hostility
- Feels powerless and unable to see alternatives
- Inability to accept positive reinforcement
- Lack of eye contact
- Lack of follow-through
- Nonparticipation in treatment
- Passivity
- Hesitancy to ask for help
- Self-neglect
- Social isolation

Expected Outcomes/Goals

The patient will
- identify the source of threat to self-esteem as evidenced by verbalizing past/present events leading to decreased feelings of self-worth.
- experience emotional support while dealing with the threat to self-esteem as evidenced by verbalizing statements of self-acceptance and worth.
- explore perception of self and feelings as evidenced by verbalizing a realistic self-perception and expressing emotions.
- explore own strengths and past coping mechanisms as evidenced by
  - identifying own skills, resources
  - discussing results of past coping strategies.
- develop new coping as necessary as evidenced by
  - exploring new coping options
  - discussing potential consequences
  - choosing one or two new options to implement.

Content appearing in this typeface is additional information not included in the NANDA nursing diagnoses.

Nursing Orders with Rationale

- Assess and monitor for presence/absence/changes in assessment findings outlined above *in order to detect any change in status.*

- Establish a trusting, open relationship:
  - offer unconditional acceptance.
  - listen to patient.
  - encourage discussion of thoughts and feelings.
  - respond nonjudgmentally.
  - convey to the patient that she or he is a valued person who is both responsible for and able to help self.
    A trusting relationship will help to reduce the threat that the medical staff poses and to build rapport for intervention (Davies & Janosik, 1991).

- Assist patient to identify the specific source of threat to self-esteem; explore distortions in perceptions, possibility of misinformation/lack of correct information.
  Unrealistic expectations and distorted perceptions can result in disappointment, anxiety, and negative self-appraisal.

- Correct distorted perceptions patient has about self/others; lend perspective to situation.
  Offering a broader and more accurate perspective to a situation lowers anxiety, promotes realistic problem solving and constructive coping.

- Provide a safe, supportive environment:
  - reduce level of anxiety (refer to nursing care plan "Anxiety").
  - approach patient in a respectful way.
  - discourage patient from isolating self.
  - give positive reinforcement.
    The patient needs some degree of external support for self-control and integration.

- Provide openings for the patient to express feelings by validating your observations (e.g., "You look sad today.").
  Expressing feelings reduces anxiety, clarifies the situation, and promotes feelings of well-being.

- Explore the patient's positive and negative coping responses to own situation:
  - contrast positive and negative responses.
  - explore pros and cons of alternative coping responses.
  - explore past coping mechanisms, abilities, consequences.

> help to generalize adaptive coping from the past to the present.
>> *Examining coping skills will allow the patient to make better decisions about his or her behavior.*

➤ Practice with patient to change negative self-talk (e.g., "I feel I am no longer a good person.") to a positive statement (e.g., "People like me the way I am.").
>> *Continuous derogatory thoughts have harmful effects on a person's self-image; positive affirmations eliminate negative self-talk (Miller, 1983).*

➤ Give positive reinforcement for statements and behaviors that indicate good self-esteem.
>> *Reinforcement increases the possibility of a behavior becoming integrated into the person's personality.*

➤ Involve family/significant others in supporting patient.
>> *When a relationship is disrupted, insecurity and lowered self-esteem result.*

Charting Components

➤ Behaviors indicative of increasing self-esteem
>> attention to grooming and appearance
>> smiling
>> relaxed posture
>> interacting with others
➤ Behaviors indicative of low self-esteem
>> indecisiveness
>> lack of eye contact
>> lack of self-care
>> refusal to look in mirror
>> unable to ask for help
➤ Cognitive distortions identified
➤ Effectiveness of past/current coping strategies
➤ Feelings expressed
➤ Statements of low or increasing self-esteem
➤ Techniques taught to increase self-esteem

4. Personal Identity Disturbance

Definition

Inability to distinguish between self and nonself

Related to

➤ Severe child abuse
➤ Lack of adequate role models

➤ Lack of adequate mirroring, consoling, empathy of self
➤ Immaturity
➤ Lack of autonomy
➤ Disturbance in object relations
➤ Incapacity to tolerate stress

Characteristics/Assessment Findings

Major
➤ Asking "Who am I?"
➤ Uncertainty about several life issues (e.g., self-image, long-term goals, career choice, sexual orientation, moral values)
➤ Chronic feelings of emptiness and boredom
➤ Intense and unstable relationships, emotional intensity
➤ Fear of abandonment, avoidance of being alone
➤ Marked mood shifts
➤ Excessive and impulsive expressions of anger/rage
➤ Lack of impulse control
➤ Suicidal threats
➤ Self-mutilating behaviors
➤ Inability to integrate aspects of the self into a relatively coherent and acceptable sense of self

Minor
➤ Pessimistic outlook
➤ Contradictory personality traits
➤ Irritability, anxiety
➤ Depression
➤ Gender confusion
➤ Inability to empathize with others
➤ Absence of moral code
➤ Lack of authenticity
➤ Unrealistic idealized self
➤ Self-doubt, doubt about the future
➤ Difficulty in making choices
➤ Cognitive disorganization under stress (e.g., diminished ability to process information, distortion of meaning or significance of an event, partial amnesia)
➤ Brief psychotic regression

Content appearing in this typeface is additional information not included in the NANDA nursing diagnoses.

Expected Outcomes/Goals

The patient will

➤ demonstrate a sense of self as evidenced by
  ▷ articulating self-insights and awareness
  ▷ choosing positive alternatives with certainty
  ▷ answering the question "Who am I?" with certainty.

➤ clarify own choices about career, friendships, moral values as evidenced by
  ▷ choosing and pursuing a career
  ▷ developing relationships with chosen others
  ▷ expressing values and religious beliefs.

➤ improve social and role competence as evidenced by
  ▷ establishing a stable relationship
  ▷ modulating mood shifts
  ▷ expressing a decrease in feelings of emptiness and boredom
  ▷ taking responsibility for own emotions and reactions.

➤ demonstrate strong ego boundaries as evidenced by
  ▷ being able to say "no" to others
  ▷ controlling angry outbursts
  ▷ tolerating being alone.

Nursing Orders with Rationale

➤ Assess and monitor for presence/absence/ changes in assessment findings outlined above *in order to detect any change in status.*

➤ Assess patient for degree of identity disturbance by inquiring about goals, values, plans, importance of friends, religious beliefs; discern if patient can tell you anything substantial about him- or herself.
  Patients with a personality disturbance (i.e., a borderline patient) are experienced by others as "chameleon-like" because they act "as if" they were other people by taking on the characteristics of whomever they are with (Platt-Koch, 1982).

➤ Provide a "holding environment" for patient by building a trusting alliance with him or her; give soothing and comforting measures as tolerated.
  These patients lack the capacity for self-soothing and the ability to calm themselves (Hickey, 1985).

➤ Modulate the amount of warmth shown to the patient.
  Too much warmth and closeness frightens the patient and stimulates rage and destructive feelings (Kernberg, 1984).

➤ Recognize when the patient is devaluing or idealizing you/staff; when you gratify the patient you will be seen as wonderful, and when you frustrate the patient you will be seen as hateful.
  Borderline patients alternate between idealization and devaluation of others (Kernberg, 1984).

➤ Learn to tolerate the patient's rage/verbal assaults without retaliating or withdrawing.
  By this process, the patient's hostility can be examined and understood as part of a more general pattern of relating to important others (Kaplan, 1986).

➤ When patients are acting hostile and angry toward you, ask who treated them with hostility in the past.
  Reflecting on past feelings and behaviors helps the patient see that there is a historical reason for the rage.

➤ Establish a connection between the patient's actions and feelings in the present; help to see that she or he communicates by action as a defense against uncomfortable feelings.
  In borderline patients, action is a primary defense against the awareness of uncomfortable affect. Awareness of this defense is essential to developing autonomy and self-control (Kaplan, 1986).

➤ Help patients understand the nature of their self-destructive behaviors and their influence on others by consistently and repeatedly drawing attention to the consequences of such behaviors (e.g., drug abuse, sexual promiscuity, emotional outbursts); focus on the consequence of the behavior rather than on the motive.
  Borderline patients have a great investment in remaining unaware of the self-destructive nature of actions that gratify certain wishes and allay anxiety (Kaplan, 1986).

➤ Recognize that the quality of depression is empty and lonely, and persons with an identity disturbance are frequently left out of genuine human interactions; spend time with the patient in a warm and authentic way, particularly when she or he is acting out.
  The emptiness stems from the patient's lack of identity. This leaves a frightening inner void that the individual tries to fill with impulsive, self-destructive acting out (e.g., sex, gambling, substance abuse, suicidal gestures) (Platt-Koch, 1982).

➤ Help patient to discuss feelings of depersonalization (feeling unreal or strange) and derealization (the sense that the environment is unreal and strange).

> *Much wrist-cutting and multiple superficial incisions are done to counteract these feelings. The panic experienced in states of depersonalization leads to extreme behavior in order to feel "something" (Kernberg, 1984).*

➤ Work with patients on limiting acting-out behaviors that are self-mutilating or destructive toward others or self by
  ▷ helping them recognize cues that precede the behavior.
  ▷ teaching them to develop self-dialogue to reverse automatic response (e.g., thought stopping, thought insertion, mental rehearsal techniques).

> *Cognitive disorganization frequently occurs under stress, which causes increased emotional intensity. The acting-out behavior provides a release of internal stress (Gallop, 1988).*

➤ Characterize and label the difficulties that the patient experiences in relationships, occupational settings (e.g., "Your emotional intensity seems to create difficulty for you in your work setting."); help to recognize early warning signals that emotions are beginning to intensify too rapidly.

> *Labeling the type of difficulty helps the patient to be able to place his or her troubles within some general category. This helps to demystify the thing and reduce it to more manageable proportions (Gallop, 1988).*

➤ Assist the patient in setting up a control plan of what to do when emotions are getting out of control:
  ▷ anticipate the difficult situation.
  ▷ steer the interaction away from the troublesome area.
  ▷ have someone who can be telephoned when situations are overwhelming.
  ▷ examine impulses and intense emotions rather than acting so quickly.

> *Such a plan will help the patient learn control, avoid self-destructive acting out, and learn to deal with emotions differently (Gallop, 1988).*

➤ Build the patient's sense of self and self-esteem by providing consistent, caring, nonpunitive interactions; refer to nursing care plan "Chronic Low Self-Esteem" for more interventions.

> *The capacity to know, esteem, and love oneself can be developed only when there are adequate experiences of being known, esteemed, and loved by a significant other (Hickey, 1985).*

➤ Provide clear limits and enforce them consistently.

> *Consistent limit-setting counteracts the patient's divisive attempts to split staff into "all good" and "all bad" people (Platt-Koch, 1982).*

➤ Establish a stable framework for all interactions and activities (e.g., groups, therapy sessions, mealtime):
  ▷ schedule regular appointment times.
  ▷ begin and end sessions on time.
  ▷ make clear expectations for each activity.
  ▷ confront deviations from the framework.
    > *The framework provides a sense of security, boundaries, and containment.*

➤ Contain and prevent regression by telling patient what is not acceptable and what is expected, i.e.,
  ▷ she or he will be held accountable for all behavior.
  ▷ suicidal behavior will result in being transferred to a closed unit.
  ▷ assaultive behavior will result in discharge.
  ▷ substance abuse will result in disciplinary action.
    > *Hospitalization fosters regressive behavior, which normally includes demanding behavior, suicide threats, and destructive acts (Platt-Koch, 1982).*

➤ Emphasize "here-and-now" interpretations concerning dangerous behaviors that disrupt the patient's life; explore past developmental history as it relates to current behavior.

> *Patients often get lost in the past and self-rumination on their victimization rather than deal with current behaviors that are destructive (Hickey, 1985).*

➤ Pay attention to countertransference feelings, particularly feelings of aversion and malice.
   The nurse needs to be able to tolerate the uncomfortable feelings that the patient projects onto staff. In order to get better, the patient needs to experience both love and hate for the therapist. These patients work hard at keeping good and bad separate, and their estimation of the nurse can change from week to week, from hour to hour, or from minute to minute (Platt-Koch, 1982). Refer to nursing care plan "Risk for Self-Mutilation" for more interventions.

Charting Components

➤ Ability to calm and soothe self
➤ Ability to regulate emotions
➤ Feedback given regarding relationships/work
➤ Feelings of emptiness expressed rather than acted out
➤ Genuine feelings expressed
➤ Goals regarding life, work, relationships
➤ Impulsive acting out, patient's insight into motive
➤ Level of regression
➤ Limits set, patient's response
➤ Occurrence of splitting in staff
➤ Outbursts of rage and anger
➤ Plans for implementing more control of feelings/ behavior
➤ Quality of relationships with other patients/staff
➤ Self-destructive and self-mutilating behaviors
➤ Time spent alone, how well tolerated

Additional Nursing Orders for
THE PATIENT WITH A DISSOCIATIVE IDENTITY DISORDER

➤ Provide a safe and trusting environment for the multiple-personality patient.
   The patient has rarely, if ever, had a trusting relationship with anyone. Without the basic building blocks of trust, safety, and acceptance the patient will be unable to progress in treatment (Kluft, 1984).

➤ Discuss with patient the dynamics of a multiple-personality disorder (MPD) and why the dissociative aspects exist:
   ▷ MPD develops due to a defensive process called "dissociation." A child blocks out feelings, memories, and behaviors and forms other parts or "alters" to help cope with the traumatic events (Wilbur, 1984).
   ▷ usually the original personality has no knowledge or awareness of the existence of any other personalities.
   ▷ physical and sexual abuse are prevalent in MPD.
      Accepting the diagnosis and learning to cope with the consequences of having alter personalities necessitate a clear understanding of what is happening and why (Wilbur, 1984).

➤ Realize that the original personality may have amnesic barriers concerning the presence and behavior of alter personalities, which result in the patient waking up from a blank spell in unfamiliar surroundings, not knowing how she or he got there.
   When different personalities are in conscious control, the presenting personality becomes amnesic during the time when the others are "out" (Anderson, 1988).

➤ Draw a map or keep a chart of the patient's personality system that is available to the staff; include each alter ego's name, age, function, degree of power, and amnesic barriers.
   Mapping provides a practical way of understanding the personality system and the different alters, and it helps organize data (Anderson, 1988).

➤ Be empathic with each personality; refuse to take sides with any of the personalities but oppose efforts of any of them to do harm to themselves, the other personalities, or other individuals.
   Evenhanded gentleness, with respect for all personalities, helps the patient to experience and integrate overwhelming feelings and events from the past (Kluft, 1984).

➤ Encourage the patient to write and dialogue with the various personalities
   to facilitate internal communication back and forth.

➤ Videotape the personalities talking about themselves

> *to illustrate the various personalities to the part that is amnesic. Breaking down amnesic barriers enables the parts to become co-conscious with one another and is a step toward integration (Wilbur, 1984).*

➤ Allow the patient to express feelings and memories from the past that may have contributed to the splitting off of aspects of self (e.g., screaming, hiding in a closet, curling up under a table); provide support and reassurance that these experiences happened in the past and that the patient is now safe.

> *Abreaction facilitates integration of aspects of the self.*

➤ Use behavioral techniques to deal with aggressive or threatening personalities who are acting out.

> *Each part or personality usually deals with a set of conflicts and emotions related to abuse. Usually one personality will be angry or persecutory (Anderson, 1988).*

Additional Charting Components

➤ Degree of amnesia between personalities
➤ Level of trust demonstrated toward staff/therapist
➤ Memories recalled, feelings experienced
➤ Number and nature of different personalities
➤ Techniques used to facilitate integration (e.g., writing, videotape)

B. SENSORY/PERCEPTUAL

1. Sensory/Perceptual Alterations

Definition

A state in which an individual experiences a change in the amount or patterning of oncoming stimuli accompanied by a diminished, exaggerated, distorted, or impaired response to such stimuli

Related to

➤ Altered environmental stimuli: excessive or insufficient
➤ Altered sensory reception: transmission or integration
➤ Chemical alterations: endogenous (e.g., electrolyte), exogenous (e.g., drugs)
➤ Psychological stress
➤ Psychological exhaustion
➤ Inadequate reality testing
➤ Extreme anxiety, panic
➤ Structural diseases of the sensory organs

Characteristics/Assessment Findings

➤ Disoriented to time, persons, and place
➤ Altered abstraction
➤ Altered conceptualization
➤ Change in problem-solving abilities
➤ Reported or measured change in sensory acuity
➤ Change in behavior pattern
➤ Anxiety
➤ Apathy
➤ Change in usual response to stimuli
➤ Indication of body-image alteration
➤ Restlessness
➤ Irritability
➤ Altered communication patterns
➤ Drug-related chemicals in lab tests
➤ Withdrawal from alcohol or sedatives/hypnotics
➤ Nutritional deficits

Other Possible Characteristics

➤ Complaints of fatigue
➤ Alteration in posture
➤ Change in muscular tension
➤ Inappropriate responses
➤ Hallucinations

Expected Outcomes/Goals

The patient will
➤ respond appropriately to incoming stimuli as evidenced by
   ▷ accurately stating time, place, person, situation
   ▷ clarifying reality- versus nonreality-based phenomena
   ▷ controlling impulse behavior when experiencing perceptual disturbances.
➤ Identify situations that exacerbate/stimulate sensory misinterpretations as evidenced by recalling events that occurred before the sensory disturbance.

Content appearing in this typeface is additional information not included in the NANDA nursing diagnoses.

Nursing Orders with Rationale

➤ Assess and monitor for presence/absence/ changes in findings outlined above
in order to detect any change in status.

➤ Approach patient with a calm, confident, and firm manner.
This attitude is therapeutic and will help calm the patient (Brunner & Suddarth, 1988).

➤ Provide patient with a safe and quiet environment.
Patients experiencing sensory disturbances will benefit from a low-stimulation environment (Hyman, 1984).

➤ Establish an alliance (sense of trust) with the patient in a one-to-one, nurse-patient relationship.
Patients who form positive alliances with their caregivers are more likely to achieve better outcomes (Frank & Gunderson, 1990).

➤ Be an active listener; allow patient to verbalize fears, emotions, ideas, anxieties.
This is a way to reduce tension, improve self-image and self-confidence, and establish a sense of identity.

➤ Call patient directly by name and ask to look at you when suspecting hallucinations.
This helps to focus the patient's attention on the environment rather than internally.

➤ Structure amount/type of incoming stimuli patient receives in an attempt to gain the patient's full attention and decrease hallucinations.
The structure present in the materials used for stimulation and its attention-commanding properties are what may determine the occurrence of hallucinating phenomena (Asaad & Shapiro, 1986).

➤ Monitor patient to determine if she or he is responding to internal stimuli (e.g., appears to be listening when no one is speaking, conversing when no one is there, bizarre gesturing, inappropriate affect).
Command or visual hallucinations may precede bizarre, destructive, or suicidal behavior (Asaad & Shapiro, 1986).

➤ Do not reinforce patient's hallucinations by treating them as real; instead, acknowledge that the patient is having hallucinations and state that you are not experiencing them; explore the hallucination with the patient.
Acknowledging what the patient is experiencing and exploring what might have triggered the experience are the first steps toward diffusing the sensory alteration (Clark, 1984).

➤ Determine if patient is having auditory or vivid visual hallucinations; assess if the auditory hallucinations seem to be coming from the environment or from within the individual.
Vivid visual hallucinations and auditory hallucinations that seem external are often associated with organic factors.

➤ Do not give the hallucinations special status; refer to them as the "so-called voices"; stay with patient and direct him or her to tell the "so-called voices" to go away; repeat often, in a matter-of-fact manner when patient appears to be responding to internal stimuli.
Patients may learn to self-control hallucinations when given repeated instructions and permission by a trusted person.

➤ Instruct patient to sing a simple, pleasing song when hallucinations begin.
Temporary relief from hallucinations can be obtained by giving them competition.

➤ Administer medications as ordered; monitor therapeutic benefits and negative side effects; teach patient self-monitoring skills.
Neuroleptics are the most effective medication for psychotic conditions (American Psychiatric Association, 1989). Nursing observations are critical in determining the effectiveness of any psychiatric medication (Townsend, 1990).

➤ Watch for signs of physical and neurological side effects (e.g., sedation: postural hypotension, dry mouth, visual blurring; endocrine: skin rashes, seizures, dystonia, pseudoparkinsonism, akathisia).
Neuroleptics are beneficial for the patient with sensory alterations, but they are not without related side effects (Schatzberg & Cole, 1986).

➤ Help patient obtain quality sleep by providing uninterrupted time periods.
> *When patients get an adequate amount of sleep,
> they will experience less physical and psycho-
> logical stress and fewer mental status alter-
> ations (Helton, Gordon, & Nunnery, 1980).*

➤ Obtain a complete history of drug use/abuse from
the patient; as well as from friends, family, and
significant others.
> *Symptoms of altered perception may be caused
> by acute ingestion of drugs, chronic ingestion
> (especially amphetamines), or withdrawal
> (Hyman, 1984).*

➤ Maintain patient's homeostasis; provide for physical needs; monitor vital signs when appropriate.
> *Systematic nursing assessment will alert the
> nurse of a change in the patient's functional state
> and to the need for prompt and further observa-
> tion/intervention (Brunner & Suddarth, 1988).*

➤ Provide prompt feedback to patients regarding
their unusual bizarre behavior.
> *Patients who experience sensory alterations have
> a specific difficulty using central feedback to
> monitor their own actions (Frith & Done, 1989).*

➤ Assess elderly patient's nutrient and vitamin intake.
> *Vitamin deficiency is associated with a number
> of psychiatric disturbances (Burns, Marsh, &
> Bender, 1989).*

➤ Involve family/significant others in treatment
plans so that a sense of security and continuity is
maintained for the patient.
> *Families wish to be able to use their strengths to
> help treatment and to learn management tech-
> niques that will help the patient recover (Cole &
> Jacobs, 1989).*

➤ Help patient to reorient to reality (i.e., to time,
place, person, situation) in a concrete way by using large clocks, calendars, clearly printed room
signs indicating occupant's name, calling patient
by name, etc.
> *Direct nursing interventions toward helping the
> patient function in the environment (Stuart &
> Sundeen, 1987).*

➤ Help patient to participate in appropriate/avail-
able activities in order to decrease the possibility
of acting on sensory/perceptual misinterpretations.
> *When the patient's energies are redirected to
> more acceptable activities, the chance of inap-
> propriate behavior is reduced.*

Charting Components

➤ Adaptations required and made
➤ Any abnormal change in patient's physical/emo-
tional status
➤ Disorientation
➤ Diversionary activities
➤ Effects/side effects of medications
➤ Expressions of fears, emotions, anxieties
➤ Extent and degree of limit setting required to re-
lieve anxiety and decrease acting-out behavior
➤ Hallucinations: type, patient's response
➤ Level of anxiety
➤ Participation in ADL, milieu
➤ Quantity/quality of sensory alterations noted
➤ Sleep patterns
➤ Patient/family teaching, response

C. MEANINGFULNESS

1. Hopelessness

Definition

A state in which an individual sees limited or no alternatives or personal choices available and is unable to mobilize energy on own behalf

Related to

➤ Prolonged activity restriction creating isolation
➤ Failing or deteriorating physiological conditions
➤ Long-term stress
➤ Abandonment
➤ Lost belief in transcendent values/God
➤ Altered body image
➤ Feelings of being abandoned, of despondency, despair, depression
➤ Lack of future orientation
➤ Loss of emotional and caring support systems
➤ Multiple physical and functional losses
➤ Perceived powerlessness, helplessness
➤ Unrealistic self-expectations, feelings of incompetence, sense of failure

Characteristics/Assessment Findings

Major
➤ Passivity, decreased verbalization
➤ Decreased affect
➤ Verbal cues (despondent content, "I can't," sighing)

Minor
➤ Lack of initiative
➤ Decreased response to stimuli
➤ Decreased affect
➤ Turning away from speaker
➤ Closing eyes
➤ Shrugging in response to speaker
➤ Decreased appetite
➤ Increased/decreased sleep
➤ Lack of involvement in care/passively allowing care
➤ Emotional negativism
➤ Impaired decision making
➤ Impaired verbal/nonverbal communication
➤ Inability to set future-oriented goals
➤ Lack of motivation
➤ Lethargy
➤ Negative expectations
➤ Sleep disturbances
➤ Withdrawn social behavior

Expected Outcomes/Goals

The patient will
➤ identify and verbalize feelings of hopelessness as evidenced by
  ▷ verbal cues (e.g., "I can't see the light at the end of the tunnel." "There is no hope.")
  ▷ expression of despair
  ▷ inability to see a positive future or available choices.
➤ demonstrate ability to mobilize energy on own behalf as evidenced by
  ▷ verbalizing alternatives available
  ▷ setting own short-term goals
  ▷ describing and planning for future-oriented outcomes
  ▷ implementing plans to reach identified goals.

Content appearing in this typeface is additional information not included in the NANDA nursing diagnoses.

➤ participate in self-care activities as evidenced by
   ▷ making decisions related to care/treatment
   ▷ assuming control for aspects of ADL.
➤ seek support groups for assistance as evidenced by
   ▷ sharing feelings and emotional needs with family or friends
   ▷ using community resources, counseling, social services, family, significant others.

Nursing Orders with Rationale

➤ Assess and monitor for presence/absence/ changes in assessment findings outlined above
   in order to detect any change in status.

➤ Discuss the meaning of illness with patient, how it is necessary to feel the depth of suffering before a renewed hope and faith can emerge.
   Acknowledging the presence of despair allows the patient to express feelings and to feel an increased sense of hope.

➤ Provide another point of view by discussing other meanings to the situation; help patient redefine priorities
   Patients can find inner strength, peace, and hope by finding meaning in their situations.

➤ Identify feelings of guilt or self-blame reflected in statements such as, "If only I had . . . "; help patient to practice self-forgiveness, to make amends, and to release self-blame.
   Diminishing guilt and resentment can increase hope.

➤ Convey acceptance by acknowledging patient's right to feel sadness, anger, grief (e.g., "It's natural to feel angry when you have experienced so many losses.")
   It is healing to experience and express emotions.

➤ Affirm that good things can still take place no matter what the magnitude of the loss; instill hope and support patient's faith; provide examples of how other people have dealt with similar situations.
   Faith diminishes fear and raises hope.

➤ Acknowledge patient's capacity to struggle with issues and to reach a positive resolution (e.g., "You can do it. I believe in your capacity to find the answer that is right for you.")
   Believing in people helps people believe in themselves.

➤ Assist patient to find hope in short-term goals, pleasure and meaning in everyday events; discuss how others have found hope and strength in similar situations.
   Hope is something that an individual seeks, desires, or wants; having hope can make a significant impact in coping with major illness and loss; in some cases it can make the difference between survival and death (Carson, Soeken, & Grimm, 1988).

➤ Encourage to verbalize feelings regarding disappointment and grief, lost hope, expectations, desires.
   The greatest therapeutic resource for people in emotional or spiritual pain is listening, and listening long enough for the person to share emotional pain and to release its tension (Dugan, 1987).

➤ Provide an atmosphere of open communication by giving empathy, using reflections (e.g., "It must be difficult to face so many losses all at once"), and clarifying.
   Being heard, acknowledged, and empathized within a nonjudgmental framework is basic to instilling hope.

➤ Help define reachable goals.
   People usually have a mix of time-specific and non-time-specific hopes (e.g., hoping for positive outcome of diagnosis, hoping to live long enough to see a granddaughter married in June).

➤ Help to focus on what patient can accomplish:
   ▷ make menu choices, eat balanced meals.
   ▷ take medications on schedule.
   ▷ participate in pain control.
   ▷ exercise regularly; practicing biofeedback, visualization, relaxation techniques.
   ▷ keep a journal of feelings and daily thoughts.
      Patients who become comanagers of their care develop and maintain self-esteem (Stryker, 1977). Feeling helpless and a victim of circumstances means one cannot feel hopeful.

➤ Have patient describe past situations in which hopes were fulfilled; find out how patient coped with unfilled hopes and expectations.
   Memories of fulfilled hopes are ways to reinforce reasons to be hopeful (Dufault & Martocchio, 1985). Past coping with disappointment may provide clues to current positive adaptation to situation.

➤ Assess patient support systems; encourage to use those available (e.g., social services, individual or group members of patient's occupational or social network, community groups such as those for breast cancer, AIDS).

> *Hope does not exist in a vacuum, but rather in shared experiences with others.*

➤ Use clergy and spiritual/religious resources; refer to nursing diagnosis "Spiritual Distress" for more interventions dealing with despair.

> *Hope is positively linked to spiritual well-being (Carson et al., 1988).*

Charting Components

➤ Feelings expressed
➤ Goals set, ability to reach them
➤ Participation in ADL
➤ Statements of hope or faith
➤ Support given by family/significant other
➤ Patient/family teaching, response

2. Powerlessness

Definition

The perception that one's own action will not significantly affect an outcome; a perceived lack of control over a current situation or immediate happening.

Related to

➤ Healthcare environment (e.g., restrictions of hospitalization)
➤ Interpersonal interaction
➤ Illness-related regimen
➤ Life-style of helplessness
➤ Acute or chronic disease process
➤ Inability to perform ADL
➤ Lack of knowledge
➤ Progressive debilitating disease

Content appearing in this typeface is additional information not included in the NANDA nursing diagnoses.

Characteristics/Assessment Findings

Severe

➤ Verbal expressions of having no control or influence over situation, outcome, self-care
➤ Depression over deterioration that occurs despite patient compliance with regimen
➤ Apathy

Moderate

➤ Nonparticipation in care or decision making when opportunities are provided
➤ Expressions of dissatisfaction and frustration over inability to perform previous tasks or activities
➤ Does not monitor progress
➤ Expression of doubt regarding role performance
➤ Reluctance to express true feelings
➤ Fears alienation from caregivers
➤ Passivity
➤ Inability to seek information regarding care
➤ Dependence on others that may result in irritability, anger, resentment, and guilt
➤ Does not defend self-care practices when challenged

Low

➤ Expressions of uncertainty about fluctuating energy levels

Expected Outcomes/Goals

The patient will
➤ identify factors that can be controlled by self as evidenced by
  ▷ verbalizing an interest in participating in own care
  ▷ expressing hope
  ▷ identifying specific situations that present a degree of control and choice
  ▷ identifying areas that are realistically out of own control (e.g., other person's decisions, health, life).
➤ make decisions regarding own care as evidenced by
  ▷ participating in ADL at level possible
  ▷ discussing future plans, including discharge.

Nursing Orders with Rationale

➤ Assess and monitor for presence/absence/ changes in assessment findings outlined above *in order to detect any change in status.*

➤ Identify factors that can contribute to the patient's sense of powerlessness (e.g., impaired functioning, decreased physical strength, altered self-image, lack of knowledge).
   Helplessness is a psychological state that results when circumstances are uncontrollable. Identifying situations in which patient has no control will help patient to control own expectations.

➤ Assess patient's positive strengths.
   Nursing strategies involving repeated identification, development, and recognition of positive experiences through positive feedback help the patient to construct an increased acceptance of self (Thompson, McFarland, Hirsch, Tucker, & Bower, 1989).

➤ Assess patient's weaknesses and assist in exploring adaptive ways to cope.
   Realistically identifying areas of weakness and ways to supplement these deficiencies allows for realistic planning of strategies to ensure success for the patient.

➤ Assess patient's coping mechanisms and capitalize on positive strategies (e.g., seeking information, praying, expressing feelings, social activities).
   Adaptive coping enables the patient to deal with the powerlessness.

➤ Work with patient to set mutually agreed-on goals for care
   to allow the individual to assume responsibility for own behavior and the outcomes of own decisions.

➤ Clarify those things that are not under the individual's control (e.g., other person's health, life); encourage patient to grieve for those things that cannot be.
   Recognizing one's limitations in controlling others is, paradoxically, a beginning to finding one's strengths.

➤ Clarify patient's expectations and correct distorted perceptions about self, others, illness, or treatment.
   Powerlessness is a perception that one's own actions will not affect an outcome. The perception may be inaccurate and amenable to correction (Miller, 1983).

➤ Collaborate with patient to identify issues under patient's control; provide opportunities for the patient to make decisions in these areas whenever feasible; make patient aware of alternatives and consequences.
   Realistically identifying those things over which patient has control can help to reappraise patient's own sense of power. Making own decisions and taking responsibility for the outcomes is a beginning in accepting own limits of control and power.

➤ Help patient to recognize, accept, and develop an internal sense of self-esteem by promoting positive use of first person ("I") statements (e.g., "I can do this.")
   Assertiveness techniques can be very helpful for the person who feels powerless.

➤ Teach problem-solving skills
   to help reduce ambiguity and feelings of loss of control (Wykle, 1983).

➤ Involve significant other(s) in plans as possible.
   This involvement extends a message of caring to the patient, enhances a sense of control, and reduces feelings of helplessness and isolation.

➤ Encourage patient to seek information about illness and illness-related modifications in habits, diet, etc.
   The approach that is most successful in dealing with illness is seeking information, being attentive to details of care and symptoms, and asking questions about treatment (Carpenito, 1989).

➤ Provide explicit written directions for patient to follow.
   Information can help patients to know what is happening and to have a say in decision making (Moorhouse, Geissler, & Doenges, 1987).

➤ Allow and encourage patient to do as much for self as possible; document in care plan what patient is capable of doing.
   Carrying out self-care activities can enhance feelings of control and self-worth (Roberts, 1986).

➤ Provide for primary nurse as much as possible.
   Consistency helps establish rapport between patient and caregiver and provides a supportive climate (Carpenito, 1989). The relationship allows for predictability and comfort within acceptable limits and permits adaptation to occur.

➤ Keep patient informed about condition, treatments, and progress.

Keeping patient up-to-date regarding own care can help patient to feel more hopeful about the situation (Moorhouse et al., 1987).

➤ Explain all procedures, hospital rules, and options; review periodically.

Knowledge is power and allows for choices (Roberts, 1986). It allows patient to become more independent in developing informed choices regarding care issues.

➤ Increase effective communication with patient by allowing time for questions and providing answers.

Feeling heard and understood increases the patient's sense of being in control and having a say in own care (Carpenito, 1987).

➤ Be an active listener; allow patient to verbalize concerns and feelings of hostility, anger, helplessness; assess areas of concern; use open-ended questions to elicit thoughts, feelings.

Expressing feelings can be helpful in moving toward a more hopeful outlook (Moorhouse et al., 1987).

➤ Spend time exploring the meaning of feelings with the patient; ascertain the meaning of verbal and nonverbal communication

to allow the patient to develop adaptive coping strategies by using own strengths, interests, and abilities (Miles, 1986).

➤ Discuss with patient the need to accept the unacceptable when faced with permanent losses and altered life-style; suggest using prayer, meditation.

Patients can gain inner strength from spiritual practices, which can assist in dealing with illness (Miller, 1983).

Charting Components

➤ Decisions made by patient, implementation and results
➤ Expressions of dissatisfaction or frustration with current situation
➤ Passivity, activity
➤ Patient participation in self-care
➤ Plans after discharge
➤ Strategies used to decrease patient's sense of powerlessness, patient's response
➤ Verbal expressions of feelings, sense of control
➤ Verbalizations of having no control or influence over life
➤ Patient/family teaching, response

VIII. Knowing

A. KNOWING

1. Knowledge Deficit

Definition

Inadequate understanding of information or inability to perform skills needed by an individual to practice health-related behaviors (Taylor & Cress, 1988)

Related to

- Lack of exposure
- Lack of recall
- Information misinterpretation
- Cognitive limitation
- Lack of interest in learning
- Unfamiliarity with information resources
- Absence of similar experience in past
- Absence of learned information, skill, or attitude
- Inability to transfer similar information or skill to current situation
- Moderate to severe situational/chronic anxiety
- Lack of motivation
- Inability to process information
- Loss of short- or long-term memory
- Severe depression, psychomotor retardation

Content appearing in this typeface is additional information not included in the NANDA nursing diagnoses.

Characteristics/Assessment Findings

- Verbalization of the problem
- Inaccurate follow-through of instruction
- Inaccurate performance of test
- Inappropriate or exaggerated behaviors (e.g., hysterical, hostile, agitated, apathetic)
- Inability to verbalize knowledge appropriate for self-care
- Performance of inappropriate or incorrect self-care skills
- Verbalization of incorrect healthcare knowledge
- Verbalization of health beliefs that are counter-productive to appropriate self-care
- Inability to focus on knowledge or skills appropriate for self-care
- Failure to adhere to treatment regimen
- Unwillingness to set goals
- Failing to learn new skills

Expected Outcomes/Goals

The patient/family will

- demonstrate adequate knowledge regarding the illness, hospitalization, and follow-up care as evidenced by
  - verbalizing accurate information relative to the healthcare problem
  - performing skills in the appropriate sequence and with correct methods to accomplish safe self-care
  - verbalizing health beliefs that are productive toward appropriate self-care (Redman, 1988).
- understand mental illness as a mental/emotional/biological dysfunction that becomes aggravated under conditions of stress as evidenced by
  - adherence to the treatment regimen
  - minimizing environmental stressors.

➤ develop an empathic understanding of their own/family member's experience in living with severe mental illness as evidenced by
  ▷ demonstrating compassion and patience with self/relative
  ▷ verbalizing limitations with acceptance.
➤ understand the current treatments for mental illness and learn how to access available resources for care and rehabilitation as evidenced by
  ▷ making sound judgments based on facts about treatment options
  ▷ contacting appropriate community resources and exploring self-help groups, classes, books, etc.
  ▷ participating in programs designed to facilitate rehabilitation of mental illness.

Nursing Orders with Rationale

➤ Assess and monitor for presence/absence/changes in assessment findings outlined above *in order to detect any change in status.*

➤ Assess baseline attitudes, skills, and knowledge related to the healthcare problem in order to identify what patient/family already knows or can do.
These baseline data help the nurse to build on previous experience and to maintain self-esteem of the adult learner (Ford, 1987; Rankin & Duffy, 1983). It also discloses the patient's level of anxiety, which may be interfering with ability to focus on learning new information or using known skills (Ford, 1987).

➤ Assess the needs of the potential learners; ascertain patient/family's knowledge of
  ▷ mental illness
  ▷ why patients behave as they do
  ▷ available resources and treatments
  ▷ appropriate expectations and prognosis
  ▷ feelings of guilt and anxiety about illness.
    A systematic process of determining goals can be achieved by assessing the needs of the learner.

➤ Assess patient's/family's prior knowledge about the subject; organize the new material in a way that includes what the individual already knows.
Isolated answers and bits of unrelated information are not meaningful. If new material is learned in isolation from what is already known, even substantive passages may not be retained (Hatfield, 1990).

➤ Assess readiness and ability to learn; if patient has a physical deficit that limits cognitive or psychomotor ability or influences the affective component of insight for making decisions, teach a primary caregiver (e.g., family, friend); if no primary caregiver is available or willing to assume such responsibility, then other resources must be obtained for the patient (e.g., home health services, skilled nursing facility placement).
Learning will only take place when readiness and motivation are evidenced (Ford, 1987).

➤ Assess learners' motivation for learning; do not assume that you know their needs by promising patient improvement and inducing fear or guilt.
Families of the mentally ill give practical reasons for learning about the patient's illness. Adult learners look for real substance in what is taught (Hatfield, 1990).

➤ Assess patient's language skills and preferred learning style; individualize the learning plan based on patient's preferred style (e.g., self-paced learning with literature or audiovisual media, one-to-one counseling, group settings: either formal classes or informal support groups); provide information using the patient's visual sense, for both cognitive and psychomotor learning.
Teaching must be focused appropriately to the patient's language level and reading ability when using both verbal and written language (Rankin & Duffy, 1983). Multisensory learning has been shown to be more effective, especially if tailored to the patient's preferences (Ford, 1987).

➤ Preplan what you want to accomplish; evaluate how best to meet your goal.
Only after becoming clear about what you hope to achieve can materials be selected, teaching strategies developed, and information sequenced properly (Hatfield, 1990).

➤ Translate patient/family needs for knowledge into behavioral goals that will help them to develop increasing competence to cope with the mental illness and its consequences; take into account the need for cognitive learning, problem solving, and attitudinal change.
Stating goals in terms of behavioral or performance objectives stresses to the learners what they will be expected to do, and makes evaluation more objective (Hatfield, 1990).

➤ Base the teaching on your mutually agreed-upon goals and assessment factors; tell patient/family what they will be able to do (e.g., learn to relax by using breathing techniques); state situations that need to be reported to physician/clinic.

Involving the patient/family in goal setting helps them to obtain realistic goals and facilitates learning.

➤ Include behavioral and content components in objectives

to guide the teaching/learning plan toward specific outcomes.

➤ Provide patient/family with a solid knowledge base of mental illness—its nature, causes, prognosis, and treatment.

Families with knowledge can develop reasonable expectations and realistic hope. They can understand the patient's limitations and plan realistically for both short- and long-term goals (Hatfield, 1990).

➤ Reflect and restate patient's/family's point of view and beliefs about the issue before presenting a different perspective.

Affective problems (e.g., lack of interest in learning, definite but erroneous ideas, lack of confidence) can be diminished by taking the patient's point of view (Redman, 1988).

➤ Identify patient/family cultural health beliefs related to current health problem.

Matching teaching to learned value systems will enhance acceptance of new information/skills and will increase compliance with self-care practices (Rankin & Duffy, 1983; Redman, 1988). Relevance to the patient's needs and priorities will enhance the effectiveness of learning (Ford, 1987).

➤ Organize new material in a hierarchical order: teach concepts and generalizations first, then specific items of information.

New information is not stored in long-term memory randomly; rather, it is stored systematically and in hierarchical order. Good organization provides cognitive hooks on which to hang new information (Hatfield, 1990).

➤ Present information in a sequenced manner, giving general material before more detailed information.

The general information will serve as a structure to anchor the more specific ideas.

➤ Present key concepts clearly; keep the number of concepts to a minimum; help the learner to differentiate between the key ideas and related and supporting information of lesser importance.

The number of concepts that any individual can fully comprehend in a session is very few; trying to cover too much exceeds the pace of learning beyond that which a person can grasp and integrate into existing knowledge (Hatfield, 1990).

➤ Teach patient/family that the information can be used to develop solutions to new problems in life situations.

Transfer of learning is based on relevance, meaningfulness, clarity, and ability to integrate the originally learned material (Hatfield, 1990).

➤ Ensure transfer of learning to other situations:
  ▷ use a variety of examples in the learning situation.
  ▷ point out both differences and similarities in contexts.
  ▷ find common elements in several contexts.
  ▷ develop generalizations or principles that can be applied in various situations.
  ▷ identify task similarity and make linkages between ideas presented and what goes on at home.

The transferability of learning depends on the extent to which the learning situation illustrates how to apply the new concept to as many specific contexts as possible (Hatfield, 1990).

➤ Provide patient with a variety of learning stimuli (e.g., audiovisual and literature resources; discussion and demonstration; self-testing exercises; practice with models, supplies, and equipment; peer counseling).

A variety of input stimulates interest and provides examples of practical application (Rankin & Duffy, 1983; Redman, 1988).

➤ Use strategies to provide the patient as much control over each learning situation as possible; e.g.,
  ▷ seek out individual motivating factors and incorporate them as incentives to learn.
  ▷ use respected sources of information such as peers, professional literature (Ford, 1987).
  ▷ use bargaining on occasion, especially where the patient is not convinced of the efficacy of a particular regimen.

Building short-term success will often convince the patient to continue the learned procedures. Bargaining is thus a helpful change-agent process (Rankin & Duffy, 1983).

➤ Reinforce all efforts at learning new skills, knowledge, etc.
Positive reinforcement helps to shape and strengthen new learning.

➤ Use repetition and visual aids when teaching patients with a cognitive impairment.
Some cognitive limitations can be overcome with use of concrete, simple concepts, repetition, use of strategically placed reminder signs in the patient's environment, pictures, diagrams, comparison to those things with which the patient is familiar, etc. (Ford, 1987; Redman, 1988).

➤ Be creative in your approach when teaching patients with psychomotor limitations; teaching aids can enhance motivation and retention.
Psychomotor limitations can also be overcome with some creative planning (e.g., using large print for visually impaired older adults, headphones for the hearing impaired patient who must view a videotape, multiple return demonstrations, assistive devices (Ford, 1987).

➤ Provide referrals to additional sources of learning (e.g., home health agencies, libraries, ancillary services, voluntary health organizations, classes, self-help groups, etc.); include in discharge planning.
Learning may not be completely achieved during normal course of interaction with patients because of shorter inpatient stays and cost-containment requirements (Rankin & Duffy, 1983; Redman, 1988). Learning in the acute care setting must be aimed at the patient's safety and survival needs (Rankin & Duffy, 1983). Patients' learning must continue after discharge from hospital and after short contact with healthcare providers in outpatient settings.

➤ Consider doing group teaching (e.g., a medication group).
A group provides the opportunity for patient to become aware that other patients have the same effects/problems as they are experiencing (Farkas, 1990).

➤ Assess the effectiveness of the educational interventions by comparing the patient's progress to the predetermined goals and objectives (Ford, 1987).
Continual evaluation helps healthcare providers give appropriate feedback and provides an opportunity to redirect the plan, enlist the assistance of family/other health professionals on the team, refer to community resources, etc. (Ford, 1987; Rankin & Duffy, 1983; Redman, 1988).

Charting Components

➤ Attitudes/feelings about learning
➤ Content of instruction
➤ Dates of teaching
➤ Knowledge/skills learned, learning level achieved by patient/family/primary caregiver
➤ Learning aids used
➤ Level of existing knowledge
➤ Problems with learning
➤ Readiness and ability to learn
➤ Referrals made
➤ Sensory, physical, or emotional limitations to learning; acceptance of necessary adjustments

B. THOUGHT PROCESSES

1. Acute Confusion

Definition

The abrupt onset of a cluster of global, transient changes and disturbances in attention, cognition, psychomotor activity, level of consciousness, or sleep/wake cycle

Related to

- Alcohol or drug abuse
- Delirium
- Toxicity/poisoning
- Nutritional/metabolic disorders
- Cerebral edema
- Traumatic head injury
- Sensory overload or deprivation
- Sleep/wake cycle disturbance
- Sundown syndrome
- Renal/liver failure
- Severe chemical withdrawal syndromes
- Exchange problems
  - metabolic or electrolyte disturbances
  - high fever
  - autonomic hyperactivity
  - ischemia
  - hypoglycemia
  - postoperative states
  - anticholinergic syndrome
  - severe infection

Characteristics/Assessment Findings

- Fluctuation in cognition
- Fluctuation in sleep/wake cycle
- Fluctuation in level of consciousness
- Fluctuation in psychomotor activity
- Increased agitation or restlessness
- Misperceptions
- Lack of motivation to initiate or follow through with goal-directed or purposeful behavior
- Hallucinations (e.g., tactile, visual, olfactory, auditory)
- Physiological manifestations (e.g., elevated vital signs, vomiting)
- Perceptual disturbances (incoherent speech)
- Anxiety and fear
- Excessive talkativeness
- Overalertness
- Clouding of consciousness

Expected Outcomes/Goals

The patient will

- have confusion self-limited on successful treatment of cause as evidenced by
  - orientation to time, place, and person
  - no clouding of consciousness
  - vital signs within normal limits
  - sleep/wake cycle normalized
  - no hyperactivity
  - ability to attend to and complete ADL
  - no perceptual disturbances

Nursing Orders with Rationale

- Assess and monitor for presence/absence/changes in assessment findings outlined above *in order to detect any change in status.*

- Assess for early signs of confusion in the older adult.
  Susceptibility for delirium increases with age because of physiological changes, heightened sensitivity to drugs and infections, and imbalances in blood chemistry (Stolley, 1995).

Content appearing in this typeface is additional information not included in the NANDA nursing diagnoses.

➤ Assess for cumulative anticholinergic effects of medications such as belladonna alkaloids, tricyclic antidepressants, quinidine, hypnotics, and general anesthetics.

Central anticholinergic blockage may result in confusion, disorientation, agitation, and visual hallucinosis. In extreme causes, delirium may result. This is caused by disturbance in the CNS muscarinic transmission of acetylcholine antagonists or lack of acetylcholine (Marchlewski, 1994).

➤ Conduct a mental status examination or a minimental state examination to establish baseline objective data on cognitive functioning.

In delirium there is mental status fluctuation that needs to be constantly updated against baseline data.

➤ Replace fluid loss as ordered by the physician *to maintain adequate circulating volume and tissue perfusion (Clochesy, 1988).*

➤ Minimize confusion and disorientation.

Confusion and disorientation are not the same as delirium. The delirious patient may be confused or disoriented; however, not all confused or disoriented patients are delirious (Luckmann & Sorensen, 1987).

➤ Assess for the underlying cause of the confused/delirious state.

Accurate assessment is imperative when a patient's level of consciousness changes because a state of delirium is considered a medical emergency (Carrieri, Lindsey, & West, 1986).

➤ Appraise the pharmacodynamics and toxic reactions of medications, especially in the elderly.

Decreased ability to metabolize medications can result in adverse reactions. Often the elderly consume numerous medications that have the potential for dangerous drug interactions (Eliopoulos, 1987).

➤ Assess effectiveness of medications.

Patients who are in acute withdrawal from alcohol or other CNS depressants may be prescribed long-acting benzodiazepines to reduce agitation and prevent seizure (Bennett & Woolf, 1991).

➤ Assign the same nurse for several consecutive days.

The confused patient needs consistency. This patient finds everything bewildering, a situation made worse by the presence of many different people.

➤ Explain to patient what you are doing in the way of care and talk to the patient in a calm voice using simple sentences while proceeding.

The nurse strives to include rather than exclude the patient. Simple concrete explanations serve to facilitate orientation and lessen confusion.

➤ Provide normal aids to orientation, such as clocks, calendars, watch, newspapers, radio, TV.

Everyday clues such as clocks and calendar reinforce reality and give the patient feedback regarding the current situation and events.

➤ Have patient's family bring in familiar objects from home.

The confused patient often feels depersonalized.

➤ Regulate the physical environment: adequate light that varies between day and night, use of night lights, lighting adjusted to prevent shadow, excessive noise decreased.

Confused patients need assistance in adjusting to normal sleep-wake cycles. Shadows and poor lighting can add to confusion and contribute to visual hallucinations. A noisy environment may increase hyperactivity.

➤ Encourage patient to use the toilet and give the patient adequate fluids; supervise patient during mealtimes.

The acutely confused patient is not capable of meeting his or her own basic needs without assistance from the nursing staff.

➤ Reassure the patient frequently and speak quietly, slowly, and concretely.

This helps reduce anxiety, which can contribute to hyperactivity.

➤ Ensure patient safety by providing a sitter or one-to-one care or by putting side rails up. Do not restrain the patient with cloth or leather restraints.

Delirious patients cannot control their behavior and may be unpredictable, irrational, and impulsive. The patient needs to be protected from accidents and injury (Stolley, 1995).

➤ Monitor level of consciousness, pupillary responses, and vital signs.

The symptoms probably most indicative of increasing cerebral dysfunction are a lowering level of consciousness and a change in pupillary equality and reactivity. Vital signs are an indication of autonomic hyperactivity.

➤ Ensure open airway; observe for aspirations, obstruction, or decreased level of consciousness.
  Partial airway obstruction typically manifests itself through noisy respirations or obvious efforts in breathing.

➤ Refer to nursing care plan "Fluid Volume Deficit" and "Potential for Injury: The Patient with Seizures."
  Delirium may lead to seizures.

Charting Components

➤ Indications of decreased tissue perfusion
➤ I&O
➤ Skin integrity
➤ Positioning
➤ Vital signs, peripheral pulses
➤ Orientation
➤ Level of consciousness
➤ Pupil reactions
➤ Infections
➤ Perceptual disturbances
➤ Hyperactivity
➤ Nutritional status
➤ Motor and sensory functioning
➤ Reflexes
➤ Safety precautions used

Additional Characteristics/Assessment Findings for
THE PATIENT WITH SUNDOWN SYNDROME

➤ Usually more than 75 years of age
➤ Recurring confusing and exacerbation of disruptive behavior and agitation occurring late in the afternoon and evening
➤ Wandering
➤ Nocturnal awakening

Related to

➤ Relocation
➤ Stress, fear, isolation
➤ Sensory overload or deprivation
➤ Circadian rhythm disruption
➤ Dehydration
➤ Cardiovascular disorders
➤ Drugs
➤ Brain hypoxia

Additional Nursing Orders

➤ Assess elderly patient on admission for high risk for sundown syndrome.
  Sundowning is a temporary condition but is disruptive and dangerous when it occurs (Ebersole & Hess, 1994). Patients with a history of delirium or sundowning, cardiovascular or cerebrovascular disease, polypharmacy and paradoxical excitation, or electrolyte imbalance are particularly at risk for sundown syndrome.

➤ Avoid additional relocation once the patient is admitted
  to prevent further confusion.

➤ Use soft music or socialization opportunities in evening; keep patient near nurse's station where patient is visible to staff.
  This disrupts the cycle that initiated confusion (e.g., diminished environmental cues and energy in afternoon hours).

➤ Turn lights on before dark
  to increase safety. Bright lights in evening may alter sleep/wake cycle disturbance (Satlin, Volicer, & Ross, 1992).

➤ Monitor frequently
  for safety.

➤ Provide environmental cues: calendar, clock, sign on bathroom door, sign to room, bathroom light on at night.
  Signs or symbols of time and place may remind a confused person of the familiar when his or her memory fails to do so. Success of this intervention is minimal.

➤ Allow familiar person at bedside as much as possible
  who can protect from injury and provide meaningfulness to the unfamiliar situation.

➤ Use short-term neuroleptics cautiously.
  Elderly patients are especially susceptible to the neurological effects of psychotropic medications, which are thought to relate to specific structural changes in the basal ganglia. These changes render some patients particularly susceptible to neuroleptic-induced Parkinsonism (Figel, Kirshman, Doraiswany, & Nemeroff, 1991).

Additional Charting Components

➤ Time of behavior changes
➤ Examples of behavior changes
➤ Causative factors present

➤ Successful interventions
➤ Safety precautions taken
➤ Frequency of observation
➤ Family assistance requested
➤ Time of resolution

2. Chronic Confusion

Definition

An irreversible, long-standing or progressive deterioration of intellect and personality characterized by decreased ability to interpret environmental stimuli, decreased capacity for intellectual thought processes and manifested by disturbances of memory, orientation, and behavior

Related to

➤ Alzheimer's disease
➤ Korsakoff's psychosis, Huntington's chorea, Pick's disease
➤ Multi-infarct
➤ Dementia, presenile and senile
➤ Cerebrovascular accident
➤ Head injury
  ▷ Organic brain syndrome
  ▷ Prolonged substance abuse
  ▷ Prolonged malnutrition
  ▷ Cerebral arteriosclerosis
  ▷ HIV virus

Characteristics/Assessment Findings

Major
➤ Clinical evidence of organic impairment
➤ Altered interpretation/response to stimuli
➤ Progressive/long-standing cognitive impairment
➤ No change in level of consciousness
➤ Impaired socialization
➤ Impaired memory (short term progressing to long term)
➤ Altered personality
➤ Altered meaningfulness
➤ Altered judgment
➤ Altered self-concept

➤ Language disability
➤ Potential for anxiety, fear, violence
➤ Loss of intellectual functioning
➤ Disorientation
➤ Loss of abstract reasoning

Early Stage
➤ Inability to concentrate
➤ Difficulty coordinating complex ideas
➤ Strenuous effort to understand
➤ Strenuous effort to cover up disorientation
➤ Beginning personality changes
➤ Short-term, recent memory loss
➤ Losing way, direction
➤ Losing things
➤ Mild depression
➤ Word-finding difficulty

Middle Stage
➤ Inability to focus attention
➤ Inability to sequence and complete activities
➤ Emotional shallowness, lability
➤ Loss of social skills
➤ Suspiciousness
➤ Disorientation
➤ Repetitive behavior
➤ Need for frequent reassurance
➤ Loss of initiative
➤ Inability to acquire new knowledge
➤ Problem-solving disability
➤ Outbursts of anger
➤ Deterioration of personal hygiene
➤ Increasing dependency
➤ Wandering, agitation
➤ Psychomotor retardation

Late Stage
➤ Global cognitive impairment
➤ Loss of personality
➤ Loss of judgment
➤ Incontinence of bowel and bladder
➤ Loss of inhibition
➤ Violence or total passivity
➤ Forgets to eat or cannot sequence getting food from plate to mouth to swallowing
➤ Long-term memory impairment
➤ Loss of personal identity

Content appearing in this typeface is additional information not included in the NANDA nursing diagnoses.

Expected Outcomes/Goals

The patient will
- ➤ attain a feeling of security as evidenced by
  - ▷ indication of trust in caregiver
  - ▷ short-term periods of orientation to self, location, time, or persons
  - ▷ restfulness in imaginary circumstances
  - ▷ activity/rest cycles in physiologically safe amounts.
- ➤ experience success at attempted tasks and self-expression as manifested by
  - ▷ ability to make needs known
  - ▷ ability to make fears known
  - ▷ attempts at social interaction
  - ▷ attempts at self-care and familiar routines
  - ▷ signifying pleasure when praised.
- ➤ receive adequate bodily comfort as manifested by
  - ▷ freedom from complications of immobility and self-care disability (e.g., UTI, decubiti, stool impaction, pneumonia, temperature deregulation).

Nursing Orders with Rationale

- ➤ Assess and monitor for presence/absence/changes in assessment findings outlined above *in order to detect any change in status.*

- ➤ Assess contributing environmental stimuli. *Stable environment and consistent routine enhance functional abilities in confused persons (Hall, 1988).*

Early Stage

- ➤ Encourage medical evaluation for possible acute causes of confusion or disease simulating dementia. *Illnesses simulating dementia (e.g., depression, medication hypersensitivity) are treatable. MRI can now demonstrate changes indicative of early stage Alzheimer's (Shankle, 1994).*

- ➤ Assess need for medication. *Controlling depression will help rule it out as cause of confusion or as aggravating coexisting problem. Hypersensitivity to psychotropic and other drugs can simulate dementia. Many investigational drugs are showing promise in treating chronic confusion (Miller, 1995).*

- ➤ Arrange for supervised transportation and home maintenance *to allow patient to maintain independence and social supports for as long as possible.*

- ➤ Provide a stable environment and consistent schedule; provide security through personal or telephone contact *to maintain safety and security.*

- ➤ Assist to set up memory support strategies (e.g., medication box prearranged for each day, eyeglass container where glasses are always placed, light over stove always turned on when stove is on, *to maintain safety and security.*

Middle Stage

- ➤ Decrease environmental stimuli by using paste/bland color schemes; avoiding furniture location changes; using television and radio only for focused purpose, quiet at other times; using consistent place at table for meals, consistent place for sleep; following consistent routine for bathroom activities; and limiting number of caregivers as much as possible. *Loss of abilities to focus, interpret, and coordinate, lead to sensory overload with even minimal stimulation.*

- ➤ Provide repetitive activities (e.g., folding towels, wiping tables, rolling ball of yarn) and give meaning to activity; provide physical activities (e.g., dancing, gardening in home environment with familiar person). *Patients with dementia do well in environments with reduced stimuli and enhancement of the familiar (Hepburn, Severence, Gates, & Christensen, 1989).*

- ➤ Assess need for medication *to provide safety for patient and caregivers. Loss of inhibition and misinterpretation of stimuli can be manifested in violent behavior.*

- ➤ Orient to person, place, time, and situation on every interaction *to enable patient to bring the objective situation into their subjective world, thereby giving security (Rantz & McShane, 1995).*

- ➤ Praise for small accomplishments to provide frequent momentary pleasure. *Behavioral modification techniques do not cause or maintain symptomatic improvement.*

➤ Manage delusions by accepting the need to substitute past reality that is less distressing or disconcerting than the one they were perceiving.
  Accepting the need to substitute past preality reduces anxiety in confused adults because that is how they are framing their current world. Helping them express the need or idea adds to the feeling of being understood. Slowly overlaying the past with the present brings them up to the present while reducing confusion (Brooke, 1994).

➤ Realize that sometimes confusion can be positive.
  Positive effects of confusion include individuals are unaware of betrayal of their bodies; some find security in imagining they are in a secure place; some augment their sense of belonging; some distortions become symbols of meaning, of making peace, of roaming in spiritual territories (Ebersole & Hess, 1994).

➤ Toilet on schedule before the patient voids
  to prevent shame and skin breakdown.

➤ Collaborate with family to establish schedule of activities, stability of environment, and respite care.
  Disruptive behaviors and agitation, which often escalate to physical abuse, result in severe impact on caregivers (George & Gwyther, 1986).

Late Stage

➤ Provide respite for caregivers
  because exhaustion of caregivers usually leads to institutionalization of the confused patient.

➤ Mobilize patient
  to prevent hazards of immobility.

➤ Speak directly to patient in simple phrases
  to obtain optimum understanding without necessity to interpret extensively.

➤ Protect from wandering, falls, and other potentially dangerous behaviors (e.g., using matches).
  Altered perception of the objective world places patient at risk for injury.

➤ Assess for and treat infection, malnutrition, and wasting.
  These are common causes of death in Alzheimer's disease patients.

Charting Components

➤ Effective/ineffective interventions
➤ Participation in personal care
➤ Participation in socialization with one or more persons
➤ Activities capable of, for example, setting table, playing bingo, dressing self
➤ Stimuli leading to distress
➤ Response to medications
➤ Family coping strategies
➤ Indications requiring safety precautions (e.g., wandering)

Additional Nursing Orders for THE PATIENT WITH CATASTROPHIC REACTION

➤ Remove precipitant/person from each other
  for the safety of both.

➤ Distract and divert attention (e.g., assist in walking or exercise)
  to dispel energy.

➤ Avoid physical restraints
  because this agitates the patient more.

➤ Stay with patient for some time after incident
  to relieve distress.

➤ Evaluate further for medical problems.
  Episodes can be related to infection, electrolyte imbalance, dehydration.

➤ Learn predictive causes/patterns (e.g., complex tasks, instability in environment, restlessness, refusals more than usual) that precede catastrophic reactions
  to intervene immediately and prevent reactions.

Additional Charting Components

➤ Nature of the catastrophic reaction
➤ Precipitating event
➤ Resolution of problem
➤ Any medical problems

Additional Nursing Orders for
THE PATIENT WITH PSEUDODEMENTIA

➤ Assess carefully for the difference between dementia and depression in the elderly.

Depression may be misdiagnosed as dementia in the elderly. In the depressed elderly, there are several symptoms that suggest dementia (e.g., disorientation, memory loss, distractibility, apathy, difficulty in concentration, inattentiveness [Wilson, Kneisl, & Kneisl, 1992]. However, depression usually has an abrupt onset, and dependency, despondency, and somatic complaints are more apparent in the client with depression (Antai-Otong, 1995).

➤ Assess whether there is a history of depression or a recent history of a stressful event.

These factors are more likely to be present in someone suffering from depression.

➤ Conduct a mental status exam to determine the depth of memory loss, cognitive impairment, and orientation.

People with dementia will have impaired orientation, with greater impairment in recent than in remote memory, and will minimize or try to conceal impairments. The depressed person will simply answer "I don't know." Cognitive impairment for the depressed person will fluctuate, while the client with dementia will have constant impairment (Antai-Otong, 1995).

➤ Assess for the mood, affect, behavior, and appearance of the client.

The client with depression will present with a depressed affect consisting of tearfulness, irritability, and excessive concern with physical symptoms. The depressed person's mood may be anxious, fearful, or depressed. The client with mild dementia will also be anxious and depressed as awareness of deteriorating faculty is acknowledged (Wilson, Kneisl, & Kneisl, 1992).

➤ Observe response to medications to determine whether condition improves with antidepressants.

Clients with dementia will not experience a response to antidepressant while depressed clients will.

➤ Observe behavior of client to determine if he or she struggles to perform tasks or puts little effort into performing even simple tasks.

Clients with depression do not care enough to try to look good, while clients with dementia will try to conceal their impairments (Antai-Otong, 1995).

➤ Do not draw attention to or connect obvious confabulation

which is used to preserve self-esteem.

➤ Monitor for signs of improvement over time.

Depression is usually self-limiting and can be successfully treated with medication or ECT. Reversibility in dementia depends on the extent of structural damage to the brain (Wilson, Kneisl, & Kneisl, 1992).

Additional Charting Components

➤ Presence of precipitating factor for depression
➤ Abruptness or gradualness of onset
➤ History of depression
➤ Mood and affect
➤ Response to medications
➤ Degree of concealment of symptoms

3. Altered Thought Processes

Definition

A state in which an individual experiences a disruption in cognitive operations and activities

Related to

➤ Biological factors
➤ Biochemical/neurophysical imbalances
➤ Chemical alterations, endogenous factors (e.g., electrolytes), exogenous factors (e.g., drugs)
➤ Sensory deprivation or overload
➤ Persistent feelings of extreme anxiety, guilt, or fear
➤ Cerebral atrophy and degeneration/deterioration
➤ Disintegration of think processes
➤ Sleep disturbances

Content appearing in this typeface is additional information not included in the NANDA nursing diagnoses.

Characteristics/Assessment Findings

- ➤ Inaccurate interpretation of environment
- ➤ Cognitive dissonance
- ➤ Distractibility
- ➤ Memory deficit/problems
- ➤ Egocentricity
- ➤ Hypo/hypervigilance

Other Possible Characteristics
- ➤ Inappropriate, nonreality based thinking

Severe
- ➤ Presence of primary or secondary delusional thinking
- ➤ Displaying uncontrolled actions (compulsions) or experiencing uncontrollable ego-alien thoughts (obsessions)
- ➤ Disorganization of thoughts and emotions
- ➤ Disorientation to time, person, or place

Moderate
- ➤ Inappropriate nonreality-based thinking
- ➤ Confusion
- ➤ Occasional magical or autistic thinking
- ➤ Anxiety, panic
- ➤ Loss of control over own thoughts or feelings
- ➤ Impaired insight or judgment

Low
- ➤ Concreteness
- ➤ Decreased problem-solving and decision-making abilities
- ➤ Restricted affect
- ➤ Ambivalence

Expected Outcomes/Goals

The patient will maintain a reality-based orientation with appropriate behavior as evidenced by
- ➤ stating correct time, place, person, situation
- ➤ establishing meaningful dialogue or communication with others
- ➤ frequently defining and reality testing environment
- ➤ maintaining self-control and working within set therapeutic limits
- ➤ developing an awareness of psychological state.

Content appearing in this typeface is additional information not included in the NANDA nursing diagnoses.

Nursing Orders with Rationale

- ➤ Assess and monitor for presence/absence/changes in assessment findings outlined above *in order to detect any change in status.*

- ➤ Establish an alliance (sense of trust) with patient in a one-to-one nurse-patient relationship. *Patients who form positive alliances with their caregivers are more likely to achieve better outcomes (Frank & Gunderson, 1990).*

- ➤ Administer medications as ordered; monitor therapeutic benefits and negative side effects; teach patient self-monitoring skills. *Neuroleptics are the most effective medication for psychotic conditions (American Psychiatric Association, 1989). Nursing observations are critical in determining the effectiveness of any psychiatric medication (Townsend, 1990).*

- ➤ Watch for signs of physical and neurological side effects (e.g., sedation: postural hypotension, dry mouth, visual blurring; endocrine effects: skin rashes, seizures, dystonia, pseudoparkinsonism, akathisia). *Neuroleptics are beneficial for the patient with sensory alterations, but they are not without related side effects (Schatzberg & Cole, 1986).*

- ➤ Maintain therapeutic communication (e.g., listening, restating, clarification, open-ended questions, silence, reflection, and focusing). *Effective communication can facilitate the development of the therapeutic nurse-patient relationship and help the patient in working through the problem-solving process (Davies & Janosik, 1991).*

- ➤ Focus on reality-based thinking; do not reinforce delusional thinking or misinterpreted thoughts; rather, try to seek out the "truth" in it; reestablish ego boundaries without confronting delusional thinking. *Acknowledging delusional thinking and searching for what might have triggered it are the first steps toward diffusing it (Clark, 1984).*

- ➤ Assess the needs the delusional system may be fulfilling. *The need most commonly expressed through the language of delusions is self-esteem. Other common ones are for sexuality and release of hostility.*

➤ Cast doubt on the patient's delusion without arguing about the content.

> *This helps the patient see the nurse's reality but does not threaten the patient's delusional system (denial, projection, rationalization), which would reinforce the need to rigidly hold on to the false beliefs.*

➤ Structure the environment to establish a flexible, therapeutic milieu using nursing skills.

> *This may vary among defining reality for the patient, handling patient control, strengthening the patient's self-image, and strengthening interpersonal relationships (Burgess & Lazare, 1990).*

➤ Help patient to reorient to reality in a concrete fashion by using large clocks, calendars, clearly printed room signs indicating patient's name; calling the patient by name; introducing self when addressing patient.

> *Direct nursing intervention toward helping patient to function in the environment (Davies & Janosik, 1991).*

➤ Be an active learner; allow patient to express concerns, fears, and anxieties

> *to reduce tension, to improve self-image and self-confidence, and to establish a sense of identity.*

➤ Provide patients with opportunities to master own self-care and ADL; allow patient to make own choices (when appropriate).

> *Making decisions allows patient a degree of control, which will improve self-esteem and develop a sense of contentment and self-acceptance; this results from patient's appraisal of own worth, significance, competence, and ability to satisfy own aspirations (Robson, 1989).*

➤ Promote quality sleep and provide for uninterrupted sleep as much as possible.

> *When patients get an adequate amount of sleep, they will experience less physical and psychological stress and fewer mental status alterations (Helton, Gordon, & Nunnery, 1980).*

➤ Help patient to decrease feelings of anxiety and to reestablish own capacity for self-management and self-control by setting realistic, appropriate limits when needed.

> *It is nontherapeutic to let the patient escalate. The nurse must provide clear, concise, and consistent limits for the patient who is unable to set own limits (Burgess & Lazare, 1990).*

➤ Provide opportunities for patient to enhance problem-solving skills and to make own decisions.

> *The cognitive manifestations of patients with altered thought processes include symptoms involved with decision making. The patient typically vacillates and is indecisive. Encouraging the patient to make own decision enhances problem-solving skills (Beck, 1982).*

➤ Promote the patient's self-esteem by offering support and positive, genuine feedback.

> *Respecting the patient and giving emotional support can help him or her to incorporate positive feelings and to feel good about self (Burgess & Lazare, 1990).*

➤ Maintain homeostasis of patient; monitor vital signs when appropriate; provide for patient's physical needs.

> *Systematic nursing assessment will alert the nurse of a change in patient's functional state and to the need for prompt and further observation/intervention (Brunner & Suddarth, 1988).*

➤ Encourage patient to interrelate with other patients in the milieu.

> *When patient is able to "stay present" in the conversation, the patient will experience an increase in self-worth/achievement and will demonstrate an improved ability in cognitive functioning.*

Charting Components

➤ Adaptations required and made
➤ Any abnormal change in patient's physical/emotional status
➤ Cognitive level, mental status
➤ Delusions
➤ Disorientation
➤ Diversionary activities
➤ Effects/side effects of medications
➤ Improvements/deterioration in self-control/self-management
➤ Level of anxiety
➤ Participation in ADL, milieu
➤ Problem-solving skills
➤ Referrals made
➤ Sleep patterns
➤ Patient/family teaching, response

IX. Feeling

A. COMFORT

1. Chronic Pain

Definition

A state in which the individual experiences pain that continues for a period longer than six months

Related to

➤ Chronic physical/psychosocial disability
  ▷ ineffective coping
  ▷ ineffective treatment of back problems
  ▷ conversion symptoms
  ▷ hypochondriasis
  ▷ intestinal spasms or inflammation
  ▷ joint degeneration or inflammation
  ▷ muscle spasms
  ▷ myofacial pain syndrome
  ▷ neuralgia, neuropathy
  ▷ phantom limb pain
  ▷ over-/underactivity
  ▷ trauma/injury
  ▷ tumors/neoplasms
  ▷ depression
  ▷ fear
  ▷ positive reinforcement of pain behaviors by significant others

Content appearing in this typeface is additional information not included in the NANDA nursing diagnoses.

Characteristics/Assessment Findings

Major
➤ Verbal report or observed evidence of pain experienced for more than six months

Minor
➤ Fear of reinjury
➤ Physical and social withdrawal
➤ Altered ability to continue previous activities
➤ Anorexia
➤ Weight changes
➤ Changes in sleep patterns
➤ Facial mask
➤ Guarded movement

Other Possible Characteristics
➤ Atrophy and weakness of muscles associated with painful part
➤ Decreased ability to concentrate
➤ Decreased movement of painful part
➤ Depression/anger about situation
➤ Fatigue
➤ Grimacing
➤ History of repeatedly seeking help from health professionals (e.g., multiple surgeries)
➤ Increased strength in nonpainful parts due to compensatory use
➤ Inflammatory changes at site (e.g., redness, heat, swelling)
➤ Loss of interest in social activities
➤ Preoccupation with medications and treatments
➤ Restlessness, irritability
➤ Rigidity
➤ Rhythmic or rubbing body movement
➤ Self-focusing on pain
➤ Signs of progressive physical deterioration
➤ Vocalizations (e.g., crying, moaning, sighing, whimpering, gasping, screaming)
➤ Withdrawal from usual activities
➤ Dependency on prescribed medication or self-medication

Expected Outcomes/Goals

The patient will

➤ attain/maintain increased comfort status as evidenced by
  ▷ decreased complaints of pain
  ▷ descriptions of reduced intensity and duration of painful episodes
  ▷ decreased manifestations of pain behaviors
  ▷ reduction of aggravating and mitigating factors
  ▷ use of improved coping mechanisms
  ▷ use of pain-relief measures
  ▷ demonstration of preplanning activities.
➤ decrease focus on pain as evidenced by
  ▷ not participating in activities based on presence of pain
  ▷ maintaining an accurate record or graph of progress in exercise and activities.

Nursing Orders with Rationale

➤ Assess and monitor for presence/absence/ changes in assessment findings outlined above *in order to detect any change in status.*

➤ Assess pain experience and how the patient has coped with the pain in the past; include
  ▷ location
  ▷ onset and duration
  ▷ quality (e.g., throbbing, burning)
  ▷ intensity: ask patient to rate the pain at its best and worse; use a word scale (e.g., none, mild, moderate, severe, unbearable) or a number scale (e.g., 0 = no pain, 10 = the worst pain imaginable)
  ▷ aggravating and mitigating factors
  ▷ effects of pain on ADL (e.g., sleep, appetite, physical activity)
  ▷ effects of pain on relationships with others
  ▷ secondary gains obtained from pain behaviors
  ▷ what specifically reduces the intensity or increases pain
  ▷ support systems, coping mechanisms.
    A thorough assessment allows the nurse to establish a baseline, to determine effectiveness of interventions, and to promote a supportive nurse-patient relationship (Meinhart & McCaffrey, 1983).

➤ Assess patient's knowledge and use of preventive measures to avoid intense and severe pain; teach preventive approaches such as time-contingent rather than pain-contingent administration of medication, taking medication immediately when pain begins.
  Chronic pain can be managed more easily if a preventive approach is used.

➤ Collaborate with healthcare team in detoxifying patient from narcotics; if appropriate
  ▷ include patient and family in making a plan.
  ▷ use double-bind preparation, if ordered, where neither the nurse nor the patient is aware of the exact dosage of narcotic being administered.
  ▷ monitor for signs of withdrawal (e.g., diaphoresis, shaking, abdominal cramping, tachycardia).
    Narcotics are not the drug of choice (except in terminal illnesses) in chronic pain because of tolerance and side effects (Davis, 1984).

➤ Assess current use of analgesics, degree of relief obtained, and need to alter medication.
  Medication may need to be changed to reduce common side effects, increase potential, synergistic effects of nonnarcotic and narcotic drugs, and decrease pain level.

➤ Evaluate patient's use of and success with nonpharmacological pain-relief measures:
  ▷ *cutaneous stimulation* (e.g., hot/cold packs, massage, transcutaneous electrical nerve stimulation [TENS], mentholated rubs, acupressure, acupuncture)
  ▷ *relaxation techniques* (e.g., slow rhythmic breathing) and rest periods
  ▷ *guided imagery* (using one's imagination to create sensory images that decrease the intensity of pain or become a substitute for pain)
  ▷ *distraction* (focusing attention on stimuli other than on the pain; e.g., reciting a rhyme, listening to music, watching television)
  ▷ *hypnosis, biofeedback, physical exercises* designed to reduce muscle spasms, etc.

➤ Refer to appropriate healthcare professionals to increase use of nonpharmacological techniques; e.g.,
  ▷ *hypnotherapy:* uses principle similar to guided imagery; offers acceptance of ideas, use of imagination, increases concentration
  ▷ *biofeedback:* provides information about body functions; how to reduce muscle tension; encourages use of relaxation techniques (McCaffrey, 1979)

▷ *physical therapy/occupational therapy:* guides patient in increasing flexibility, endurance, co-ordination, strength (Sirancusano, 1984) to reduce muscle spasms and relieve the disuse syndrome that occurs with many chronic pain patients; helps the patient focus on function rather than on pain, and can help relieve the monotony that accompanies chronic pain.

> *Nonpharmacological measures influences the sensory, motivational, affective, and cognitive components of the perception of pain; manipulating any one of these factors will influence the person's pain experience (Abu-Said & Tesler, 1986; McCaffrey, 1979).*

➤ Provide measures that help patient cope with the effects of chronic pain on activities and social life:

▷ encourage to accept pain but not the disability that occurs with it; if pain relief will occur, it won't be until the disability is alleviated (Meilman, 1984).

▷ encourage optimistic behavior (e.g., teach to say "I can" instead of "I can't").

▷ assist with appropriate goal setting in physical exercise, vocational and recreational activities (Meilman, 1984):

• include subgoals to aim for along the way.

• include goals for social contacts—chronic pain patients often let friendships slip (e.g., contact two friends every week) (Philips, 1988).

• give positive reinforcement for goal setting and achievement.

• encourage to refrain from making pain the basis of carrying out activities (e.g., teach to avoid making statements like, "I'll mow the lawn this weekend if my back doesn't hurt.").

• teach to record and graph progress in activities and exercises.

• encourage participation of family and friends in exercise programs.

> *Chronic pain can overwhelm all aspects of the patient's life, leaving the patient without resources to cope with these changes and resulting disability (Nursing Now, 1985).*

➤ Assess for degree of depression.

> *There is a high correlation between depression and chronic pain. On the MMPI, the depression and hypochondriac scale scores decreased when patients felt they could control the pain (Shealy, 1976).*

➤ Assess for effectiveness and side effects of antidepressant medication

> *to monitor the degree of success in replacing narcotics with a different medication.*

➤ Encourage regular exercise that does not involve muscle strain (e.g., brisk walking, stretching); gradually increase time and amount daily as tolerated.

> *Exercise promotes flexibility, improves mental outlook, and reduces stiffness.*

➤ Help to increase compliance, promote communication and stress-management skills:

▷ help patient to differentiate between complaining and ventilating; encourage the latter.

▷ encourage assertive rather than aggressive or passive-aggressive behavior.

▷ teach to address doubt of others openly.

▷ teach others the consequences of doubt (i.e., it encourages patient to continue exhibiting pain behaviors to "prove" the pain is real, which leads to continuation of the disabling effects of pain) (McCaffrey, 1979).

▷ encourage patient and significant others to relate to each other when pain is not the focus of attention.

▷ help patient to recognize and manage depressive moods and tendencies toward irritability.

▷ provide support to family members who are often drained by giving prolonged emotional support, financial assistance, and help with physical activities, which often leads to deterioration in relationships (McCaffrey, 1979).

▷ monitor family's adjustment to role changes as patient improves; this may be difficult for family members who have adapted to the life-style the chronic pain has provided (e.g., the loss of someone to protect and fuss over) (Philips, 1988).

▷ refer to family therapy if appropriate.

▷ assess for other nursing diagnoses that often occur in chronic pain patients (e.g., powerlessness, hopelessness, ineffective individual/family coping); plan interventions accordingly.

> *Lack of communication and tension can contribute to increased pain (Meilman, 1984).*

➤ Develop a teaching plan geared toward the patient and significant others; include
  ▷ meaning, prognosis of pain
  ▷ factors that may influence the pain experience (e.g., fatigue may increase pain)
  ▷ explanations of diagnostic procedures using sensory information
  ▷ use of preventive approach in pain management
  ▷ use of medications (including side effects)
  ▷ use of nonpharmacological relief measures
  ▷ importance of planning activities
  ▷ increasing patient and family awareness of pain behaviors (e.g., videotaping the patient's activities and reviewing the film with them)
  ▷ difference between chronic pain and acute pain model.
    Chronic pain does not serve the purpose of preventing injury that acute pain does. Gaining this knowledge increases the patient's pain-coping strategies and reduces fear and anxiety regarding the pain experience. Including the family helps to validate patient's pain, reduces misconceptions they may have about the pain, and increases the resources available to the patient on discharge. Chronic pain imposes stresses on the entire family (Abu-Said & Tesler, 1986).

Charting Components

➤ Aggravating and mitigating factors
➤ Characteristics of pain, including where it radiates to, accompanying signs and symptoms
➤ Coping strategies used
➤ Effects/side effects of analgesics
➤ Emotional responses to pain
➤ Nonpharmacological relief measures tried, effectiveness
➤ Pain behaviors exhibited
➤ Patient's self-record of exercise, activities
➤ Patient's willingness and ability to try relief measures
➤ Progress in activities and exercises
➤ Significant others' response to pain behaviors
➤ Patient/family education, response

Additional Nursing Orders for THE PATIENT WITH CHRONIC LOW-BACK PAIN

➤ Teach patient to notify physician of any change in ability to defecate or urinate.
    This could be an emergent situation indicating spinal cord compression (Meinhart & McCaffrey, 1983).

➤ Collaborate with physical therapist to encourage exercise program and to use proper body mechanics; have patient attend a back school if available.
    An educational program covering exercise theory, body mechanics, posture, and the need for daily workouts is especially useful (Sirancusano, 1984).

➤ Administer cutaneous stimulation to an around site (e.g., hot/cold packs, TENS).
    Cutaneous stimulation can reduce pain intensity and help relieve muscle spasms (McCaffrey & Beebe, 1989).

➤ Encourage use of relaxation and stress-management techniques, hypnosis, biofeedback.
    These techniques have been shown to be particularly helpful to patients with chronic pain and low-back pain (McCaffrey & Beebe, 1989).

➤ Emphasize importance of preplanning (e.g., carrying lumbar support or foot rest when traveling).
    Pacing activities allows the patient to be active without exacerbating the pain (McCaffrey & Beebe, 1989).

Additional Charting Components

➤ Activity pacing
➤ Change in ability to urinate, defecate
➤ Compliance with exercise regimen

Additional Nursing Orders for
THE PATIENT WITH INTRACTABLE PAIN

➤ Provide patient and family with emotional and psychological support; help to explore coping mechanisms.

> *The patient and family need support and increased coping skills to deal with pain that persists despite treatment (McCaffrey & Beebe, 1989).*

➤ Emphasize to patient that the pain may persist, but the disability that occurs with intractable pain can be reduced.

> *This patient must reject the disability in order to build up to participate in activities again (Meilman, 1984).*

➤ Encourage patient to try various combinations of the relief measures discussed in the generic care plan above.

> *It may take practicing the methods several times before obtaining relief from them; measures that do not work alone may work in combinations (e.g., progressive relaxation and guided imagery). Keep trying (McCaffrey, 1979).*

➤ Refer to pain clinic or pain specialists as appropriate to have patient on a regular program of pain management with support.

> *When pain becomes the central focus of a person's life, specialized help is needed (McCaffrey & Beebe, 1989).*

➤ Assess for suicidal risk, document findings; inform physician and make appropriate referral; refer to nursing care plan "Potential for Violence: Self-Directed" for additional interventions.

> *The risk for suicide is high in patients with prolonged, uncontrolled, severe pain (McCaffrey & Beebe, 1989).*

Additional Charting Components

➤ Disability status
➤ Referrals made
➤ Suicide risk
➤ Support systems, coping mechanisms

B. EMOTIONAL INTEGRITY

1. Dysfunctional Grieving

Definition

Prolonged unresolved grief experienced by an individual, group, or family, which results in unsuccessful adaptation to the loss

Related to

➤ Actual or perceived loss (object loss is used in the broadest sense); object may include
  ▷ people (as in divorce; relocation causing separation from family, significant other, friends; children leaving home; entering a nursing home)
  ▷ possessions
  ▷ job
  ▷ status (e.g., change in social role)
  ▷ home
  ▷ ideals
  ▷ socially unspeakable loss (e.g., suicide)
  ▷ uncertainty over loss (e.g., person missing in action)
  ▷ need to be strong and in control
  ▷ ambivalence over lost object or person
  ▷ overwhelmed by multiple losses
  ▷ reawakened, old, unresolved grief

Characteristics/Assessment Findings

➤ Verbal expression of distress at loss
➤ Denial of loss
➤ Expression of guilt
➤ Expression of unresolved issues
➤ Anger
➤ Sadness
➤ Crying
➤ Difficulty in expressing loss
➤ Alterations in eating habits, sleep patterns, dream patterns, activity level, libido
➤ Idealization of lost object
➤ Reliving of past experiences
➤ Interference with life functioning
➤ Developmental regression
➤ Labile affect
➤ Alterations in concentration or pursuits of tasks
➤ Extremely low self-esteem
➤ Suicidal ideation
➤ Prolonged panic attacks
➤ Prolonged depression
➤ Engaging in self-detrimental activities
➤ Psychotic-like features
➤ Inability to remove possessions of the deceased
➤ Somatic distress (usually intermittent)
  ▷ gastrointestinal problems (e.g., weight loss or gain, anorexia, constipation, diarrhea, nausea and vomiting, indigestion, epigastric pain)
  ▷ tightness in throat, choking, shortness of breath, sighing, empty feeling in abdomen
➤ Self-neglect (e.g., inattentiveness to appearance)
➤ Excessive, distorted, exaggerated, or delayed emotional reaction
➤ Protracted social withdrawal
➤ Severe feelings of loss of identity
➤ Excessive self-blame or self-reproach
➤ Denial of the loss

Content appearing in this typeface is additional information not included in the NANDA nursing diagnoses.

Expected Outcomes/Goals

The patient will
- resolve blocks to adaptive mourning as evidenced by
  - expressing feelings of anger, sorrow, guilt
  - verbalizing acknowledgment and meaning of the loss
  - using nondestructive coping mechanisms
  - discussing positive and negative aspects of the loss.
- achieve a state of acceptance of the loss as evidenced by
  - demonstrating increased self-esteem
  - reduced feelings of guilt and self-blame for the loss
  - involvement with others
  - increased interest in living
  - making plans for the future
  - speaking comfortably about the loss.

Nursing Orders with Rationale

- Assess and monitor for presence/absence/changes in assessment findings outlined above
  in order to detect any change in status.

- Refer to nursing care plan "Anticipatory Grieving" for interventions dealing with normal grief.
  It is important and necessary to implement these along with specific interventions for dysfunctional grief.

- Monitor for suicidal ideation; refer to nursing care plan "Potential for Violence: Self-Directed" for interventions.

- Assess the loss experienced, how long ago, initial reactions, and the meaning the loss represents to the person and family/significant other.
  These data will identify where the person is "stuck" in the grieving and adaptation process.

- Identify if the grieving process is prolonged beyond what is expected for the type of loss incurred.
  Prolonged grief and mourning over a real or imagined loss should be recognized as depression and responded to as such (Davies & Janoski, 1991).

- Differentiate between normal states of mourning and depression; determine if the person is denying the loss or acknowledging it; assess if the attachment to the loss object/person is "normal" or "inordinate."
  The depressed individual regresses more deeply and fully in response to the loss; there is a fall in self-esteem in the depressed person that is not always seen in grief reactions (Beck, Rawlins, & Williams, 1987).

- Explore previous losses and how the patient reacted and went through the grief and mourning process; discuss feelings, coping used, and outcomes of all significant losses.
  Grief is affected by many factors such as personality, previous losses, and past unresolved grief, which can be restimulated with each new loss.

- Provide positive reinforcement of behaviors indicative of effective coping.
  This strengthens past coping methods that were beneficial and may be beneficial now, and encourages patient to use them.

- Observe for a lack of obvious signs of grieving when an actual loss has occurred, or a retarding of the grieving process once it has begun, or both.
  Persistent absence of any emotion may signal an undue delay in the work of mourning or a delayed grief reaction (Davies & Janosik, 1991).

- Assess for indications of delayed grief reactions (e.g., grieving stimulated years later by the anniversary of the original loss).
  The underlying emotions associated with the loss may be triggered by a spontaneous occurrence in the patient's life (Beck et al., 1988).

- Encourage patient to express feelings (e.g., anger, fear, guilt, sadness); use statements such as, "Would you like to talk about it?" "Tell me about your grief." "I'd like to try to understand what this experience is like for you."; give permission to grieve.
  Expressing feelings and repressed emotions will help patient work through excessive, distorted, and delayed emotional reactions.

- Offer support and reassurance that grieving is normal and painful, and that she or he has the capacity to withstand these feelings without harm.
  This helps the patient to accept the need to experience sadness and suffering as part of the normal grief process.

➤ Expect the patient to fulfill his or her own responsibilities and support patient for doing so; withdraw your attention when the patient does not fulfill them (i.e., do not have therapeutic interaction when the patient has refused to participate in an activity).

> *This strategy will decrease secondary gain from depression and facilitate ability to express and deal with feelings (Schultz & Dark, 1986).*

➤ Discourage shielding the grieving process with medications or other temporary relief outlets
> *to prevent delay in working through the loss.*

➤ Discourage rumination on only one aspect of the grief process (e.g., guilty feelings); after listening to the patient's feelings, ask about other feelings such as helplessness, sadness, and anger.

> *Rumination prevents the person from experiencing and working through deeper feelings that are unacceptable and frightening.*

➤ Facilitate the patient's progression through the stages of grieving by discussing the patient's fear of being overwhelmed by feelings; explore the belief that feelings are destructive or harmful and need to be pushed away.

> *Grief can precipitate a flood of emotions that threaten to overwhelm the person's sense of control. Oftentimes when powerful emotions erupt the individual feels as if she or he is going crazy (Schultz & Dark, 1986).*

➤ Determine the degree to which the loss and grief affects the person's self-esteem; refer to nursing care plans "Chronic Low Self-Esteem" and "Situational Low Self-Esteem" for specific interventions.

> *Dysfunctional grief often results in chronic depression and lowered self-esteem (Davies & Janosik, 1991).*

➤ Evaluate progress in the grieving process; plan appropriate interventions as needs change.

> *Grieving follows specific stages (i.e., denial, anger, bargaining, depression, acceptance) that require different interventions (Kübler-Ross, 1970).*

➤ Analyze our own feelings and beliefs regarding grief, and your success or lack of success in resolving significant losses.

> *One's ability to facilitate grieving with others is related to their own comfort with feelings of grief and resolution of personal losses.*

➤ Identify appropriate community resources and refer patient/family to them (e.g., grief groups, Emotional Anonymous, spiritual and religious resources, community hot lines)

> *to provide group support from others who have experienced a similar loss.*

Charting Components

➤ Absence of crying or verbal expression of loss
➤ Adaptive coping skills used
➤ Availability/use of support systems
➤ Behaviors indicating grieving
➤ Changes in eating, sleeping, activity patterns
➤ Expressions of hopelessness, hope
➤ Feelings expressed about loss
➤ Isolation of patient
➤ Lack of interest in living, suicidal ideation
➤ Level of self-esteem
➤ Self-destructive behaviors
➤ Statements of persistent guilt regarding loss
➤ Statements reflecting adaptation to changes

2. Anticipatory Grieving

Definition

The process by which an individual, group, or family begins to grieve and mourn a real or perceived significant loss

Related to

➤ A potential real or perceived loss as in
  ▷ change in life-style from social role; divorce; relocation causing separation from family, significant other, friends; children leaving home; entering a nursing home; child born with birth defect
  ▷ death of self or significant other
  ▷ loss of body part (e.g., limb, breast, uterus, lung)
  ▷ loss of financial assets (e.g., job, money, home, treasured possessions)
  ▷ loss of physical or mental capabilities (as from cancer, AIDS, Alzheimer's disease, other debilitating nervous system/mental disorders)

Content appearing in this typeface is additional information not included in the NANDA nursing diagnoses.

Characteristics/Assessment Findings

➤ Potential loss of significant object
➤ Expression of distress at potential loss
➤ Denial of potential loss
➤ Guilt
➤ Anger
➤ Sorrow
➤ Choked feelings
➤ Changes in eating habits
➤ Alterations in sleep patterns
➤ Alterations in activity level
➤ Altered libido
➤ Altered communication patterns
➤ Somatic distress (usually intermittent)
  ▷ gastrointestinal problems (e.g., weight loss/gain, anorexia, constipation, diarrhea, nausea and vomiting, indigestion, epigastric pain)
  ▷ insomnia or sleeping more than usual
  ▷ fatigue; may have increased or decreased activity level
  ▷ tightness in throat, choking, shortness of breath, sighing, empty feeling in abdomen
  ▷ complaints of loss of muscle power, tension or pain, headache
➤ Psychological distress
  ▷ altered communication patterns
  ▷ avoiding the source of the potential loss (e.g., spouse, friend, work, pet)
  ▷ denial of potential loss
  ▷ inability to concentrate (short attention span), recurring thoughts of the potential loss
  ▷ overt expressions of reaction to potential loss ranging from incessant crying to withdrawn behavior, inability to cry, apathy
  ▷ restlessness; stays busy but accomplishes less than usual
  ▷ self-neglect (e.g., inattentiveness to appearance)
  ▷ verbalized feelings of shock, disbelief, sadness, depression, anger, fear, guilt
➤ Separation anxiety
  ▷ clinging
  ▷ nightmares
  ▷ unrealistic worry of harm to self/significant other

Content appearing in this typeface is additional information not included in the NANDA nursing diagnoses.

Expected Outcomes/Goals

The patient will
➤ grieve adaptively as evidenced by
  ▷ expressing anger, sadness, guilt
  ▷ verbalizing anticipated changes
  ▷ seeking support from others.
➤ use nondestructive coping mechanisms while dealing with the potential loss as evidenced by
  ▷ searching for appropriate support system
  ▷ maintaining regular health and social routine
  ▷ guarding against excessive use of alcohol, drugs, food.
➤ progress through the grieving process without exhaustion and induced illness as evidenced by
  ▷ dissipation of somatic and psychological symptoms of grief
  ▷ describing how the loss will impact own life situation.
➤ plan how to continue life after the loss as evidenced by identification of satisfactory replacements or substitutes for what may be lost.

Nursing Orders with Rationale

➤ Assess and monitor for presence/absence/changes in assessment findings outlined above *in order to detect any change in status.*

➤ Identify the cause of the anticipatory grief and the meaning the potential loss represents to the patient. *This information is needed to plan appropriate interventions.*

➤ Assess for indications of dysfunctional grieving (e.g., ambivalence, low self-esteem, overattachment).
  Grief is affected by many factors such as personality, previous losses, and past unresolved grief, which can be restimulated with each new loss (Carpenito, 1989).

➤ Establish a trusting relationship with patient *to help patient feel comfortable expressing feelings that are difficult to express or accept.*

➤ Encourage patient to express feelings (e.g., anger, fear, guilt, sadness); use statements such as "Would you like to talk about it?" "Tell me about your grief." "I'd like to try to understand what this experience is like for you."; give permission to grieve.
  Expressing feelings and repressed emotions will help patient to work through excessive, distorted, and delayed emotional reactions.

➤ Reflect and paraphrase responses.
   This assures patient that you received the information correctly.

➤ Ask patient how loss will affect his or her life; problem solve how to adapt to necessary changes.
   Provides opportunity for patient to become aware of the impact of the loss, and lays foundation for making plans to adapt to changes.

➤ Provide privacy during times of emotional ventilation
   to protect patient's sense of dignity.

➤ Observe interaction with family/significant other and willingness to accept help/support
   the identify potential support available from them.

➤ Involve family/significant other (to degree they are willing) in helping to provide care and emotional support for the patient; explain all procedures and treatments to them
   to assist them to understand what the patient is experiencing and to plan how they can help.

➤ Be sensitive to patient's need to be with others and to be left alone; do not assume a grieving person wants only to be left alone.
   Many factors influence coping methods of individuals (e.g., past experience with family, cultural mores, religious beliefs). These need to be considered when determining whether a person prefers solitary grieving or wishes family/significant other to participate in the grieving process (Thompson, McFarland, Hirsch, Tucker, & Bowers, 1989).

➤ Evaluate progress in the grieving process; plan appropriate interventions as needs change.
   Grieving follows specific stages (i.e., shock, developing awareness, resolution) that require different interventions (Carpenito, 1989).

➤ Explore patient's/family experience with grief and methods used to cope with it in the past; provide positive reinforcement for adaptive behaviors; help patient to identify or suggest new ones that can be tried.
   This is a time for patient to use previous successful coping strategies. If these are not available, new ones need to be developed.

➤ Direct the patient to differentiate between wants and needs (e.g., the patient "needs" support in accepting the loss or changes but may "want" a different but unrealistic outcome)
   to facilitate acceptance of reality and what is possible to hope for and receive.

➤ Discourage shielding patient from the grieving process with medications or other temporary relief outlets.
   Medications will only delay working through the loss.

➤ Evaluate patient's progress through the grieving process; discourage rumination (e.g., if patient ruminates over own guilt, listen, then tell patient you are willing to talk about other aspects of grieving such as the fears of being overwhelmed by feelings and of feelings being destructive or harmful [Schultz & Dark, 1986]).
   The nurse can facilitate the patient's process through the stages of grieving by not letting the patient dwell on negative aspects of the loss and by eliciting and coping with any underlying fears.

➤ Provide information to patient/family that grieving is normal and painful, that a variety of feelings is expected and usual.
   This information can help them to experience sadness and suffering and to understand why many feelings exist.

➤ Assess somatic and psychological symptoms of reaction to grief; teach patient that these symptoms are frequently manifested when grieving.
   This information will help patient to understand that the symptoms are not unique but are expected responses from anyone in a similar situation.

➤ Determine the degree to which the potential loss and grief threatens the person's self-esteem
   to identify when referral to professional counseling needs to be made.

➤ Identify appropriate community resources and refer patient to them (e.g., grief groups, Reach to Recovery, hospice, stroke or ostomy clubs, widowers and widows clubs, spinal cord rehabilitation centers)
   to provide group support from others who have experienced a similar loss.

Charting Components

➤ Adaptive coping used
➤ Anxiety
➤ Availability, use of support systems
➤ Behaviors reflecting positive adaptation to loss
➤ Changes in eating, sleeping, activity patterns
➤ Expressions of hope, hopelessness
➤ Feelings expressed
➤ Indications of psychological distress
➤ Somatic responses
➤ Stage of grieving
➤ Patient/family teaching, response

3. Potential for Violence: Self-Directed

Definition

A state in which an individual experiences behaviors that can be physically harmful

Related to

➤ Antisocial character
➤ Battered women
➤ Catatonic excitement
➤ Child abuse
➤ Manic excitement
➤ Organic brain syndrome
➤ Panic states
➤ Rage reactions
➤ Suicidal behavior
➤ Temporal lobe epilepsy
➤ Toxic reactions to medication
➤ Childhood history of abuse, incest, substance abuse
➤ Hormonal disturbance (e.g., PMS)
➤ Recent/severe losses/life changes (e.g., family death, major accidents, financial losses)
➤ Stimulants (i.e., cocaine withdrawal)

Characteristics/Assessment Findings

➤ Presence of risk factors
  ➢ body language (e.g., clenched fists, tense facial expression, rigid posture, tautness indicating effort to control)
  ➢ hostile threatening verbalizations (e.g., boasting to or prior abuse of others)
  ➢ increased motor activity (e.g., pacing, excitement, irritability, agitation)
  ➢ overt and aggressive acts (e.g., goal-directed destruction of objects in environment)
  ➢ possession of destructive means (e.g., gun, knife, weapon)
  ➢ rage
  ➢ self-destructive behavior, active aggressive suicidal acts
  ➢ suspicion of others, paranoid ideation, delusions, hallucinations
  ➢ substance abuse/withdrawal

Other Possible Characteristics

➤ Increasing anxiety levels
➤ Fear of self or others
➤ Inability to verbalize feelings
➤ Repetition of verbalizations (e.g., continued complaints, requests, demands)
➤ Anger
➤ Provocative behavior (e.g., argumentation, dissatisfaction, overreaction, hypersensitivity)
➤ Vulnerable self-esteem
➤ Depression (specifically active, aggressive, suicidal acts)
  ➢ stated desire to harm self
  ➢ history of actual or attempted harm to self (e.g., history of past trouble with impulse control)
  ➢ statements of depression, despair, hopelessness
  ➢ withdrawn, isolated behavior (vegetative signs of depression)
  ➢ purposeful accidents
  ➢ omission of therapeutic measures
  ➢ limited educational/family/community/religious resources
  ➢ recent severe disfiguring accident/illness or severe exacerbation of past illness
  ➢ recent knowledge of own terminal illness

Content appearing in this typeface is additional information not included in the NANDA nursing diagnoses.

Expected Outcomes/Goals

The patient will

➤ verbalize fears of loss of impulse control to others as they occur as evidenced by daily report of precursors to feelings of hopelessness/helplessness.

➤ demonstrate impulse control in a variety of settings as evidenced by talking about losses/sadness without acting out suicidal feelings.

➤ verbalize a new perspective on life situation as evidenced by verbal self-reports and abandonment of access to suicide means (e.g., gives up gun, pills, other "secrets" to staff).

➤ assume responsibility for own portion of health-care contract as evidenced by compliance with regimen, requests.

➤ communicate assertively with staff/family/peers as evidenced by family report and staff observations.

➤ practice self-care/stress-management techniques (e.g., deep breathing, journal keeping, exercise) as evidenced by patient record keeping and staff observations.

➤ report decrease in tension state as evidenced by
  ▷ self-report
  ▷ decreased blood pressure, pulse, respirations
  ▷ decreased neck, jaw, back muscle tension.

Nursing Orders with Rationale

➤ Assess and monitor for presence/absence/changes in assessment findings outlined above *in order to detect any change in status.*

➤ Assess
  ▷ cause of patient hopelessness; identify "last straw" and meaning of event to patient
  ▷ patient's coping strategies and what has been done in the past when these feelings surface.
    Critical assessment of the patient's past and current coping skills is a nursing responsibility (Barry, 1984).

➤ Monitor suicidal ideation/behavior (e.g., question expressions of despair, disregard for personal safety, driving recklessly, hoarding medications); maintain hourly contact/observation with patient; be sure patient takes all medication.
  Close observation of suicidal patients is the most important nursing intervention with the depressed (Barry, 1984).

➤ Provide safety measures:
  ▷ Ask patient directly: "Do you have a plan? What is it? When do you plan on carrying it out?"
  ▷ Report/record all suicidal behavior to staff; ensure open staff communication so that patient cannot keep information from any staff members.
  ▷ Remove patient from source of unmanageable anxiety when needed; provide one-to-one observation at these times.
  ▷ Give permission for patient to express angry feelings in a safe environment (rather than choosing suicide to express anger).
  ▷ Remove dangerous items (e.g., knives, razor blades) from setting; during acute danger, provide safe setting (e.g., locked windows, one-to-one observation).
    Providing safety measures is a primary nursing responsibility. The nurse's role is to represent life during the patient's period of hopelessness (Aguilera, 1990).

➤ Teach patient
  ▷ methods for cognitive control of depressive thoughts/feelings/preoccupations (e.g., give examples of self-talk such as "I feel useless today but that doesn't mean I will always feel this way.").
  ▷ self-care for depression (e.g., exercise, nutrition).
  ▷ problem-solving techniques; help patient to think of at least three reasonable alternative actions.

➤ Teach family to use reflection, empathy, limit setting with suicidal member.
  Education regarding basic health-management skills and reasonable alternatives besides suicide will decrease lethality (Hatton & Valente, 1984).

➤ Use resources:
  ▷ Involve family/other resources in contracting process.
  ▷ Appeal to part of patient that wants to live; address as "Healthy part inside you. . . ."
  ▷ Help to use successful coping strategies from past crises (e.g., "The priest was helpful to you when you felt hopeless before; maybe he could be of help to you now.").
    Success in reducing suicide lethality hinges on getting the patient to a network of resources where personal feelings of isolation and worthlessness diminish (Hatton & Valente, 1984).

➤ Structure problem solving:

   ▷ Assist patient to continue daily activities and purposeful activity (e.g., "Call your children," "Continue your classes.").

   ▷ Make a verbal/written contract with patient regarding suicide, stating that patient will call someone (designate who) before a suicide attempt.

       A structured contract creates boundaries for patient, provides message that nurse takes the matter very seriously, and engages the healthy part of the patient in the problem-solving process (Cassey, 1985).

   ▷ Assign structured tasks (e.g., "Call your brother at 10 A.M.); include simple and detailed directions; begin by giving few choices; later provide patient with more latitude in planning a structured day.

       Helping patient to structure the day harnesses the patient's own coping devices (Hatton & Valente, 1984).

   ▷ Include family members in problem-solving phase; do not keep secrets from patient/family; provide a new perspective on the problem, another way to view the situation.

       Providing a new perspective is one way that nurses can inspire hope in hopeless situations (Miller, 1985).

Charting Components

➤ Compliance with medical regimen
➤ Examples of progress in ability to use cognitive skills to stop violent impulses
➤ Expression of suicidal ideation, feelings of hopelessness
➤ Feelings of grief, fear, guilt, helplessness
➤ Interactions with family/staff/peers
➤ Progress with self-care skills
➤ Signs/symptoms of alcohol/drug abuse
➤ Specific examples of patient's ability to communicate assertively
➤ Statements indicating a different perspective
➤ Patient/family teaching, response

4. Potential for Violence: Directed at Others

Definition

The state in which an individual experiences behaviors that can be physically harmful, either to the self or others

Related to

➤ Antisocial personality
➤ Battered women
➤ Catatonic excitement
➤ Child abuse
➤ Manic excitement
➤ Organic brain syndrome (especially if there is decreased impulse control or agitation)
➤ Panic states
➤ Rage reactions
➤ Suicidal behavior
➤ Temporal lobe epilepsy
➤ Toxic reactions to medications
➤ Psychosis involving command hallucinations ordering violence
➤ Childhood history of abuse
➤ Adjustment disorder
➤ Paranoia
➤ Alcohol or drug abuse (especially PCP, amphetamines)
➤ Withdrawal syndrome (especially from sedatives/hypnotics)
➤ Increase in stressors within a short period of time
➤ Real or perceived threat to self
➤ Response to a catastrophic event
➤ Misperceived messages from others
➤ Dysfunctional communication patterns
➤ Acute neurological illness (e.g., toxic delirium, encephalitis), head injury
➤ Hormonal imbalance (e.g., PMS)
➤ Postpartum depression
➤ Erotomania
➤ Akathisia following haldol administration

Content appearing in this typeface is additional information not included in the NANDA nursing diagnoses.

Characteristics/Assessment Findings

➤ Presence of risk factors
  ‐ body language (e.g., clenched fists, clenched jaw, rigid posture, tautness indicating effort to control)
  ‐ hostile, threatening verbalizations (e.g., boasting of prior abuse of others)
  ‐ increased motor activity (e.g., pacing, excitement, irritability, agitation)
  ‐ overt and aggressive acts (e.g., goal-directed destruction of objects in environment)
  ‐ possession of destructive means (e.g., gun, knife, other weapon)
  ‐ rage
  ‐ self-destructive behavior, active aggressive suicidal acts
  ‐ history of assaultive behavior
  ‐ suspicion of others, paranoid ideation, delusion, hallucinations
  ‐ substance abuse/withdrawal

Other Possible Characteristics
➤ Increasing anxiety levels
➤ Fear of self or others
➤ Inability to verbalize feelings
➤ Repetition of verbalizations (e.g., continued complaints, requests, demands)
➤ Anger
➤ Provocative behavior (e.g., argumentative, dissatisfied, overactive, hypersensitive)
➤ Vulnerable self-esteem
➤ Depression (specifically active, aggressive, suicidal acts)
➤ Loud, threatening, profane speech
➤ Increased muscle tension (e.g., sitting on the edge of a chair, gripping the arms)
➤ Slamming doors, knocking over furniture
➤ Intended victims, if any
➤ Poor impulse control
➤ Perception of environment as hostile
➤ Minimal tolerance of anxiety, stress
➤ Overcontrolled with brittle defenses
➤ Hallucinations

Content appearing in this typeface is additional information not included in the NANDA nursing diagnoses.

Expected Outcomes/Goals

The patient will
➤ verbalize understanding of why behavior occurs and precipitating factors as evidenced by a willingness to explore these issues one-to-one with staff.
➤ communicate assertively and nonaggressively with staff/family/peers as evidenced by family report and staff observations.
➤ use adaptive coping mechanisms in conflicts as evidenced by talking about feelings and perceptions directly and openly.
➤ practice stress-management techniques (e.g., journal writing, talking, exercising, relaxation) as evidenced by patient record keeping and staff observations.
➤ express increased self-concept and self-esteem as evidenced by positive self-statements and a willingness to be assertive.

Nursing Orders with Rationale

➤ Assess and monitor for presence/absence/changes in assessment findings outlined above *in order to detect any change in status.*

➤ Assess level of agitation and be alert for indicators of agitation (e.g., nervousness, pacing, loud voice, demanding demeanor).
   These are signs that the anger is escalating (Rawlins & Heacock, 1988).

➤ Decrease environmental stimuli, depending on the level of agitation.
   A stimulating environment may increase agitation and provoke aggressive behavior (Doenges, Townsend, & Moorhouse, 1989).

➤ Be honest and consistent with patient; be available and show genuine positive regard.
   These behaviors promote trust, which is necessary for a relationship to be therapeutic (Doenges et al., 1989).

➤ Convey an attitude of acceptance toward the patient; make it clear that it is the behavior, not the patient, that is unacceptable.
   An attitude of acceptance promotes feelings of self-worth. These feelings are further enhanced as person and behavior are viewed separately, communicating unconditional positive regard (Doenges et al., 1989).

➤ Monitor behavior; if patient's behavior escalates, always use the least restrictive measures first; offer mediations as ordered and escort to a calmer, quieter environment; when the patient is calm, offer to talk; enlist assistance of additional staff as necessary; if patient remains agitated, follow unit protocol regarding seclusion or restraints; refer to nursing care plan "Potential for Injury/Trauma" regarding safeguards of restraints.

These measures will protect patient and others from injury and convey evidence of control over the situation to the patient (Townsend, 1988).

➤ Encourage to verbalize feelings of anger gradually; help to explore frustrations and situations that patient usually responds to with violence.

Violence often erupts around issues that could not be talked about; the violence itself may be experienced as a forbidden subject (Goodwin, 1985).

➤ Help patient to identify the internal and interpersonal factors that provoke violence or that strengthen a relationship against violence.

This is the first step in a structured violence-prevention strategy (Goodwin, 1985).

➤ Identify serious risk factors for further violence (e.g., multiple incidents, family chaos, conscious/subconscious desires that the abuse continue, specific mental or physiological disorders associated with the violent episodes, weapons, and other environmental risk factors such as legal entanglements); implement violence-prevention strategies (e.g., use calm but firm approach; raise your voice to be heard, but do not appear aggressive).

Attempts to calm and talk the patient down are used as a first approach in preventing the escalation of potentially assaultive behavior. Wherever possible, reduce the possibility of continued violence by treating the risk factors (second step in violence-prevention strategy). Inform significant others if failure is probable (Goodwin, 1985).

➤ Be aware of own body language and proximity to patient; stand at least an arm's length from patient, turn slightly to side, and have an open posture.

The face-to-face "challenge" position can provoke patients because the nurse's stance may appear hostile.

➤ Help patient to identify what support is lacking; problem solve how to achieve it; encourage patient to obtain the needed support.

Advocacy with support is the third helpful intervention for violence (Goodwin, 1985).

➤ Explore with patient alternative ways of handling frustration and pent-up anger in order to channel energy into socially acceptable behavior (e.g., physical exercise, journal writing).

Developing new ways of reacting is essential to breaking the maladaptive pattern of responding (Doenges et al., 1989).

➤ Give praise and encouragement to patient for choosing socially acceptable methods of managing anger and aggressiveness.

Positive reinforcement tends to strengthen the behavior (Rawlins & Heacock, 1988).

➤ Reinforce that patient is responsible for controlling own behavior, recognizing feelings, and choosing the method of dealing with them.

This creates a sense of responsibility in the patient for own angry feelings and helps the patient to learn that she or he has choices in ways to respond (Rawlins & Heacock, 1988).

➤ Encourage patient to request the assistance of staff when feeling a buildup of angry emotions.

This can prevent anger from escalating and helps the patient to learn to talk about anger rather than act on it (Rawlins & Heacock, 1988).

➤ Teach self-reinforcement for getting through anger-producing situations.

This helps the patient boost own self-esteem for appropriate behavior and become more autonomous, and lessens the need to rely on others for reinforcement (Rawlins & Heacock, 1988).

Charting Components

➤ Ability to maintain self-control
➤ Ability to verbalize sources of anger, rage
➤ Current coping methods, exploration of alternatives
➤ Family interaction, patient's response
➤ Identification of constructive ways to increase power, supportive people/groups in environment
➤ Intervention, patient response
➤ Mood, agitation
➤ Patient teaching regarding alternative ways of dealing with aggressive feelings

5. Risk for Self-Mutilation

Definition

A state in which an individual is at risk to perform an act on the self to injure, not kill, which produces tissue damage and tension relief

Related to

➤ Borderline personality disorder
➤ Psychotic states (e.g., delusions, command hallucinations)
➤ Eating disorders
➤ Autistic disorder
➤ Emotionally disturbed or battered children
➤ Mentally retarded and autistic children
➤ Clients with a history of self-injury
➤ History of physical, emotional, or sexual abuse
➤ Unresolved fears of abandonment
➤ Lack of impulse control
➤ Agitation, anger, hostility
➤ Cognitive impaired disorders
➤ Obsessive-compulsive disorders
➤ Substance abuse or dependence

Characteristics/Assessment Findings

➤ Inability to cope with increased psychological/physiological tension in a healthy manner
➤ Feelings of depression, rejection, self-hatred, separation anxiety, guilt, shame, and depersonalization
➤ Fluctuating emotions
➤ Command hallucinations
➤ Need for sensory stimuli
➤ Parental emotional deprivation
➤ Dysfunctional family
➤ Immaturity and insecurity
➤ Severe, bizarre, and grotesque injuries (e.g., self-enucleation, autocastration)
➤ Superficial slashing of the body, especially the limbs
➤ Recurrent suicidal threats, gestures, or behavior
➤ Self-hitting, tearing out hair, bone breaking
➤ Skin carving, burning, severe scratching, needle sticking

Content appearing in this typeface is additional information not included in the NANDA nursing diagnoses.

Expected Outcomes/Goals

The patient will

➤ not physically injure self as evidenced by no suicidal gestures or self-mutilating behaviors.
➤ identify new coping skills for managing feelings of tension as evidenced by
  ▷ identifying and describing sources of stress and anxiety
  ▷ expressing feelings related to stress and tension
  ▷ discussing alternative ways to meet demands of current situation
  ▷ demonstrating improved communication skills.

Nursing Orders with Rationale

➤ Assess and monitor for presence/absence/changes in assessment findings outlined above *in order to detect any change in status.*

➤ Assess for frequency of the behavior, the type of behavior, stressors preceding the event, the reason for behavior, and the effects on others.
  Determining baseline measurements of the behavior assists in designing interventions that are specific to the individual and more effective in diminishing the self-mutilation behavior (Fontaine & Fletcher, 1995).

➤ Secure a verbal contract from patient that he or she will seek out a staff member when the urge for self-mutilation is experienced.
  A contract places some of the responsibility for the patient's safety on him or her. Discussing feelings of self-harm provides a degree of relief for the patient.

➤ Remove all dangerous objects from the patient's environment to ensure patient safety.
  Clients can be very creative in using objects not usually considered dangerous (e.g., staple from magazine to scratch self) (Fontaine & Fletcher, 1995).

➤ Observe patient's behavior frequently without appearing suspicious.
  Close observation ensures patient's safety because early intervention is possible.

➤ Institute one-to-one supervision if the patient is highly agitated, angry, or stressed.
  Patients with borderline personality disorder suffer from extreme fears of abandonment and, when left alone, their fears may escalate and cause an increase in the level of anxiety and agitation, thus creating greater possibility of self-harm (Townsend, 1993).

➤ Care for patient's wounds in a matter-of-fact manner without criticism or sympathy.
> *Positive attention will reward unwanted behaviors. Lack of attention to the maladaptive behavior may decrease the repetition of its use (Townsend, 1993).*

➤ Encourage the patient to identify their feelings prior to the self-mutilation
> *so the patient can acknowledge the precipitating factors that led to the need for tension reduction.*

➤ Help the patient become aware of angry feelings and let the patient know it is all right to feel angry. Role model appropriate expressions of anger and reinforce positive attempts to express anger constructively.
> *Self-destructive behaviors can be a result of angry feelings turned inward against the self (Davies & Janosik, 1990).*

➤ Help patients understand the nature of their self-destructive behaviors and their influence on others by consistently and repeatedly drawing attention to the consequences of such behaviors (e.g., scars from wounds, anger from others, interruption of ADL).
> *Borderline patients have a great investment in remaining unaware of the self-destructive nature of actions that gratify certain wishes and allay anxiety (Kaplan, 1986).*

➤ Work with patients on limiting acting-out behaviors that are self-mutilating or destructive toward others or self by
> ▷ helping them recognize cues that precede the behavior
> ▷ teaching them to develop self-dialogue to reverse automatic response (e.g., thought stopping, thought insertion, mental rehearsal techniques).
>> *Cognitive disorganization frequently occurs under stress, which causes increased emotional intensity. The acting-out behavior provides a release of internal stress (Gallop, 1988).*

Content appearing in this typeface is additional information not included in the NANDA nursing diagnoses.

➤ Assist the patient in setting up a control plan of what to do when emotions are getting out of control:
> ▷ anticipate the difficult situation.
> ▷ have someone who can be telephoned when situations are overwhelming.
> ▷ examine impulses and intense emotions rather than acting so quickly.
>> *Such a plan will help the patient learn control, avoid self-destructive acting out, and learn to deal with emotions differently (Gallop, 1988).*

➤ Build the patient's sense of self and self-esteem by providing consistent, caring, nonpunitive interactions; refer to nursing care plans "Chronic Low Self-Esteem" and "Personal Identity Disturbance" for more interventions.
> *The capacity to know, esteem, and love oneself can be developed only when there are adequate experiences of being known, loved, and esteemed by a significant other (Hickey, 1985).*

Charting Components

➤ Presence or absence of self-inflicted wounds
➤ Self-destructive and self-mutilating behaviors
➤ Level of anxiety and tension
➤ Expression of genuine feelings
➤ Ability to calm and soothe self
➤ Outbursts of anger
➤ Limits set and patient's response
➤ Insight into feelings
➤ Impulsive acting out

6. Posttrauma Response

Definition

The state of an individual experiencing a sustained painful response to an overwhelming traumatic event

Related to

➤ Disasters, wars
➤ Epidemics
➤ Rape
➤ Assault
➤ Torture
➤ Catastrophic illness or accident
➤ Incest
➤ Childhood traumas
➤ Robbery, burglary

Characteristics/Assessment Findings

Major

➤ Reexperience of the traumatic event, which may be identified in cognitive, affective, or sensorimotor activities
  ▷ flashbacks
  ▷ intrusive thoughts
  ▷ repetitive dreams or nightmares
  ▷ excessive verbalization of the traumatic event
  ▷ verbalization of survival guilt
  ▷ guilt about behavior required for survival

Minor

➤ Psychic/emotional numbness
  ▷ impaired interpretation of reality
  ▷ confusion
  ▷ dissociation or amnesia
  ▷ vagueness about traumatic event
  ▷ constricted affect
➤ Altered life-style
  ▷ self-destructiveness
  ▷ substance abuse
  ▷ suicide attempt or other acting-out behavior
  ▷ difficulty with interpersonal relationships
  ▷ development of phobia regarding trauma
  ▷ poor impulse control/irritability/aggressiveness
➤ Rage (at the source, at persons associated with trauma, at those exempted from trauma)
➤ Issues of personal responsibility
➤ Sadness over loss of another person or aspects of self
➤ Discomfort over discovered personal vulnerability
➤ Fear of repetition of event
➤ Shame over helplessness or emptiness
➤ Exaggerated startle response
➤ Sleep disturbance
➤ Isolation, feelings of alienation, paranoia
➤ Addictive disorders (e.g., substance abuse to self-medicate, gambling)
➤ Somatic complaints (e.g., tension headaches, irritable colon)
➤ Underachievement, "wandering" life-style
➤ Confusion concerning values, direction, meaning in life
➤ Outbursts in antisocial activity
➤ Obsessive-compulsive behavior

Expected Outcomes/Goals

The patient will
➤ effectively cope with thoughts and feelings concerning the traumatic event as evidenced by
  ▷ absence of flashbacks and intrusive thoughts
  ▷ decreased verbalization of guilt
  ▷ decreased feelings of rage
  ▷ diminished fear of repetition of event.
➤ effectively manage maladaptive behaviors developed after the traumatic event as evidenced by
  ▷ absence of somatic complaint and symptoms
  ▷ absence of obsessive-compulsive behavior
  ▷ decrease in antisocial behavior, underachievement, confusion.
➤ reconstruct life to achieve optimal adjustment for the future as evidenced by
  ▷ establishing new goals and actively pursuing them
  ▷ participating in social events
  ▷ becoming involved in meaningful relationships.

Nursing Orders with Rationale

➤ Assess and monitor for presence/absence/changes in assessment findings outlined above *in order to detect any change in status.*

➤ Assess carefully the nature of the traumatic event: was it a single, brief incident? several, ongoing incidents? a human trauma (e.g., rape, POW) or a natural trauma (e.g., earthquake, flood)?
  Human-induced trauma and natural disasters can have different ramifications on the experiences of the survivors and the onset of psychological symptoms. Human-induced trauma victims often experience more guilt and humiliation; survivors of natural disasters experience a lessened sense of responsibility for the event because they see it as an "act of fate" (Green, Wilson, & Jacob, 1985).

➤ Differentiate whether the traumatic stressor was bereavement (loss of significant other, sadness over loss, discomfort over discovered personal vulnerability, rage) or a personal-injury trauma (fear of repetition of the event, feelings of responsibility, rage).
  There appears to be differing symptomatology among survivors of different kinds of human-induced trauma (Scurfield, 1985).

Content appearing in this typeface is additional information not included in the NANDA nursing diagnoses.

➤ Assess patient's coping attempts and reactions immediately posttrauma.

A range of behaviors possible during and after a traumatic event that later manifest posttraumatic symptoms. Denial or numbing is a universal response (Scurfield, 1985).

➤ Inquire about the role of the survivor during the trauma itself and immediately afterward: did the person act helpless, out of control, calculating? what alternatives were open to the survivor? is the perception and judgment of own behavior congruent with what really happened? what impact did the role performed have?

Answers to these questions can tell about the specific meaning and impact of the trauma to the individual at the time of the event and help identify key areas of conflict (Figley, 1985).

➤ Make a thorough assessment of functioning prior to the traumatic event; include parent-child, peer, and authority-figure relationships; behavior patterns in family, work, social life; and environmental factors.

A thorough assessment is essential to determine a premorbid personality that suggests an additional diagnosis other than posttrauma response (Scurfield, 1985).

➤ Assess the presence or absence of positive pretrauma factors (e.g., level of accomplishment, self-esteem, quality of relationships)

to determine the possible impact of the trauma on such factors and the degree of dysfunction since the event (Green et al., 1985).

➤ Explore with the person the idiosyncratic meaning of the stressor in depth.

The same stressor may have a different meaning to different individuals.

➤ Inquire about the degree of control over intrusive thoughts, the degree of preoccupation with such thoughts and images, and the severity of impact of symptoms on various areas of functioning (e.g., social relationships, work, recreation).

The degree and duration of dysfunction differentiates between a posttraumatic stress disorder and a normal stress recovery process (Rundell, Ursano, Holloway, & Silberman, 1989).

➤ Inquire about alcohol and drug use.

Chemical abuse may be a source of self-medication to suppress nightmares and to diminish autonomic activity (Rundell et al., 1989).

➤ Explore the person's shattered assumptions about invulnerability and the belief that "It can't happen to me" that occurs with the experience of victimization.

Feelings of intense anxiety and helplessness accompany the victim's lost sense of safety and security (Janoff-Bulman, 1985). There is an apprehension that anything may now happen to him or her.

➤ Discuss the question, "Why did this happen to me?"; assist the person to find meaning in the event if possible.

Victims often feel a total lack of comprehension regarding the why of their misfortune. The lack of meaning derives from an inability to understand the event, particularly if the person regards him or herself as a decent person who doesn't deserve this kind of treatment (Janoff-Bulman, 1985).

➤ Refer to nursing care plans "Situational Low Self-Esteem" and "Powerlessness" for interventions dealing with feelings of decreased self-esteem and helplessness.

The trauma of victimization activates negative self-images in the victims, who see themselves as weak, helpless, frightened, and out of control (Horowitz, 1983).

➤ Refer to nursing care plan "Rape-Trauma Syndrome" for interventions dealing specifically with rape.

➤ Assist the individual in rebuilding a conceptual system of beliefs that includes a view of the world as not totally dangerous and she or he is not unique in being a victim (e.g., "Wars have existed for thousand of years and many people have lost their lives during wars, but the world has also experienced times of peace where people prosper and are safe.").

Incorporating one's experience as a victim involves reworking one's assumptions about oneself and the world so that they "fit" with one's new personal data (Janoff-Bulman, 1985).

➤ Help the person to redefine the event by comparing his or her situation with less fortunate others, creating hypothetical worse worlds, and deriving benefits from the experience.

These self-enhancing strategies are effective for reducing the likelihood of perceiving oneself as a victim (Burgess & Holmstrom, 1979). Redefining the event minimizes the threat to one's assumptive world.

➤ Explore possible meanings for the event with the individual to help make sense of it.

> *If victimization can be viewed as serving a purpose, the victim will be able to reestablish a belief in an orderly, comprehensible world (Horowitz, 1983).*

➤ Encourage the person to take action and to change certain behaviors (e.g., get new locks on doors, move, change jobs, take a class in self-defense, get an unlisted phone number).

> *These actions can foster a sense of personal control and safety, minimize vulnerability, and maximize positive self-perceptions (Taylor, 1983).*

➤ Provide positive emotional support; direct person to groups and people who will give social support.

> *It is important that the victim reestablish psychological well-being by enhancing self-esteem and demonstrating a benevolent view of the world (Figley, 1985).*

➤ Differentiate between characterologic self-blame (e.g., "I am a stupid person to have trusted him") and behavioral self-blame (e.g., "I did a stupid thing to get in the car with a stranger.").

> *Characterologic self-blame is associated with depression. Behavioral self-blame may be an effective strategy to enable the victim to believe in his or her control over future victimizations by modifying the "blamed" behavior (Janoff-Bulman, 1985).*

➤ Suggest that the victim is not responsible for what happened, but she or he is responsible and in control of own recovery from the event.

> *People can be powerless in preventing their own victimization, but they can be powerful in learning to cope with it (Figley, 1985).*

Additional Nursing Orders for THE ADULT PATIENT WITH TRAUMA AFTER CHILDHOOD INCEST

➤ Build a trusting relationship with the patient.

> *An inability to trust others is the most prevalent and pervasive effect of childhood incest. This results in extreme ambivalence concerning intimacy, minimal self-disclosure, and a sense of worthlessness (Johnson, 1989).*

➤ Be nonjudgmental, listen attentively, and accept what the patient says.

> *This fosters trust. Nurses who can promote disclosure in a gentle, therapeutic manner have a considerable positive impact on these patients (Greenfeld, 1990). The therapeutic process can be successful only if it is based on uncovering the truth about the patient's childhood instead of denying that reality (Miller, 1984).*

➤ Recognize that symptoms of incest may be present in other problems (e.g., personality disorders, relationship problems, depression, low self-esteem, lack of trust, feelings of powerlessness or anxiety, sexual problems, alienation, self-destructive behavior).

> *These patients usually seek treatment for problems other than incest. This disguised presentation, where the history of incest remains hidden and negative effects are not available for treatment, is very common (Johnson, 1989).*

➤ Question the patient directly about abuse (e.g., ask, "Have you ever had an adverse sexual experience where someone tried to touch you or have sex with you against your will?").

> *The patient may still deny abuse, but direct questioning enables the person with a history of abuse to address the issue later when she or he feels safer (Gise & Paddison, 1988).*

➤ Provide an atmosphere of safety and protection. Be aware of and respect the amount of distance the patient needs to feel secure, how touching may feel to this patient, what you as an authority figure may represent, what your gender signifies, and the kind of eye contact that feels safe to the patient.

> *This atmosphere is integral to the patient feeling safe enough to discuss and explore this threatening issue (Greenfeld, 1990).*

➤ Encourage patient to begin to get in touch with the repressed emotions; point out that the powerful emotions connected to past experiences are not part of present reality.

> *Memories of abuse are out of conscious awareness.*

➤ Use the analogy of the "child" inside each one of us to understand the patient's feelings of vulnerability.

> *The seriously abused child is panicky and overwhelmed, trusts no one, allows no one to see the pain.*

➤ Teach patient to accept the child within and what this child feels, thinks, and remembers.

> *The child must be allowed to tell all about the past experience and not be questioned, disbelieved, or denied.*

➤ Explain that the panic attacks, physical pain, and frightening memories are simply the child reaching out.

> *Recollection of the incest can be extremely painful and can bring up feelings of guilt, anger, shame, and an intensification of symptoms. The memories can be terrifying and cause further repression if the process is not understood (Blake-White & Kline, 1985).*

➤ Reinforce that you hear what the patient says, that you believe him or her, that you will not abandon him or her, and that the feelings are a normal response to the trauma.

> *This reinforcement combats the patient's sense of shame, guilt, and helplessness, and will help him or her feel alone and more connected.*

➤ Encourage patient to explore feelings about having been abused.

> *In order to get to the origin of the feelings the patient is experiencing they must be explored and uncovered (Miller, 1984).*

➤ Support the patient when feelings of fear, anxiety, confusion, and anger surface.

> *"Closing off" and "opening up" are the two general stages of mourning after incest. Opening up begins when the patient expresses rage and anger, and is a necessary part of the healing process (Hays, 1985).*

➤ Teach patient supplementary ways of getting in touch with the feelings (e.g., journal writing, role playing, writing letters, drawing).

> *Withdrawn patients sometimes respond better to alternatives to talking as a way to break gently into dealing with their feelings.*

➤ Explore with patient how the abuse affects patient and how it impacts on patient's daily life.

> *This exploration prevents the patient from trying to keep the abuse a secret and bearing the burden alone (Rawlins & Heacock, 1988). It also helps the patient become more aware of the full extent of the effect of the trauma.*

➤ Teach patient about normal and common responses to incest.

> *This information can make the patient feel supported, less alone, and more secure with the knowledge that other victims have responded similarly.*

➤ Promote a sense of hope and confidence that in time the impact of the incest will diminish in intensity.

> *This will help to restore the patient's faith in self, others, and the world in general (Rawlins & Heacock, 1988).*

Charting Components

➤ Ability to trust
➤ Attitudes regarding sexuality
➤ Degree of anxiety
➤ Feelings expressed about incidents
➤ Relationship status
➤ Self-destructive behaviors
➤ Suicidal ideation

7. Rape-Trauma Syndrome

Definition

Forced, violent sexual penetration against the victim's will and consent; the trauma syndrome that develops from this attack or attempted attack includes an acute phase of disorganization of the victim's life-style and long-term process of reorganization of life-style

Related to

➤ Anxiety, fear
➤ Alterations in sleep patterns
➤ Anger, resentment, humiliation, self-blame, guilt, depression
➤ Emotional numbness
➤ Difficulty with relationships
➤ Negative self-image
➤ Feelings of isolation

Content appearing in this typeface is additional information not included in the NANDA nursing diagnoses.

Characteristics/Assessment Findings

➤ Acute phase
  ▷ emotional reactions (e.g., anger, embarrassment, fear of physical violence and death, humiliation, revenge, self-blame)
  ▷ multiple physical symptoms (e.g., GI irritability, GU discomfort, muscle tension, sleep-pattern disturbance)
➤ Long-term phase: change in life-style (e.g., change in residence, dealing with repetitive nightmares and phobias, seeking family support, seeking social support)
➤ Compound reaction (in addition to characteristics outlined above): reactivated symptoms of previous conditions (i.e., physical illness, psychiatric illness, reliance on alcohol or drugs)
➤ Silven reaction
  ▷ abrupt changes in relationships with men
  ▷ increase in nightmares
  ▷ increased anxiety during interview (e.g., blocking of associations, long periods of silence, minor stuttering, physical distress)
  ▷ pronounced changes in sexual behavior
  ▷ no verbalization of the occurrence of rape
  ▷ sudden onset of phobic reactions
  ▷ inadequate social support

Expected Outcomes/Goals

The patient will
➤ share feelings, issues, and concerns related to the rape as evidenced by
  ▷ verbalizing feelings of guilt, self-blame, being "out of control," anger, fear of being alone, sadness, fear of life-threatening violence
  ▷ acknowledging that these feelings and reactions are common and will decrease over time
  ▷ discussing anxieties related to resumption of sexual activity following rape (e.g., fears of being rejected by partner, intrusive memories of the attack, physical discomfort during sexual activity).
➤ resume normal activities of daily life as evidenced by
  ▷ sleeping at night without nightmares/awakening
  ▷ going back to work or school
  ▷ caring for family and household.
➤ use support system in coping with rape as evidenced by
  ▷ sharing fears, concerns, and reactions with friends or family members
  ▷ accepting attempts of others to be supportive
  ▷ contacting local rape crisis center for additional support (e.g., group, information, self-defense classes).
➤ integrate the experience of sexual assault as evidenced by
  ▷ verbalizing that she or he is not responsible for the rape
  ▷ resuming prerape functional status or demonstrating a higher level of coping skills
  ▷ expressing feelings of being "in control"; making decisions to reestablish sense of control.

Nursing Orders with Rationale

➤ Assess and monitor for presence/absence/changes in assessment findings outlined above *in order to detect any change in status.*

➤ Identify and address own learning needs and feelings related to rape.
  There are many myths and misconceptions related to rape, which can affect the quality of care given to the patient (Rose, 1989). One study reported that nurses may react negatively to a victim who demonstrated carelessness in locking a car door prior to the rape (Damrosch, Gallo, Kulak, & Whitaker, 1987).

➤ Identify the style of coping that the patient is using to deal with the trauma of rape.
  Immediately following rape, the patient may demonstrate a wide range of behaviors from calm and collected, controlled style, to acute psychic distress (Green, 1988).

➤ Provide support to the patient in a nonjudgmental fashion.
  A supportive setting allows the patient to discuss fears and concerns.

➤ Allow an opportunity for the patient to verbalize feelings related to the rape; use reflection and empathy to encourage expression of painful feelings (e.g., "It must have been terribly frightening to feel so helpless.").
  Intervening early with a rape victim can reduce the amount of psychological damage (Aguilera, 1990). Memories of other losses may be triggered by the rape.

➤ Encourage the patient to tell own story with as much detail as possible.

Telling what happened can help to "desensitize" the victim to the experience and diminish its emotional impact (Koss & Harvey, 1987). It can also help to identify what meaning the event has for the victim, and issues and concerns the victim has about rage.

➤ Provide reassurance that feelings of fear, anger/ rage, anxiety, and self-blame are reactions that are commonly seen in victims of rape.

The wide range of emotions expressed by rape victims is a normal reaction to an "abnormal" situation. Rape is a "sudden overwhelming experience for which usual coping mechanisms probably are inadequate" (Aguilera, 1990).

➤ Be particularly sensitive to the unique issues that male rape victims experience; encourage them to express feelings and beliefs about self and the situation.

The male rape victim may experience feelings of guilt and self-blame if he holds the belief that men should always be able to protect themselves from others.

➤ Provide reassurance that however the individual coped at the time of the attack was the right thing because she or he is alive to tell of the experience.

A wide range of coping behaviors is used by the victim to deal with the life-threatening situation of sexual assault (Burgess & Holmstrom, 1976).

➤ Identify the positive coping strategies used and emphasize that submission does not imply consent.

Pointing out positive coping strategies used during the rape can help lessen feelings of guilt (Katz & Burt, 1988).

➤ Assess victim's patterns of coping in past "crisis" situations, presence of social support system, and patient's "perception of the event."

Prior coping behaviors, social support systems, and perception of the event are balancing factors in the victim's successful resolution of the current crisis (Aguilera, 1990).

➤ Provide patient with information about common responses that occur after a sexual assault

to help predict and prepare the patient for possible future reactions. Phobic reactions are common following rape, especially to situations or places that have a connection to the rape or trigger memories (e.g., men wearing plaid shirts or a particular cologne).

➤ Refer patient to local rape crisis center

to provide patient with additional support in dealing with issues related to the sexual assault.

➤ Help patient to explore options but refrain from making decisions or choices for the patient.

Feelings of loss of control are a serious issue for many rape victims; restoration of this sense of control is an important step in the recovery process.

➤ Encourage patient to discuss troubling dreams or nightmares.

Two types of dreams often occur in female rape victims: dreams in which the victim "wishes to do something but then wakes before acting," and dreams in which the content evolved over time to the point where the victim achieved mastery over the assault situation (Burgess & Holmstrom, 1974).

➤ Encourage patient to maintain a regular program of exercise

to help relieve feelings of anxiety and to enhance patient's ability to sleep at night.

➤ Encourage to make whatever changes are needed in own home to make it a more secure environment (e.g., change locks on doors and windows, get a dog)

to promote feelings of safety and security, and to increase feelings of control.

➤ Encourage to discuss issues and concerns related to sexuality

to assess for patient's status and to identify problems and issues of concern to the patient.

➤ Encourage to report changes in sexual activity including a change in frequency, changes in ability to experience orgasm, and feelings related to touching and being touched.

It is common for rape victims to have difficulty resuming sexual relations. Male and female sexual partners of victims can react either positively or negatively to the victim following rape.

➤ Provide significant others opportunities to verbalize feelings related to rape and the victim.

Family members may initially experience some of the same crisis-related reactions as the victim. Often male partners of the victim experience guilt for not having been able to protect the victim. Family members may resolve their own issues related to the rape faster than the victim and become impatient with the person (Koss & Harvey, 1987).

➤ Elicit from the family what they know and believe about rape and people who get raped.

Family and friends of the victim often hold inaccurate views about rape or find their own reactions to be confused or somehow affected by the myths surrounding sexual assault (e.g., the victim did something to provoke it).

➤ Provide information to the victim's significant others about sexual assault and its aftermath.

Predicting for the family some of the psychological reactions they and the victim may experience will help "normalize" the situation for them, give a greater sense of control over the situation, and assist them in their efforts to be supportive of the victim.

➤ Discourage the family from trying to overprotect the victim.

The family may seek to protect the victim by either trying to distract him or her or by not talking about the rape. Avoiding the subject of the rape can deny support much needed by the victim (Heinrich, 1987).

➤ Discourage significant others from acting on impulses to get revenge on the assailant.

Energy placed toward getting revenge will not be available to provide support for the victim and will probably result in criminal charges.

➤ Be aware that there are many other issues that homosexual rape victims must deal with in addition to the rape.

Gay men and lesbian women are frequently targets of hate crimes or are raped "opportunistically" in an effort to degrade homosexuality. Homosexual victims may perceive the sexual assault to be punishment for their sexual orientation (Garnets, Herek, & Levy, 1990).

Charting Components

➤ Ability to make decisions
➤ Anxiety, fear
➤ Availability and use of support systems
➤ Feelings of depression/thoughts of suicide
➤ Feelings related to sense of control
➤ Measures taken by the nurse to provide supportive relationship to patient
➤ Measures taken/planned to increase sense of safety and security
➤ Referrals made

➤ Resolution (or nonresolution) of issues and concerns related to sexuality
➤ Sharing feelings with friends, family
➤ Sleep disturbances, experience of nightmares
➤ Statements of who is responsible for the rape
➤ Steps taken to resume normal daily activities; results
➤ Verbalization of feelings, fears, and reactions related to the rape
➤ Verbalizations of feeling in control

Additional Nursing Orders for
THE PATIENT WITH RAPE-TRAUMA SYNDROME: COMPOUND OR SILENT REACTION

➤ Refer to nursing care plan "Posttrauma Response" for interventions on how to deal with posttrauma stress symptoms.

There is clear evidence that most rape victims reexperience the traumatic event, have a numbing of responsiveness, and reduce involvement with the external world. They also display avoidance behaviors, hyperalertness, and intensification of symptoms when exposed to rape-related cues (Kilpatrick, Veronen, & Best, 1985).

➤ Assess for history of psychiatric or somatic symptoms or a history of substance abuse.

The victim may experience resurgence or exacerbation of physical or psychiatric symptoms following sexual assault. Additional symptoms may develop, including depression, acting-out behaviors related to sexual activity, or use of alcohol or drugs (Koss & Harvey, 1987).

➤ Explore with the patient the effect that the rape may have on other symptoms.

Increased stress can exacerbate many psychiatric symptoms. A rape victim who also has a psychotic disorder—with the associated problems of trust, ego-boundary diffusion, and social isolation— faces a complex recovery process (Rinear, 1985).

➤ Help patient to understand when his or her rights have been violated.

Patients with preexisting emotional problems or psychiatric illness may have difficulty identifying the dynamics of the rape experience (Rinear, 1985).

➤ Encourage patient to seek feedback from others related to how situations are perceived and handled.

Psychiatric patients often have impaired social skills and judgment about situations and people, which may increase their vulnerability to sexual assault. Individuals with perceptual difficulties may have diminished capacity for anticipating dangerous situations (Rinear, 1985).

➤ Assess for unresolved past sexual trauma.

Some victims have not told others about the sexual assault and are denied the social support, catharsis, or validation of their status as a victim (Koss & Harvey, 1987).

➤ Assess and monitor for anxiety, phobic reactions, difficulty in maintaining relationships with men, avoidance of sexual relationships, or continued feelings of low self-esteem or self-blame.

While the patient may not relate symptoms to unresolved sexual trauma, there will be need for assistance in integrating the sexual-trauma experience (Koss & Harvey, 1987).

➤ When appropriate, discuss special issues of vulnerability (e.g., youth, old age, physical deformity or handicap); help patient to assess own style of coping with situations, especially those that are potentially dangerous.

Rapists often choose victims because of some special vulnerability (Rinear, 1985).

➤ Make referrals to therapists experienced in dealing with issues related to sexual assault.

Additional therapy can provide patient with support in obtaining assistance needed to work through the sexual trauma.

Additional Charting Components

➤ Changes in relationships with men, sexuality
➤ History of past sexual trauma
➤ Impact of stress on psychiatric symptoms
➤ Phobic reactions
➤ Posttrauma stress symptoms
➤ Referrals made
➤ Patient/family teaching related to special vulnerabilities, response

C. EMOTIONAL STATE

1. Anxiety

Definition

A vague uneasy feeling whose source is often non-specific or unknown to the individual

Related to

- ➤ Unconscious conflicts about essential values/goals of life
- ➤ Threat to self-concept
- ➤ Threat of death
- ➤ Threat to or change in health status
- ➤ Threat to or change in role functioning
- ➤ Threat to or change in environment
- ➤ Threat to or change in interaction patterns
- ➤ **Situational or maturational crisis** (e.g., hospitalization, treatments, diagnostic tests; becoming a parent, children leaving home)
- ➤ **Interpersonal transmission/contagion**
- ➤ **Unmet needs** (emotional, physical, spiritual)
- ➤ Lack of knowledge regarding illness
- ➤ Loss of status prestige, recognition, valued possessions, significant others, economic security, control
- ➤ Powerlessness, helplessness
- ➤ Threat to financial status, life-style, family stability
- ➤ Pathological factors: food, air, water (i.e., anything interfering with basic needs)
- ➤ Situational factors: stress, noise, change, technology, society, life events
- ➤ Maturational factors: unresolved conflicts in early life stages, inconsistent limit setting, inappropriate punishment

Characteristics/Assessment Findings

Subjective
- ➤ Increased tension, apprehension
- ➤ Painful and persistent increased helplessness
- ➤ Fearful, scared, uncertainty
- ➤ Regretful
- ➤ Overexcited, rattled
- ➤ Distressed
- ➤ Jittery, shakiness
- ➤ Feelings of inadequacy
- ➤ Fear of unspecific consequences
- ➤ Expressed concerns regarding change in life events
- ➤ Worried, anxious
- ➤ Confusion
- ➤ Difficulty concentrating, poor memory
- ➤ Distorted time sense
- ➤ Narrowed perceptual field, tunnel vision
- ➤ Indecisiveness, losing control
- ➤ Oversensitivity, nervousness
- ➤ Selective inattention, inability to learn or think clearly
- ➤ Apprehension
- ➤ Inability to integrate environment with the self
- ➤ Inability to function, disorganized physical ability (e.g., frozen)

Objective
- ➤ *Sympathetic stimulation: cardiovascular excitation, superficial vasoconstriction, pupil dilation
- ➤ Restlessness
- ➤ Insomnia
- ➤ Glancing about
- ➤ Poor eye contact
- ➤ Trembling/hand tremors
- ➤ Extraneous movement (e.g., foot shuffling, hard/arm movements)
- ➤ Facial tension
- ➤ Voice quivering
- ➤ Focus on self
- ➤ Increased wariness
- ➤ Increased perspiration

Content appearing in this typeface is additional information not included in the NANDA nursing diagnoses.

*Critical.

- GI changes in bowel, eating patterns; dry mouth, indigestion, nausea
- Motor activity changes: shuffling, hand/arm movements
- Muscular changes: muscle tension, fatigue, restlessness, weakness, trembling/hand tremors
- Respiratory changes: dyspnea, hyperventilation
- Acting out, agitation
- Angry outbursts, irritability
- Asking same question repeatedly
- Crying, complaining
- Cold clammy hands
- Pressured speech, rumination
- Refusing treatments
- Self-criticism and depreciation
- Statements that reflect inability to cope
- Dilated pupils
- Personality disorganization (in panic attacks)
- Difficulty communicating

Expected Outcomes/Goals

The patient will

- recognize own behaviors of anxiety as evidenced by telling nurse when she or he is feeling anxious.
- gain insight regarding precipitating factors as evidenced by linking precipitating events with anxious feelings.
- reduce anxiety at least one level as evidenced by exhibiting a decrease in anxious behavior.
- become aware of usual coping methods and effectiveness as evidenced by stating past coping techniques and evaluating degree of effectiveness.
- learn and demonstrate alternative methods of coping as evidenced by demonstrating at least two new effective coping mechanisms.

Nursing Orders with Rationale

- Assess and monitor for presence/absence/ changes in assessment findings outlined above *in order to detect any change in status.*

- Assess the patient's perception of threat, precipitating factors and current stressors, physiological factors that may be contributing to the anxiety.
  The intensity of the patient's anxiety is related to the severity of the threat, the accuracy of the perception, and the person's ability to cope with all the factors and feelings (Beck, Rawlins, & Williams, 1988).

- Identify recent changes and their meaning to patient.
  Change signifies the loss of something and can precipitate feelings of being unable to cope, overwhelmed (Carpenito, 1989).

- Determine the degree of perceived disruption, defense and coping mechanisms used.
  Coping mechanisms can be effective in reducing anxiety.

- Identify and examine patterns of coping; reinforce effective and constructive coping mechanisms; teach alternative methods (e.g., relaxation techniques, guided imagery, deep breathing, talking it out).
  People develop a repertoire of coping behaviors that can be adaptive or maladaptive.

- Prevent anxiety from escalating by providing reassurance, comfort; give brief factual information.
  Information and the presence of another person provide a sense of security.

- Assess the level of anxiety being experienced and plan interventions according to the level of anxiety (e.g., moderate, severe, panic) that is being exhibited.
  Anxiety occurs at different levels of intensity and requires more specific controls when it escalates (Beck et al., 1988).

Content appearing in this typeface is additional information not included in the NANDA nursing diagnoses.

Additional Nursing Orders for THE PATIENT EXHIBITING MODERATE ANXIETY

➤ Assist to recognize anxiety by exploring the feelings that precede anxious behavior.

> *Recognition of anxiety and precipitating events promotes future problem solving to prevent anxiety.*

➤ Evaluate the perceived threat by exploring what the expectations of the situation were: was this realistic? what needs are unmet?

> *Unrealistic expectations and unmet needs precede anxiety (McFarland & Wasli, 1986).*

➤ Provide a new perspective on the situation by helping the patient "redefine" the problem in a way that is solvable.

> *Correcting distorted perceptions increases the possibility of finding workable solutions to a problem.*

➤ Give information regarding diagnosis, treatment, expected outcomes; discuss patient's fears and perceptions of these events.

> *Health teaching and factual information regarding patient's illness ensure accurate perceptions, alternatives, and reassurance for the patient (Carpenito, 1989).*

➤ Give feedback about present reality, how you perceive the situation, the patient's expectations, and possibilities for getting needs met.

> *Feedback helps to focus the individual on the broader aspects of the situation and to take more factors into account (McFarland & Wasli, 1986).*

➤ Encourage descriptions of feelings and events without asking, "Why?"

> *Questions tend to increase anxiety and frustration (McFarland & Wasli, 1986).*

➤ Monitor your own reactions to patient's anxiety; use deep breathing and quiet pauses to maintain own equilibrium.

> *Anxiety is contagious (Carpenito, 1989).*

➤ Administer antianxiety medication as ordered; evaluate the effects/side effects.

> *Uncontrolled anxiety may require minor tranquilizers (Haber, Hoskins, Leach, & Sideleau, 1987).*

➤ Redirect attention from rumination to concrete tasks and activities that do not require concentration.

> *Activity uses energy and dissipates the physical responses to anxiety. Repetitive actions are helpful in concentrating attention.*

➤ Teach the signs and symptoms of anxiety and the importance of recognizing escalating anxiety before it reaches the panic stage.

> *The goal is to prevent anxiety from mounting and becoming uncontrollable.*

➤ Identify with patient-specific coping techniques to use in the moment to lower anxiety (e.g., deep breathing, verbalization of the feeling of anxiety to someone).

> *Adaptive coping behaviors can prevent escalation of anxiety.*

➤ Teach assertive techniques, problem solving, and stress management.

> *These strategies help to promote future problem solving to prevent anxiety.*

Additional Nursing Orders for THE PATIENT EXHIBITING SEVERE ANXIETY/PANIC

➤ Lend perspective as needed to correct distortions, reestablish realistic expectations, open up tunnel vision.

> *High anxiety affects the individual's ability to see a broader perspective (Beck et al., 1988).*

➤ Recognize the need for outlet of high anxiety through physical activities such as walking, pacing, running, yelling, punching a bag; make arrangements as needed.

> *Activity use energy and dissipates the physical responses to anxiety.*

➤ Stay with the patient; instruct to take slow, deep breaths; breathe with patient; provide comfort measures (e.g., bath, exercise, back rub, warm drink).

> *Your quiet presence and appropriate touch will convey empathy and reassurance.*

➤ Decrease sensory stimulation by providing a quiet environment.

> *Limits provide a sense of control and security.*

➤ Speak in a calm, modulated voice; use short, simple sentences.
   Anxiety is contagious; conveying a sense of calmness reduces anxiety (Haber et al., 1987).

➤ Give precise directions as needed without making unnecessary demands; focus on the here and now.
   Anxiety limits the ability to focus, recall information, or attend to more than one thing at a time (Haber et al., 1987).

Charting Components

➤ Effects/side effects of medications
➤ Factors contributing to anxiety
➤ Level of anxiety before and after intervention
➤ Patient's stated feeling of change in anxiety level
➤ Subjective/objective manifestations of anxiety, any changes therein
➤ Successful techniques used to decrease anxiety
➤ Patient/family teaching, response

Additional Nursing Orders for
THE PATIENT WITH OBSESSIVE-COMPULSIVE DISORDER

➤ Do not try to prevent or call attention to the patient's compulsive acts.
   This may result in increased anxiety.

➤ Acknowledge rumination, then try to redirect interaction in a positive direction; if patient continues to ruminate, withdraw attention and state when you will be back.
   Patients can learn to stop obsessive thoughts.

➤ Positively reinforce nonritualistic behavior.
   Reinforce only positive behavior that deals with anxiety.

➤ Discuss pattern of behavior with patient; focus on events that occur before the ritualistic behaviors; work with patient to identify stressors, concern, anxieties, and fears.
   Coping with anxiety and intense feelings is a learned behavior; anticipatory guidance can assist the patient to learn to identify and cope with feeling (Stuart & Sundeen, 1987).

➤ Establish reasonable time limits for doing rituals, allow adequate time to prepare for next activity
   to prevent further stress of patient harming self through neglect or repetition of a potentially harmful ritual (e.g., repetitive handwashing) (Reighley, 1988).

➤ Observe the patient's eating, drinking, elimination, and hygiene patterns; assist as necessary so patient will have time for ritualistic behavior and ADL.
   Patients with obsessive-compulsive behaviors often get too involved with rituals to do ADL (Beck et al., 1988).

➤ Use empathic responses and reflective statements to assist patient to describe own feelings.
   This will help patient to gain control of overwhelming feelings and impulses (Reighley, 1988).

➤ Encourage attendance at groups that focus on expression of feelings (e.g., assertiveness training, psychodrama, art therapy)
   to help the patient learn alternative ways to express feelings.

Additional Charting Components

➤ Level of anxiety
➤ Quality of ADL, need for assistance
➤ Rituals engaged in, frequency
➤ Success in limiting ritualistic behavior

Additional Nursing Orders for
THE PATIENT WITH PANIC DISORDER

➤ Stay with patient; offer reassurance that she or he is not dying, will not lose consciousness, that you can help.
   The most frightening aspect of a panic attack is the loss of control, altered awareness of surroundings, and the fear of having a heart attack or losing one's mind (Beck et al., 1988).

➤ Have patient take long, deep breaths; breathe with the person to facilitate compliance.
   Slow, deep breathing quickly reduces panic to a manageable level of anxiety.

➤ Reassure with calmness and short sentences that patient is experiencing the physical symptoms of anxiety, not a physical illness.
   People having a panic attack are convinced that the physiological symptoms are indicative of a stroke, heart attack, or impending death (Beck et al., 1988).

➤ Ask the patient, "What are you afraid of during an attack?" "Can you identify any specific feelings that preceded the attack?"
   Physiological sensations usually occur first, followed by autonomic thoughts of "I'm losing my grip." "I'm going out of my mind." "I'm having a stroke." (Beck et al., 1988).

➤ Help patient to see the connection between the physical sensations and his or her interpretation of them as harmful and dangerous; suggest other possibilities (e.g., anxiety causes sensations similar to a heart attack).

> *Cognitive distortions of the meaning of events leads to mental blocking, confusion, and escalates the anxiety.*

➤ Refer to interventions below for "Generalized Anxiety Disorder" for cognitive techniques to reduce anxiety.

➤ Give beta-adrenergic blocker drugs as prescribed by physician.

> *These drugs reduce tachycardia, faintness, freezing, and tremors associated with panic attacks (Beck et al., 1988).*

Additional Charting Components

➤ Behavior during an attack
➤ Effects/side effects of medication
➤ Precipitants to the panic attack
➤ Techniques that diminish the fear and anxiety

Additonal Nursing Orders for
THE PATIENT WITH GENERALIZED ANXIETY DISORDER

➤ Introduce patient to the principles of cognitive therapy by communicating that anxiety is maintained by mistaken or dysfunctional appraisal of a situation; that it is a result of exaggerated, automatic thinking.

> *The cognitive model of anxiety is used as a basis for intervention and is explicitly given as the rationale for treatment (Beck et al., 1988).*

➤ Explain the symptoms of anxiety in detail.

> *Understanding the symptoms will decrease the patient's excessive concern for them.*

➤ Discuss physiological symptoms of anxiety as a natural bodily reaction to threat; explain the fight-flight-freeze response and the difference between the parasympathetic and sympathetic systems in dealing with stress.

> *Explanations can normalize much of the mystery attached to a symptom (Haber et al., 1988).*

➤ Stay focused on manageable problems when instituting a course of cognitive therapy; keep it simple, specific, and concrete; stress doing homework as a chance of getting better fast.

> *The typical course of cognitive therapy for anxiety is from 5 to 20 sessions. Specific performance anxieties or mild anxiety states may be alleviated in a few sessions (Beck et al., 1988).*

➤ Ask questions that expand the patient's constricted thinking:

▷ Where is the evidence that this is true?
▷ Where is the logic?
▷ What do you have to lose?
▷ What do you have to gain?
▷ What would be the worst thing that could happen?
▷ What can you learn from this experience?
▷ Are you thinking in all-or-nothing terms?
▷ Is your information source reliable?
▷ Are your judgments based on feelings rather than facts?

> *Good questions can clarify the patient's statements, awaken the patient's interest, open up a previously closed system of logic, help the patient to think in a new way about his or her problem, and enhance the patient's ability to observe self (Beck et al., 1988).*

➤ Generate alternative interpretations; help the patient to consider other possibilities besides dire predictions; provide realistic information

> *to enable the person to reassess the potential of danger.*

➤ Enlarge the perspective by looking at some of the positive attributes to the anxiety (e.g., a way to teach acceptance, increasing tolerance of frustration).

> *The anxious patient has tunnel vision of a situation and is unable to see the broader perspective.*

➤ Teach the patient to recognize distorted automatic thoughts (e.g., use of words like *should, never, always*) and how to respond to distorted thoughts with logic, reason, and empirical testing (i.e., asking questions).

> *Recognition of distorted thinking allows the possibility of developing more balanced thoughts based on reality.*

➤ Teach the patient to replace "why" am I anxious to "how " she or he is creating the anxiety.
Focusing on "how" switches a person out of the thinking self to the observing self. Asking "why" elicits more thinking and less awareness (Beck et al., 1988).

➤ Have patient comment on own anxiety, behavior, and thoughts by referring to self by first name (e.g., "John seems to be scared, his heart is beating." "John is concerned about what people are thinking about him.")
A patient can increase self-awareness by voluntarily choosing to distance self from own anxiety (Beck et al., 1988)

➤ Have the patient count own thoughts during those times when he cannot slow down his mind enough to correct his distortions
  ▷ count specific types of anxiety-producing thoughts
  ▷ count thoughts in the midst of an anxiety attack (may help person to gain mastery over situation)
  ▷ count at random time periods of 10 minutes
  ▷ count during selected time periods (e.g., from 5 P.M. to 7 P.M.)
    Counting allows patient to distance self from own thoughts, gain a sense of mastery over them, and recognize their automatic quality (Beck et al., 1988).

➤ Use the turnoff technique with patients who are reliving a traumatic event or experiencing repeated fantasies of danger to help them gain mastery over the fantasy:
  ▷ clap your hands when the patient is having the fantasy.
  ▷ teach patient to clap own hands whenever the fantasy starts.
  ▷ instruct family members to clap when patient's fantasy occurs.
  ▷ practice hand clapping until the patient is able to stop the fantasy and reduce the anxiety.
    Increasing sensory input and using distraction can eliminate intrusive thoughts and fantasy (Beck et al., 1988).

➤ Inquire about feelings of shame over having anxiety; help the patient to express feelings.
Shame about having anxiety in front of others stems from belief that she or he is being judged as childish, weak, foolish for exhibiting anxiety (Beck et al., 1988).

➤ Instruct patients to act as if they are not anxious; encourage to increase their tolerance for anxiety (e.g., saying "I'm strong enough to take this.").
Getting the patient to act as normally as possible lessens anxiety symptoms. Increased tolerance decreases the anxiety about having anxiety (Beck et al., 1988).

➤ Check to see that medical reasons for the patient's symptoms have been ruled out.
The patient's symptoms may be caused by a physical illness that she or he interprets as anxiety.

Additional Charting Components

➤ Amount of practicing of techniques and exercises
➤ Behavioral techniques implemented
➤ Cognitive techniques taught
➤ Distorted thoughts identified
➤ Level of anxiety before and after treatment
➤ Techniques that reduced anxiety
➤ Willingness to do cognitive restructuring

2. Fear

Definition

A feeling of dread related to an identifiable source that the person validates

Related to

➤ Early experiences of losses in life
➤ Pain or disappointment that are denied by person
➤ Feelings of powerlessness in life
➤ Lack of trust
➤ Low self-esteem
➤ Disabling or long-term/terminal illness
➤ Hospitalization
➤ Knowledge deficit
➤ Loss of function or body part
➤ Relinquishing roles
➤ Loss of job
➤ Separation from support system
➤ Sudden noise, darkness, pain
➤ Threat of death
➤ Treatments and invasive procedures
➤ Unfamiliar surroundings

Content appearing in this typeface is additional information not included in the NANDA nursing diagnoses.

Characteristics/Assessment Findings

➤ Ability to identify object of fear

Subjective
➤ Afraid, frightened, terrified, suspicious
➤ Feeling a loss of control and power
➤ Hypervigilance
➤ Increased alertness/concentration on source of fear
➤ Nightmares
➤ Panicky, jittery

Objective
➤ Constant questioning or repeating same question (i.e., ruminating)
➤ Demanding, aggressive behavior
➤ Inability to carry out ADL
➤ Social isolation
➤ Avoids being alone in public places (e.g., crowds, tunnels, public transportation)
➤ Pacing and other psychomotor disturbances
➤ Diaphoresis
➤ Increased verbalization
➤ Muscle tension, fatigue
➤ Refusing treatments
➤ Tachycardia, tachypnea

Expected Outcomes/Goals

The patient will
➤ identify the fear and its cause as evidenced by verbalization of the feared object or situation.
➤ focus on eliminating or reducing the source of the fear as evidenced by
  ▷ talking about the fear directly
  ▷ discussing ways to reduce the fear.
➤ learn and use adaptive coping and problem solving to manage fear as evidenced by
  ▷ implementing coping mechanisms to deal with the fear
  ▷ identifying past coping that has been helpful
  ▷ verbalizing reduced feelings of fear.
➤ comply with medication regimen in the hospital as evidenced by
  ▷ taking all medications
  ▷ allowing staff to check for possible cheeking (if suspected).

Content appearing in this typeface is additional information not included in the NANDA nursing diagnoses.

Nursing Orders with Rationale

➤ Assess and monitor for presence/absence/ changes in assessment findings outlined above *in order to detect any change in status.*

➤ Approach the patient frequently for interaction *to establish trusting relationship.*

➤ Identify the specific source of the fear, using indirect, open-ended questions (e.g., "What concerns you most about being hospitalized?").
Fear is a response to a specific external threat that is identifiable (Carpenito, 1989).

➤ Assess the degree of fear, the reality of the perceived threat, the extent to which fear interferes with functioning.
Fear can lead to disequilibrium, affecting the patient's ability to cope, make decisions, or perceive the situation accurately (Carpenito, 1989).

➤ Ensure patient understands hospital schedule, procedures, treatments by giving careful explanations at the patient's level of understanding; prepare patient for what to expect; have patient repeat in own words what she or he comprehends about the events that will occur.
Information about the unknown provides a sense of adequacy in confronting the fear.

➤ Spend time with patient each day; direct the conversation toward responses to hospitalization; reinforce discussion on reactions and questions concerning diagnosis and treatment.
Fear is reduced when thoughts and feelings are expressed.

➤ Acknowledge the fears inherent in repeated hospitalizations and concerns for the unknown.
Fear is a natural response to illness, hospitalization, unpredictable outcomes (Beck, Rawlins, & Williams, 1984).

➤ Be nonthreatening and calm in all approaches to the patient; answer all questions honestly, avoiding vague or evasive remarks.
These strategies will help to decrease sense of threat, feelings of hostility and aggression.

➤ Encourage patient to face the fear by talking about it; correct distorted perceptions; direct patient to question physician regarding prognosis and expected outcome of hospitalization.
Fear is reduced when the reality of a situation is confronted (Haber, Hoskins, Leach, & Sideleau, 1987).

➤ Do not allow patient to ruminate or ramble indefinitely about fears; redirect to talk about feelings regarding fears.
Rumination only increases anxiety.

➤ Engage the patient in one-to-one activities at first, then activities in small groups, and gradually activities in large groups.
Increasing activity with others will decrease isolation, help patient join milieu, and develop relationships with other patients and staff.

➤ Observe patient for expression of fears; try to note environmental factors that precipitate or escalate symptoms.
Manipulating the environment can decrease or control some fears.

➤ Observe patient closely for agitation; decrease stimuli or move to less stimulating area; seclude if appropriate.
Taking control of the patient's environment can reduce fear considerably.

➤ Place patient in a room near the nursing station or where she or he can be easily observed; avoid placing patient in a room near the exit or stairwell
to decrease fear and to increase sense of security.

➤ Stay with patient or make arrangements for someone to be there when fear is acute.
Fear can become anxiety that can escalate to panic and disorganization (McFarland & Wasli, 1986).

➤ Assess for history of suicidal behavior or present suicidal ideation or plans; closely supervise use of potentially dangerous objects.
The fearful patient might want to defend him- or herself by striking out at others or harming self.

➤ Be aware of and in control of own emotions and reactions to patient's fears.
Fear in the nurse can intensify the patient's feelings that no one is in control (McFarland & Wasli, 1986).

➤ Implement specific and immediate interventions when the fear seems to be overwhelming or out of control (e.g., "Take a deep breath and relax. I will take care of this right now.").
Action will establish firm control of the situation and reduce patient's fears.

➤ Promote patient control of situation as soon as possible; delineate choices available.
A sense of control in dealing with the situation diminishes fear (Beck et al., 1988).

➤ Do not make decisions for the patient; rather, teach problem-solving techniques of identifying the problem, what the options are, the advantages/disadvantages of each option.
The ability to problem solve promotes a sense of adequacy and competency to cope (Carpenito, 1989).

➤ Use soft lights, music, touch as tolerated, and deep breathing when patient is faced with fearful situation.
Specific relaxation techniques enhance patient's control and lessen fear (Beck et al., 1988).

➤ Support usual adaptive coping mechanisms; discuss alternative coping strategies if usual mechanisms are maladaptive.
Successful coping with a dreaded situation decreases fear and increases self-confidence and a sense of mastery.

➤ Encourage expression of other feelings; anger and sorrow are often present, and need to be released along with the fear.
Anger may be an adaptive response to fear.

➤ Involve and give information to significant others so they may reinforce the teaching you have done.
Reinforcement of information is necessary because fear reduces the patient's ability to concentrate, recall, and learn information (Beck et al., 1988).

➤ Allow family and friends to express their fears about the patient's illness so they will be able to support patient and now withdraw.
Unexpressed fear can cause an intensification of feelings and withdrawal from the source of the fear.

Charting Components

➤ Adaptive coping mechanisms used and encouraged
➤ Behavioral/physiological responses to fear
➤ Nursing interventions that decreased patient's fear
➤ Patient's sense of fear increasing, decreasing
➤ Source of patient's fear
➤ Patient/family teaching, response

Additional Nursing Orders for
THE PATIENT WITH PHOBIAS

➤ Differentiate between realistic and unrealistic fears to determine the presence of a phobia.

The main quality of a phobia is that it involves the appraisal of a high degree of risk in a situation that is relatively safe (Beck & Emery, 1985).

➤ Realize that phobias are an exaggerated and often disabling fear whereby anxiety is experienced when the individual is exposed to the feared situation.

The concept of danger arises from the possible consequences of contact with the feared object or situation (Beck & Emery, 1985).

➤ Adjust the patient's initial ADL routine to minimize contact with feared object or situation (e.g., if patient is phobic about eating with others, allow to eat alone in own room).

Patients who have choices can establish some control over the anticipated future danger and avoid it if possible (Reighley, 1988).

➤ Do not attempt to counsel the patient out of the phobia by use of reason.

Recognition or education of the unreasonableness of a fear does not modify it—the appraisal of the fear is caused by cognitive distortions (Beck & Emery, 1985).

➤ Ask the patient what are the feared consequences (both subjectively and objectively) of contacting the object or situation (e.g., a fear of flying may be a fear of dying if the plane crashes).

When the specific content of a fear is elicited, that fear becomes more readily understandable.

➤ Identify the type of phobia and the initial onset of symptoms.

This will help to differentiate between traumatic phobias, which develop as a result of an unpleasant or injurious experience; fixation phobias (fear developed in early childhood that has not been outgrown); and specific phobias (e.g., social rejection, agoraphobia, being cut or bleeding, fear of heights or closed spaces) (Beck & Emery, 1985).

➤ Question the person with multiple phobias about what his or her fear of consequences is for each phobia; try to find a central theme or common denominator.

Many phobic individuals fear more than one object or situation; however, the patient generally fears the occurrence of similar consequences in dissimilar situations (Beck & Emery, 1985).

➤ Point out to the patient that what she or he really fears is his or her feelings and sensations, not the object or situation itself; describe the two levels of fear.

The first level of fear is of the primary danger: fear of public humiliation, dying, of being alone. The second level is fear of the symptoms of anxiety (Beck & Emery, 1985).

➤ Give the patient some concrete ways to handle the second level of fear; refer to nursing care plan "Anxiety" for specific methods.

Cognitive and behavioral techniques can be very helpful in reducing anxiety and fear.

Additional Nursing Orders for
THE PATIENT WITH AGORAPHOBIA

➤ Assess readiness of patient to participate in a program of systematic desensitization if indicated as a therapeutic measure.

Behavior changes can be made with a systematic method of confronting anxiety while in a relaxed state.

➤ Plan carefully how to implement the three separate sets of operation that are required in systematic desensitization.

The goal of systematic desensitization is to help the patient to change his or her response to threatening stimuli (Davies & Janosik, 1991).

➤ Begin with step one: "training in relaxation" by implementing the following techniques:
  ▷ Tell the patient that ordinary relaxing can produce noticeable calming effect, that you are going to teach him or her some methods to relax.
  ▷ Start with the arm: ask patient to grip arm chair tightly, feel the tightness, then gradually relax, noticing the difference in sensations.
  ▷ Have patient describe sensations of tightness and relaxation.
  ▷ Assign patient to practice for two 15-minute periods a day, or guide practice if necessary.
  ▷ Focus on the face muscles in session two; teeth for session three; neck and shoulders for session four; back, abdomen, and thorax for session five; feet and legs for session six.

Relaxation techniques are useful when the patient's level of stress interferes with the ability to function and to be productive.

- Continue with program by implementing step two, "the construction of hierarchies":
  - Identify patient's fears by asking patient to list all disturbing, fearful, and embarrassing situations, thoughts, or feelings (e.g., fear of walking any distance, being alone).
  - Classify the fears into themes of the sources of anxiety (e.g., fear of physical trauma, dying).
  - Have patient rank anxiety-provoking situations from least threatening to most threatening; e.g.,
    - being alone in a library
    - consciousness of being looked at by a girl
    - reading in the library, two men walk by
    - sitting at a table and four people sitting down
    - standing in line to check out a book and several people standing in front and behind.
      The patient can learn to recognize when and how own body responds to stress, and can initiate relaxation exercises accordingly (Wolpe, 1985).

- Implement step three, "counterposing relaxation and anxiety-evoking stimuli from the hierarchies":
  - Relax patient, using above techniques.
  - Use guided imagery to have patient experience the least threatening scene.
  - Have patient describe own feelings.
  - Continue the relaxation training and proceed to the next scene of the hierarchy.
  - Continue through all the scenes until the patient can imagine being in the most threatening one without anxiety.
    The principle of reciprocal inhibition says that two opposing feelings (i.e., anxiety and relaxation) cannot be experienced at the same time (Wolpe, 1985).

- Refer to nursing care plan "Anxiety (Generalized Anxiety Syndrome)" for cognitive techniques to decrease anxiety.

Additional Charting Components

- Degree of impairment due to phobia
- Degree of success with relaxation exercises
- Description of subjects experience of anxiety
- Hierarchy of feared scenes
- Identified cognitive beliefs
- Level of anxiety during and after desensitization program

Appendixes

Contents

NANDA-Approved Nursing Diagnostic Categories

This list represents the NANDA-approved nursing diagnoses for clinical use and testing (1994).

Pattern 1: Exchanging

	1.1.2.1	Altered Nutrition: More than Body Requirements
	1.1.2.2	Altered Nutrition: Less than Body Requirements
	1.1.2.3	Altered Nutrition: Potential for More than Body Requirements
*	1.2.1.1	Risk for Infection
*	1.2.2.1	Risk for Altered Body Temperature
	1.2.2.2	Hypothermia
	1.2.2.3	Hyperthermia
	1.2.2.4	Ineffective Thermoregulation
	1.2.3.1	Dysreflexia
	1.3.1.1	Constipation
	1.3.1.1.1	Perceived Constipation
	1.3.1.1.2	Colonic Constipation
	1.3.1.2	Diarrhea
	1.3.1.3	Bowel Incontinence
	1.3.2	Altered Urinary Elimination
	1.3.2.1.1	Stress Incontinence
	1.3.2.1.2	Reflex Incontinence
	1.3.2.1.3	Urge Incontinence
	1.3.2.1.4	Functional Incontinence
	1.3.2.1.5	Total Incontinence
	1.3.2.2	Urinary Retention
	1.4.1.1	Altered (Specify Type) Tissue Perfusion (Renal, cerebral, cardiopulmonary, gastrointestinal, peripheral)
	1.4.1.2.1	Fluid Volume Excess
	1.4.1.2.2.1	Fluid Volume Deficit
*	1.4.1.2.2.2	Risk for Fluid Volume Deficit
	1.4.2.1	Decreased Cardiac Output
	1.5.1.1	Impaired Gas Exchange
	1.5.1.2	Ineffective Airway Clearance
	1.5.1.3	Ineffective Breathing Pattern
	1.5.1.3.1	Inability to Sustain Spontaneous Ventilation
	1.5.1.3.2	Dysfunctional Ventilatory Weaning Response (DVWR)
*	1.6.1	Risk for Injury
	1.6.1.1	Risk for Suffocation
*	1.6.1.2	Risk for Poisoning
*	1.6.1.3	Risk for Trauma
*	1.6.1.4	Risk for Aspiration
*	1.6.1.5	Risk for Disuse Syndrome
	1.6.2	Altered Protection
	1.6.2.1	Impaired Tissue Integrity
	1.6.2.1.1	Altered Oral Mucous Membrane
	1.6.2.1.2.1	Impaired Skin Integrity
*	1.6.2.1.2.2	Risk for Impaired Skin Integrity
#	1.7.1	Decreased Adaptive Capacity: Intracranial
#	1.8	Energy Field Disturbance

Pattern 2: Communicating

	2.1.1.1	Impaired Verbal Communication

Pattern 3: Relating

	3.1.1	Impaired Social Interaction
	3.1.2	Social Isolation
#	3.1.3	Risk for Loneliness
	3.2.1	Altered Role Performance
	3.2.1.1.1	Altered Parenting
*	3.2.1.1.2	Risk for Altered Parenting
#	3.2.1.1.2.1	Risk for Altered Parent/Infant/Child Attachment
	3.2.1.2.1	Sexual Dysfunction
	3.2.2	Altered Family Processes

*Diagnoses with modified label terminology in 1994. (This change was recommended by the NANDA Taxonomy Committee and adopted to remain consistent with the ICD.)

#New diagnoses added in 1994 classified at level 1.4 using new Criteria for Staging.

	3.2.2.1	Caregiver Role Strain
*	3.2.2.2	Risk for Caregiver Role Strain
#	3.2.2.3.1	Altered Family Process: Alcoholism
	3.2.3.1	Parental Role Conflict
	3.3	Altered Sexuality Patterns

Pattern 4: Valuing

	4.1.1	Spiritual Distress (Distress of the Human Spirit)
#	4.2	Potential for Enhanced Spiritual Well-Being

Pattern 5: Choosing

	5.1.1.1	Ineffective Individual Coping
	5.1.1.1.1	Impaired Adjustment
	5.1.1.1.2	Defensive Coping
	5.1.1.1.3	Ineffective Denial
	5.1.2.1.1	Ineffective Family Coping: Disabling
	5.1.2.1.2	Ineffective Family Coping: Compromised
	5.1.2.2	Family Coping: Potential for Growth
#	5.1.3.1	Potential for Enhanced Community Coping
#	5.1.3.2	Ineffective Community Coping
	5.2.1	Ineffective Management of Therapeutic Regimen (Individuals)
	5.2.1.1	Noncompliance (Specify)
#	5.2.2	Ineffective Management of Therapeutic Regimen: Families
#	5.2.3	Ineffective Management of Therapeutic Regimen: Community
#	5.2.4	Ineffective Management of Therapeutic Regimen: Individual
	5.3.1.1	Decisional Conflict (Specify)
	5.4	Health Seeking Behaviors (Specify)

Pattern 6: Moving

	6.1.1.1	Impaired Physical Mobility
*	6.1.1.1.1	Risk for Peripheral Neurovascular Dysfunction
#	6.1.1.1.2	Risk for Perioperative Positioning Injury
	6.1.1.2	Activity Intolerance
	6.1.1.2.1	Fatigue
*	6.1.1.3	Risk for Activity Intolerance
	6.2.1	Sleep Pattern Disturbance
	6.3.1.1	Diversional Activity Deficit
	6.4.1.1	Impaired Home Maintenance Management
	6.4.2	Altered Health Maintenance
	6.5.1	Feeding Self-Care Deficit
	6.5.1.1	Impaired Swallowing
	6.5.1.2	Ineffective Breastfeeding
	6.5.1.2.1	Interrupted Breastfeeding
	6.5.1.3	Effective Breastfeeding
	6.5.1.4	Ineffective Infant Feeding Pattern
	6.5.2	Bathing/Hygiene Self-Care Deficit
	6.5.3	Dressing/Grooming Self-Care Deficit
	6.5.4	Toileting Self-Care Deficit
	6.6	Altered Growth and Development
	6.7	Relocation Stress Syndrome
#	6.8.1	Risk for Disorganized Infant Behavior
#	6.8.2	Disorganized Infant Behavior
#	6.8.3	Potential for Enhanced Organized Infant Behavior

Pattern 7: Perceiving

	7.1.1	Body Image Disturbance
	7.1.2	Self-Esteem Disturbance
	7.1.2.1	Chronic Low Self-Esteem
	7.1.2.2	Situational Low Self-Esteem
	7.1.3	Personal Identity Disturbance
	7.2	Sensory/Perceptual Alterations (Specify) (Visual, Auditory, Kinesthetic, Gustatory, Tactile, Olfactory)
	7.2.1.1	Unilateral Neglect
	7.3.1	Hopelessness
	7.3.2	Powerlessness

Pattern 8: Knowing

	8.1.1	Knowledge Deficit (Specify)
#	8.2.1	Impaired Environmental Interpretation Syndrome
#	8.2.2	Acute Confusion
#	8.2.3	Chronic Confusion
	8.3	Altered Thought Processes
#	8.3.1	Impaired Memory

Pattern 9: Feeling

	9.1.1	Pain
	9.1.1.1	Chronic Pain
	9.2.1.1	Dysfunctional Grieving
	9.2.1.2	Anticipatory Grieving

---

*Diagnoses with modified label terminology in 1994. (This change was recommended by the NANDA Taxonomy Committee and adopted to remain consistent with the ICD.)

#New diagnoses added in 1994 classified at level 1.4 using new Criteria for Staging.

---

*Diagnoses with modified label terminology in 1994. (This change was recommended by the NANDA Taxonomy Committee and adopted to remain consistent with the ICD.)

Diagnosis Qualifiers

Category 1

Actual: Existing at the present moment; existing in reality

Potential: Can, but has not yet, come into being; possible

Category 2

Ineffective: Not producing the desired effect; not capable of performing satisfactorily

Decreased: Smaller; lessened; diminished; lesser in size, amount, or degree

Increased: Greater in size, amount, or degree; larger, enlarged

Impaired: Made worse, weakened; damaged, reduced; deteriorated

Depleted: Emptied wholly or partially; exhausted of

Deficient: Inadequate in amount, quality, or degree; defective; not sufficient; incomplete

Excessive: Characterized by an amount or quantity that is greater than is necessary, desirable, or usable

Dysfunctional: Abnormal; impaired or incompletely functioning

Disturbed: Agitated; interrupted; interfered with

Acute: Severe but of short duration

Chronic: Lasting a long time; recurring; habitual; constant

Intermittent: Stopping and starting again at intervals; periodic; cyclic

References

Abu-Said, H., & Tesler, M. (1986). Pain. In V. Carrieri, A. Lindsey, & C. West (Eds.), *Pathophysiological phenomena in nursing.* Philadelphia: Saunders.

Aguilera, D. (1990). *Crisis intervention: Theory and methodology* (6th ed.). St. Louis, MO: Mosby.

American Nurses' Association. (1980). *Nursing: A social policy statement.* Kansas City, MO: Author.

American Psychiatric Association. (1994). *Diagnostic and statistical manual of mental disorders* (4th ed.). Washington, DC: Author.

American Psychiatric Association. (1989). *Treatments of psychiatric disorders: A task force report of the American Psychiatric Association.* Washington, DC: American Psychiatric Association Press.

Ames, S., & Kneisl, C. (1986). *Adult health nursing.* Menlo Park, CA: Addison-Wesley.

Anderson, G. (1988). Understanding multiple personality disorder. *Journal of Psychosocial Nursing, 26*(7), 26–30.

Annon, J. (1975). *The behavioral treatment of sexual problems: Brief therapy* (Vols. I and II). Honolulu, HI: Enabling Systems.

Antai-Otong, D. (1995). *Psychiatric nursing: Biological and behavioral concepts.* Philadelphia: Saunders.

Arnold, E., & Boggs, K. (1989). *Interpersonal relationships: Professional communication skills for nurses.* Philadelphia: Saunders.

Asaad, G., & Shapiro, B. (1986). Hallucinations: Theoretical and clinical overview. *American Journal of Psychiatry, 143*, 1088–1097.

Baer, C., & Bradley, W. (1992). *Clinical pharmacology and nursing* (2nd ed.). Philadelphia: Springhouse.

Baker, A. (1989). How families cope. *Journal of Psychosocial Nursing and Mental Health Services, 27*(1), 31–35.

Baker, D. (1984). Ten years of TPN at home. *American Journal of Nursing, 84*, 1248–1249.

Barry, P. (1984). *Psychosocial nursing assessment and intervention: Care of the physically ill person* (2nd ed.). Philadelphia: Lippincott.

Bartol, M. (1979). Non-verbal communication in patients with Alzheimer's disease. *Journal of Gerontological Nursing, 73*(12), 21–31.

Beck, A. (1982). *Depression: Causes and treatments.* Philadelphia: University of Pennsylvania Press.

Beck, A., & Emery, G. (1985). *Anxiety disorders and phobias: A cognitive perspective.* New York: Basic Books.

Beck, C., Rawlins, R., & Williams, S. (1988). *Mental health-psychiatric nursing: A holistic life-cycle approach* (2nd ed.). St. Louis, MO: Mosby.

Bennett, G., & Woolf, D. (Eds.). (1991). *Substance abuse* (2nd ed.). New York: Delmar.

Bjorntorp, P. (1983). Physiological and clinical aspects of exercise in obese persons. *Exercise and Sports—Science Preview, 11*, 159–180.

Blackburn, C. (1981). Caloric-nitrogen relationship in total parental nutrition. In *Proceedings of 67th Annual Clinical Congress of the American College of Surgeons. Pre- and Postoperative Care: Nutritional Support in Abnormal Metabolic States.*

Blake-White, J., & Kline, C. (1985). Treating the dissociative process in adult victims of childhood incest. *Social Casework: The Journal of Contemporary Social Work, 66*, 394–402.

Blum, K., Noble, E., Sheridan, P. (1991). Association of the a1 allele of the D2 dopamine receptor gene with severe alcoholism. *Alcohol, (8)*, 409–416.

Bomar, P., (1989). *Nurses and family health promotion: Concepts, assessments, and interventions.* Baltimore: Williams & Wilkins.

Bonder, B. (1990). Disease and dysfunction: The value of Axis V. *Hospital and Community Psychiatry, 41*(9), 959–960, 964.

Bowen, M. (1978). *Family therapy in clinical practice.* New York: Jason Aronson.

Brenners, D., & Weston, P. (1987). Managing manic behavior. *American Journal of Nursing, 87*, 620–623.

Brooke, V. (1994). *Problematic issues in the care of the elderly, Instructor's guide: Program 3, Behavioral problems associated with dementia.* Philadelphia: Lippincott.

Brownell, K. (1984). The psychology and physiology of obesity: Implications for screening and treatment. *Journal of Dietetic Association, 84*, 406–413.

Brunner, L., & Suddarth, D. (1988). *Textbook of medical-surgical nursing* (6th ed.). Philadelphia: Lippincott.

Burckhardt, C. (1987). Coping strategies of the chronically ill. *Nursing Clinics of North America, 22,* 543–549.

Burgess, A., & Holmstrom, L. (1979). Adaptive strategies and recovery from rape. *American Journal of Psychiatry, 133,* 413–417.

Burgess, A., & Holmstrom, L. (1976). Coping behavior of the rape victim. *American Journal of Psychiatry, 133,* 413–418.

Burgess, A., & Holstrom, L. (1974). Rape trauma syndrome. *American Journal of Psychiatry, 131,* 981–986.

Burgess, A., & Lazare, A. (1990). *Psychiatric nursing in the hospital and the community.* Englewood Cliffs, NJ: Prentice Hall.

Burns, A., Marsh, A., & Bender, D. (1989). Dietary intake and clinical, anthropometric and biochemical indices of malnutrition in elderly patients and nondemented subjects. *Psychological Medicine, 19,* 383–391.

Caine, R., & Bufalino, P. (1987). *Nursing care planning guides for adults.* Baltimore: Williams & Wilkins.

Campbell, F. (1984). The concept of shame. *Perspectives in Psychiatric Care, 22*(2), 61–64.

Carnes, P. (1989). *Contrary to love: Helping the sexual addict.* Minneapolis: CompCare.

Carpenito, L. (1989). *Nursing diagnosis: Application to clinical practice* (3rd ed.). Philadelphia: Lippincott.

Carrieri, V., Lindsey, A., & West, C. (1986). *Pathophysiological phenomena in nursing.* Philadelphia: Saunders.

Carson, V., Soeken, K., & Grimm, P. (1988). Hope and its relationship to spiritual well-being. *Journal of Psychology and Theology, 16*(2), 159–167.

Cassey, J. (1985). The suicide prevention contract. *Perspectives in Psychiatric Care, 23*(3), 99–103.

Caulker-Burnett, I. (1994). Primary care screening for substance abuse. *Nurse Practitioner, 19*(6), 42–48.

Chenitz, C., & Swanson, J. (1989). Counseling clients with genital herpes. *Journal of Psychosocial Nursing and Mental Health Services, 89*(9), 11–17.

Christian, J., & Greger, J. (1985). *Nutrition for living.* Menlo Park, CA: Benjamin-Cummings.

Clark, B. (1984). What to do when your patient lets slip his grip on reality. *Nursing 84, 14*(8), 50–56.

Clement, J. (1993). The client with substance abuse/mental illness: Mandate for collaboration. *Archives of Psychiatric Nursing, 6*(4), 990.

Clochesy, J. (1988). *Essentials of critical care nursing.* Rockville, MD: Aspen.

Cole, F., & Rogers, B. (1984). Biological rhythms: Implications for critical care. *Critical Care Nurse, 4*(6), 30–35.

Cole, S., & Jacobs, J. (1989). Family treatment of schizophrenia. In *Treatments of psychiatric disorders.* Washington, DC: American Psychiatric Association Press.

Coleman, E. (Ed.). (1987). *Chemical dependency and intimacy dysfunction.* New York: Haworth Press.

Damrosch, S., Gallo, B., Kulak, D., & Whitaker, C. (1987). Nurses' attributions about rape victims. *Research in Nursing and Health, 10,* 245–251.

Davies, J., & Janosik, E. (1991). *Mental health and psychiatric nursing: A caring approach.* Boston: Jones & Bartlett.

Davis, J. (1988). Animal-facilitated therapy in stress mediation. *Holistic Nursing Practice, 2*(3), 45–53.

Davis, J. (1984). Analgesic and psychoactive drugs in the chronic pain patient. *Journal of Orthopaedic and Sports Physical Therapy, 5,* 315–317.

Dickinson, C. (1975). The search for spiritual meaning. *American Journal of Nursing, 75,* 1789–1793.

Doenges, M., & Moorhouse, M. (1985). *Nurse's pocket guide: Nursing diagnoses with interventions.* Philadelphia: Davis.

Doenges, M., Moorhouse, M., & Geissler, A. (1989). *Nursing care plans: Guidelines for planning patient care* (2nd ed.). Philadelphia: Davis.

Doenges, M., Townsend, M., & Moorhouse, M. (1989). *Psychiatric care plans: Guidelines for client care.* Philadelphia: Davis.

Doghramji, M. (1989). Sleep disorders: A selective update. *Hospital and Community Psychiatry, 40*(1), 29–40.

Dreyfus, J. (1988). Depression assessment and interventions in the medically ill frail elderly. *Journal of Gerontological Nursing, 14*(9), 26–35.

Dufault, K., & Martocchio, B. (1985). Hope: Its spheres and dimensions. *Nursing Clinics of North America, 20,* 379–391.

Dugan, D. (1987). Death and dying: Emotional, spiritual, and ethical support for patients and families. *Journal of Psychosocial Nursing, 25*(6), 21–29.

Ebersole, P. & Hess, P. (1994). Transcendence: Death, dying, grief and legacies. In *Toward healthy aging.* St. Louis, MO: Mosby.

Eliopoulos, C. (1987). *Gerontological nursing* (2nd ed.). Philadelphia: Lippincott.

Farkas, M. (1990). Utilizing the nursing process in the development of a medication group on an inpatient psychiatric unit. *Perspectives in Psychiatric Care, 26*(4), 12–17.

Fife, B. (1985). A model for predicting the adaptation of families to medical crises: An analysis of role integration. *IMAGE: Journal of Nursing Scholarship, 18*(4), 108–112.

Figeli, G., Kirshman, R., Doraiswany, M., & Nemeroff, C. (1991). Caudate hyperintensities in elderly depressed patients with neuroleptic induced parkinsonianism. *Journal of Geriatric Psycho Neuro, 4*(2), 86.

Figley, C. (Ed.). (1985). *Trauma and its wake: The study and treatment of post-traumatic stress disorder.* New York: Brunner/Mazel.

Fink, E.B. (1986). Magnesium deficiency in alcoholism. *Alcoholism, 10*(6), 126–129.

Fontaine, K.L., & Fletcher, J.S., (1995). *Essentials of mental health nursing* (3rd ed.). Redwood City, CA: Addison-Wesley.

Ford, R. (Ed.). (1987). *Patient teaching manual, 2.* Springhouse, PA: Springhouse.

Frank, A., & Gunderson, J. (1990). The role of the therapeutic alliance in the treatment of schizophrenia. *Archives of General Psychiatry, 47,* 228–236.

Friedman, M. (1981). *Family nursing: Theory and assessment.* Norwalk, CT: Appleton-Lange.

Frith, C., & Done, J. (1989). Experiences of alien control in schizophrenia reflect a disorder in the central monitoring of action. *Psychological Medicine, 19,* 359–363.

Funkhouser, S., & Moser, D. (1990). Is health care racist? *Advances in Nursing Science, 12*(2), 47–55.

Gallop, R. (1988). Escaping borderline stereotypes. *Journal of Psychosocial Nursing, 26,* 23–27.

Gardner, D. (1985). Presence. In G. Bulechek & J. McCloskey (Eds.), *Nursing interventions: Treatments for nursing diagnosis:* Philadelphia: Saunders.

Garnets, L., Herek, G., & Levy, B. (1990). Violence and victimization of lesbians and gay men. *Journal of Interpersonal Violence, 5,* 366–383.

Geach, B. (1987). Bedtime ceremonials. A focus for nursing. *Archives in Psychiatric Nursing, 1*(2), 98–103.

George, L.K., & Gwyther, L.P. (1986). Caregiver's well-being: A multidimensional examination of caregivers of demented adults. *The Gerontologist, 26,* 253–259.

Gettrust, K., Ryan, S., & Engleman, D. (Eds.). (1985). *Applied nursing diagnosis: Guides for comprehensive care planning.* New York: Wiley.

Gise, L., & Paddison, P. (1988). Rape, sexual abuse, and its victims. *Psychiatric Clinics of North America, 11,* 529–646.

Goodman, G., & Esterly, G. (1990). *The talk book: The intimate science of communicating in close relationships.* New York: Ballantine.

Goodwin, J. (1985). Family violence: Principles of intervention and prevention. *Hospital and Community Psychiatry, 36*(10), 1074–1079.

Gournay, K. (1988). Sleeping without drugs. *Nursing Times, 84*(11), 46–49.

Green, B., Wilson, J., & Jacob, D. (1985). Conceptualizing post-traumatic stress disorder: A psychosocial framework. In C. Figley (Ed.), *Trauma and its wake: The study and treatment of post-traumatic stress disorder.* New York: Brunner/Mazel.

Green, W. (1988). *Rape: The evidential examination and management of the adult female victim.* Lexington, MA: Lexington Books.

Greenfeld, M. (1990). Disclosing incest: The relationships that make it possible. *Journal of Psychosocial Nursing, 28*(7), 20–23.

Griffiths, W. (1981). Can human behavior be modified? *Cancer, 47,* 1221–1225.

Haber, J., Hoskins, P., Leach, A., & Sideleau, B. (1987). *Comprehensive psychiatric nursing* (3rd ed.). New York: McGraw-Hill.

Hall, G.R. (1988). Care of the patient with Alzheimer's disease living at home. *Nursing Clinics of North America, 23,* 31–45.

Hall, M. (1986). Crisis as opportunity for spiritual growth. *Journal of Religion and Health, 25*(1), 8–17.

Hall, S., & Wray, L. (1989). Codependency: Nurses who give too much. *American Journal of Nursing, 89,* 1456–1460.

Harris, E. (1988). Psych drugs: Antipsychotics. *American Journal of Nursing, 88,* 1507–1518.

Harris, M. (1983). Eating habits, restraint, knowledge, and attitudes toward obesity. *International Journal of Obesity, 7,* 274–286.

Hatfield, A. (1990). *Family education in mental illness.* New York: Guilford Press.

Hatton, C., & Valente, S. (1984). *Suicide: Assessment and intervention.* Norwalk, CT: Appleton-Lange.

Hays, K. (1985). Electra in mourning: Grief work and the adult incest survivor. *Psychotherapy-Patient, 2*(1), 45–58.

Heinrich, L. (1987). Care of the female rape victim. *Nurse Practitioner, 12*(11), 9–10, 12, 16–18.

Helms, J. (1985). Active listening. In G. Bulechek & J. McCloskey (Eds.), *Nursing interventions: Treatments for nursing diagnosis.* Philadelphia: Saunders.

Helton, M., Gordon, S., & Nunnery, S. (1980). The correlation between sleep deprivation and the intensive care unit syndrome. *Heart & Lung, 9,* 31–35.

Hepburn, K., Severence, Gates, T., & Christensen, L. (1989). Institutional care of dementia patient. *The American Journal of Alzheimer's Care and Related Disorders and Research, 4*(3), 19–23.

Hesselbrock, M., Meyer, R., & Keener, J. (1985). Psychopathology in hospitalized alcoholics. *Archives of General Psychiatry, 42,* 1050–1055.

Hickey, B. (1985). The borderline experience: Subjective impressions. *Journal of Psychosocial Nursing, 123*(4), 24–29.

Hickey, J. (1986). *The clinical practice of neurological and neurosurgical nursing* (2nd ed.). Philadelphia: Lippincott.

Hill, L., & Smith, N. (1990). *Self-care nursing: Promotion of health* (2nd ed.). Englewood Cliffs, NJ: Prentice-Hall.

Hock, C., Reynolds, C., & Kupfer, D. (1987). Sleep-disordered breathing in normal and pathologic aging. *Journal of Clinical Psychiatry, 47,* 499–503.

Hoff, L. (1984). *People in crisis* (2nd ed.). Menlo Park, CA: Addison-Wesley.

Hopson, J. (1986). The unraveling of insomnia. *Psychology Today, 20*(6), 42–45.

Horowitz, M. (1983). Stress response syndromes and their treatment. In L. Goldberger & S. Breznitz (Eds.), *Handbook of stress.* New York: Free Press.

Horsley, G. (1988). Baggage from the past. *American Journal of Nursing, 88,* 60–63.

Hover, M. (1986). If a patient asks you to pray with him. *RN, 49*(4), 17–18.

Hyman, S. (1984). *Manual of psychiatric emergencies.* Boston: Little, Brown.

Janoff-Bulman, R. (1985). The aftermath of victimization: Rebuilding shattered assumptions. In C. Figley (Ed.), *Trauma and its wake: The study and treatment of post-traumatic stress disorder.* New York: Brunner/Mazel.

Johnson, B. (1986). *Psychiatric/mental health nursing: Adaptation and growth.* Philadelphia: Lippincott.

Johnson, S. (1989). Integrating marital and individual therapy for incest survivors: A case study. *Psychotherapy, 26*(1), 96–103.

Kanfer, H., Goldstein, F., & Goldstein, A. (Eds.). (1980). *Helping people change* (2nd ed.). New York: Pergamon Press.

Kaplan, C. (1986). The challenge of working with patients diagnosed as having a borderline personality disorder. *Nursing Clinics of North America, 21,* 429–437.

Kaplan, H. (1974). *The new sex therapy.* New York: Brunner/Mazel.

Kaplan, H., & Sadock, B. (Eds.). (1985). *Comprehensive textbook of psychiatry* (4th ed.). Baltimore: Williams & Wilkins.

Katz, A., & Bender, K. (1990). *Helping one another: Self-help groups in a changing world.* Oakland, CA: Third Party Publishing.

Katz, B., & Burt, M. (1988). Self-blame in recovery from rape: Help or hindrance? In A. Burgess (Ed.), *Rape and sexual assault II.* New York: Garland.

Katzin, L. (1990). Chronic illness and sexuality. *American Journal of Nursing, 90*(1), 54–59.

Keltner, N.L., Schwecke, L.H., & Bostrom, C.E., (1995). *Psychiatric Nursing* (2nd ed.). St. Louis, MO: Mosby.

Kernberg, O. (1984). *Severe personality disorders: Psychotherapeutic strategies.* New Haven, CT: Yale University Press.

Kerr, N. (1990). The ego competency model of psychiatric nursing. *Perspectives in Psychiatric Care, 26*(1), 13–24.

Kerr, N. (1987/1988). Signs and symptoms of depression and principles of nursing intervention. *Perspectives in Psychiatric Care, 26*(2), 48–63.

Kerr, N. (1980). Pathological narcissism. *Perspectives in Psychiatric Care, 18*(1), 28–36.

Kilpatrick, D., Veronen, L., & Best, C. (1985). Factors predicting psychological distress among rape victims. In C. Figley (Ed.), *Trauma and its wake: The study and treatment of post-traumatic stress disorder.* New York: Brunner/Mazel.

Kim, M., McFarland, G., & McLane, A. (Eds.). (1987). *Pocket guide to nursing diagnoses* (2nd ed.). St. Louis, MO: Mosby.

Kinney, C., Mannetter, R., & Carpenter, M. (1985). Support groups. In G. Bulechek & J. McCloskey (Eds.), *Nursing interventions: Treatments for nursing diagnoses.* Philadelphia: Saunders.

Kinney, J., & Leaton, G. (1987). *Loosening the grip* (3rd ed.). St. Louis, MO: Mosby.

Kluft, R. (1984). Treatment of multiple personality disorder. *Psychiatric Clinics of North America, 7,* 9–29.

Kolb, D. (1974). Disturbances of body image. In S. Arieti (Ed.), *American handbook of psychiatry* (2nd ed., Vol. 4). New York: Basic Books.

Koss, M., & Harvey, M. (1987). In J. Butcher (Ed.), *The rape victim: Clinical and community approaches to treatment.* Lexington, MA: Stephen Greene Press.

Krause, M., & Mahan, L. (Eds.). (1984). The assessment of nutritional status. In *Food, nutrition, and diet therapy* (7th ed.). Philadelphia: Lippincott.

Kübler-Ross, E. (1970). *On death and dying.* New York: Macmillan.

Kuhn, M. (1994). *Pharmaco-therapeutics: A nursing process approach* (3rd ed.). Philadelphia: Davis.

Larkin, J. (1987). Factors influencing one's ability to adapt to chronic illness. *Nursing Clinics of North America, 22,* 535–542.

Lewis, J., Dana, R., & Blevins, G. (1988). *Substance abuse counseling.* Pacific Grove: Brooks/Cole.

Lion, E. (1982). *Human sexuality in nursing process.* New York: Wiley.

Luckmann, J., & Sorenson, K. (1987). *Medical-surgical nursing: A psychophysiologic approach* (3rd ed.). Philadelphia: Saunders.

Marchlewski, M. (1994). Anticholinergic syndrome. *Journal of Psychosocial Nursing, 32*(9), 22–24.

Mast, D. (1986). Effects of imagery. *IMAGE: Journal of Nursing Scholarship, 18,* 118–120.

McCaffrey, M. (1979). *Nursing management of the patient with pain* (2nd ed.). Philadelphia: Lippincott.

McCaffrey, M., & Beebe, A. (1989). *Pain: Clinical manual for nursing practice.* St. Louis, MO: Mosby.

McFarland, G., & McFarlane, E. (Eds.). (1989). *Nursing diagnosis: Theory and application.* St. Louis, MO: Mosby.

McFarland, G., & Wasli, E. (1986). *Nursing diagnoses and process in psychiatric-mental health nursing.* Philadelphia: Lippincott.

McGill, C., & Patterson, C. (1990). Former patients as peer counselors on locked psychiatric inpatient units. *Hospital and Community Psychiatry, 41*(9), 1017–1019.

McGoldrick, M., Pearce, J., & Giordano, J. (1982). *Ethnicity and family therapy.* New York: Guildford Press.

McKay, M., & Fanning, P. (1987). *Self-esteem: A proven program of cognitive techniques for assessing, improving, and maintaining your self-esteem.* Oakland, CA: New Harbinger.

McNeil, B., Padrick, K., & Wellman, J. (1986). I didn't sleep a wink. *American Journal of Nursing, 86,* 26–27.

Mechanic, D. (1986). The challenge of chronic mental illness: A retrospective and prospective view. *Hospital and Community Psychiatry, 37,* 891–896.

Meilman, P. (1984). Legitimizing chronic pain. *Journal of Orthopaedic and Sports Physical Therapy, 5,* 312–315.

Meinhart, N., & McCaffrey, M. (1983). *Pain: A nursing approach to assessment and analysis.* Norwalk, CT: Appleton-Lange.

Menikheim, M., & Loen, M. (1983). Impairment in verbal communication. In M. Snyder (Ed.), *A guide to neurological and neurosurgical nursing.* New York: Wiley.

Miles, M. (1986). Counseling strategies. In S. Johnson (Ed.), *Nursing assessment and strategies for the family at risk: High-risk parenting.* Philadelphia: Lippincott.

Miller, A. (1984). *Thou shalt not be aware.* New York: Farrar, Straus and Giroux.

Miller, C. (1995). Impaired cognitive functioning: Dementia. In *Nursing care of older adults.* Philadelphia: Lippincott.

Miller, J. (1985). Inspiring hope. *American Journal of Nursing, 85,* 22–25.

Miller, J. (1983). *Coping with chronic illness, overcoming powerlessness.* Philadelphia: Davis.

Miler, S., & Winstead-Fry, P. (1982). *Family systems theory in nursing practice.* Reston, VA: Reston.

Minuchin, S., & Fishman, H. (1981). *Family therapy techniques.* Cambridge, MA: Harvard University Press.

Mooradian, A., Morley, J., Kaiser, F., Davis, S., Viosca, S., & Korenman, S. (1989). Biweekly intravenous administration of papaverine for erectile dysfunction. *Western Journal of Medicine, 151,* 515–527.

Moorhouse, M., Geissler, A., & Doenges, M. (1987). *Critical care plans: Guidelines for patient care.* Philadelphia: Davis.

Moree, N. (1985). On patients and drug regimens. *American Journal of Nursing, 85,* 51.

Morgan, J. (1984). Nutritional assessment of critically ill patients. *Focus on Critical Care,11*(3), 28–34.

Murray, R. (1990). *The nursing process in later maturity.* Englewood Cliffs, NJ: Prentice Hall.

Neal, M., Paquette, M., & Mirch, M. (Eds.). (1990). *Nursing diagnosis care plans for DRGs.* Venice, CA: General Medical.

North American Nursing Diagnosis Association. (1990). *Taxonomy 1 revised—1990.* St. Louis, MO: Author.

Nunnally, E., Chilman, C., & Cox, F. (Eds.). (1988). *Mental illness, delinquency, addictions, and neglect* (Families in trouble series, Vol. 4). Newbury Park, CA: Sage.

Nursing Now. (1985). *Pain.* Springhouse, PA: Springhouse.

O'Brien, C. (1995). What are the uses of naltrexone in the treatment of alcoholics? *The Harvard Mental Health Letter, 12*(6), 8.

Oriol, M., & Oriol, R. (1986). Involuntary commitment and the right to refuse medication. *Journal of Psychosocial Nursing and Mental Health Services, 24*(11), 15–20.

Peterson, E., & Nelson, K. (1987). How to meet your clients' spiritual needs. *Journal of Psychosocial Nursing, 25*(5), 34–39.

Philips, H. (1988). *The psychological management of chronic pain: A treatment manual.* New York: Springer.

Pimental, P. (1986). Alterations in communication: Biopsychosocial aspects of aphasia, dysarthria, and right hemisphere syndrome in the stroke patient. *Nursing Clinics of North America, 21,* 321–336.

Platt-Koch, L. (1982). Borderline personality disorder: A therapeutic approach. *American Journal of Nursing, 82,* 1666–1671.

Potter, P., & Perry, A. (1988). *Fundamentals of nursing: Concepts, process and practice* (2nd ed.). St. Louis, MO: Mosby.

Rankin, S., & Duffy, K. (1983). *Patient education: Issues, principles, and guidelines.* Philadelphia: Lippincott.

Rantz, M., & McShane, R. (1995). Nursing interventions for chronically confused residents. *Geriatric Nursing, 16*(1), 22–27.

Rawlins, R., & Heacock, P. (1988). *Clinical manual of psychiatric nursing.* St. Louis, MO: Mosby.

Redman, B. (1988). *The process of patient education* (6th ed.). St. Louis, MO: Mosby.

Reighley, J. (1988). *Nursing care planning guides for psychiatric-mental health.* Baltimore: Williams & Wilkins.

Rinear, C. (1985). Sexual assault and the handicapped victim. In A. Burgess (Ed.), *Rape and sexual assault.* New York: Garland.

Roberts, S. (1986). *Behavioral concepts and the critically ill patient* (2nd ed.). Norwalk, CT: Appleton-Lange.

Robson, P. (1989). Development of a new self-report questionnaire to measure self-esteem. *Psychological Medicine, 19,* 513–518.

Rose, M. (1989). Rape: A subject for the curriculum. *Nursing Times, 85*(26), 62–63.

Roth, B., Stone, W., & Kibel, H. (1990). *The difficult patient in group: Group psychotherapy with borderline and narcissistic disorders.* Madison, CT: International Universities Press.

Rundell, J., Ursano, R., Holloway, H., & Silberman, E. (1989). Psychiatric responses to trauma. *Hospital and Community Psychiatry, 40*(1), 68–74.

Sanger, E., & Cassino, T. (1984). Eating disorders: Avoiding the power struggle. *American Journal of Nursing, 84,* 31–33.

Sarrel, L., & Sarrel, P. (1986). *Sexual turning points: The seven stages of adult sexuality.* New York: Paper Jacks Ltd.

Satir, V. (1983). *Conjoint family therapy* (3rd ed.). Palo Alto, CA: Science and Behavior Books.

Satlin, A., Volicer, L., & Ross, V. (1992). Bright light treatment of behavior and sleep disturbance in patients with Alzheimer's disease. *American Journal of Psychiatry, 149*(8), 1028.

Scandrett, S., & Uecker, S. (1985). Relaxation training. In G. Bulechek & J. McCloskey (Eds.), *Nursing interventions: Treatments for nursing diagnoses.* Philadelphia: Saunders.

Schatzberg, A., & Cole, J. (1986). *Manual of clinical psychopharmacology.* Washington, DC: American Psychiatric Association Press.

Schultz, J., & Dark, S. (1986). *Manual of psychiatric nursing care plans.* Boston: Little, Brown.

Sclafani, M. (1986). Violence and behavior control. *Journal of Psychological Nursing and Mental Health Services, 24*(11), 8–13.

Scurfield, F. (1985). Post-trauma stress assessment and treatment: Overview and formulations. In C. Figley (Ed.), *Trauma and its wake: The study and treatment of post-traumatic stress disorder.* New York: Brunner/Mazel.

Sederer, L., & Thorbeck, J. (1986). First do no harm: Short-term inpatient psychotherapy of the borderline patient. *Hospital and Community Psychiatry, 37,* 692–696.

Seligman, M. (1975). *Helplessness: On depression, development, and death.* San Francisco, CA: Freeman.

Shankle, W. (1994). *Alzheimer's: Researcher gives hints for slowing its progress.* Lecture given in Laguna Hills, CA.

Shannon, M., Wilson, B.A., & Steng, C. (1992). *Govoni & Hayes: Drugs and nursing implications* (7th ed.). Norwalk, CT: Appleton-Lange.

Shealy, N. (1976). *The pain game.* Berkeley, CA: Celestial Arts.

Sirancusano, G. (1984). The physical therapist's use of exercise in the treatment of chronic pain. *Journal of Orthopaedic and Sports Physical Therapy, 6,* 73–75.

Smith, P. (1985). Patient power. *American Journal of Nursing, 85,* 1260–1262.

Snyder, M. (1985). Progressive relaxation. In M. Synder (Ed.), *Independent nursing interventions.* New York: Wiley.

Speilman, A., Caruso, L., & Glovinsky, P. (1987). A behavioral perspective on insomnia treatment. *Psychiatric Clinics of North America, 10,* 541–553.

Speilman, A., Saskin, P., & Thorpy, M. (1987). Treatment of chronic insomnia by restriction of time in bed. *Sleep, 10,* 45–56.

Stolley, J. (1995). Freeing your patients from restraints. *American Journal of Nursing, 95*(2), 27–31.

Stryker, R. (1977). *Rehabilitative aspects of acute and chronic nursing care.* Philadelphia: Saunders.

Stuart, G., & Sundeen, S. (1987). *Principles and practices of psychiatric nursing* (3rd ed.). St. Louis, MO: Mosby.

Suitor, C., & Hunter, M. (1980). *Nutrition: Principles and application in health promotion.* Philadelphia: Lippincott.

Sundeen, S., Stuart, G., Rankin, E., & Cohen, S. (1989). *Nurse-client interaction: Implementing the nursing process.* St. Louis, MO: Mosby.

Talashek, M., Gerace, L., Miller, A., Lindsey, M. (1995). Family nurse practitioner clinical competencies and alcohol and substance use. *American Academy of Nurse Practitioner, 7*(2), 57–63.

Tauer, K. (1983). Promoting effective decision-making in sexually active adolescents. *Nursing Clinics of North America, 18,* 275–292.

Taylor, C. (1983). Adjustment to threatening life events: A theory of cognitive adaptation. *American Psychologist, 38,* 1161–1173.

Taylor, C., & Cress, S. (1988). *Nursing diagnosis cards.* Springhouse, PA: Springhouse.

Taylor, C., Lillis, C., & LeMone, P. (1989). *Fundamentals of nursing: The art and science of nursing care.* Philadelphia: Lippincott.

Thompson, J., McFarland, G., Hirsch, J., Tucker, S., & Bowers, A. (1989). *Mosby's manual of clinical nursing* (2nd ed.). St. Louis, MO: Mosby.

Titlebaum, H. (1988). Relaxation. *Holistic Nursing Practice, 2*(3), 17–23.

Toro, I., Thom, D., Beam, H., & Horst, T. (1996). Chemically dependent patients in recovery: Roles for the family physician. *American Family Physician, 53*(5), 1667–1673.

Townsend, M. (1990). *Drug guide for psychiatric nursing.* Philadelphia: Davis.

Townsend, M. (1988). *Nursing diagnoses in psychiatric nursing.* Philadelphia: Davis.

Townsend, M.C. (1993). *Psychiatric mental health nursing: Concepts of care.* Philadelphia: Davis.

Turner, L., Althof, S., Levine, S., Risen, C., Bodner, D., Kursh, E., & Resnick, M. (1989). Self-injection of papaverine and phentolamine in the treatment of psychogenic impotence. *Journal of Sex and Marital Therapy, 15*(3), 163–176.

Tweed, S. (1989). Identifying the alcoholic client. *Nursing Clinics of North America, 24,* 53–61.

Urbanic, J. (1989). Resolving incest experiences through impatient group therapy. *Journal of Psychosocial Nursing and Mental Health Services, 27*(9), 5–8.

Urbanic, J. (1989). Helping clients with unresolved childhood incest experiences. *Journal of Psychosocial Nursing and Mental Health Services, 25*(7), 33–35.

Vance, M. (1989). Drug withdrawal syndromes. *Topics in Emergency Medicine, 7*(3), 63–68.

Van Devanter, N., Grissaffi, J., Steilen, M., Scarola, M., & Shipton, R. (1987). Counseling HIV-antibody positive blood donors. *American Journal of Nursing, 87,* 1026–1033.

Walker, R. (1992). Substance abuse and B-cluster disorders: Understanding the dual diagnosis patient. *International Journal of Addiction, 23*(8), 797.

Wegscheider, S. (1979). *The family trap,* St. Paul: Nurturing Networks.

Wegscheider-Cruse, S. (1987). *Learning to love yourself.* Pompano Beach, FL: Health Communications.

Wehr, T., Sack, D., & Rosenthal, N. (1987). Sleep reduction as a final common pathway in the genesis of mania. *American Journal of Psychiatry, 144,* 201–204.

Whall, A. (1989). Geropsychiatry: Communicating with advanced-stage dementia patients: The application of the Sullivan theory. *Journal of Gerontological Nursing, 15*(9), 31–32.

White, J. (1988). Touching with intent: Therapeutic massage. *Holistic Nursing Practice, 2*(3), 63–67.

Wilberding, J. (1985). Values clarification. In G. Bulecheck & J. McCloskey (Eds.), *Nursing interventions: Treatments for nursing diagnoses.* Philadelphia: Saunders.

Wilbur, C. (1984). Multiple personality and child abuse. *Psychiatric Clinics of North America, 7,* 3–7.

Wilson, E. (1987). Sexual needs of psychiatric clients. *Journal of Psychosocial Nursing and Mental Health Services, 25*(7), 30–32.

Wilson, H.S., Kneisl, C., & Kneisl, R. (1996). *Psychiatric nursing* (5th ed.). Menlo Park, CA: Addison-Wesley.

Wineman, N. (1980). Locus of control, body image, weight loss, and age-at-onset. *Nursing Research, 29,* 231–237.

Winnicott, D. (1988). *The maturational processes and the facilitating environment: Studies in the theory of emotional development.* Madison, CT: International Universities Press.

Wolanin, M., & Phillips, L. (1981). *Confusion: Prevention and care.* St. Louis, MO: Mosby.

Wolpe, J. (1985). *The practice of behavior therapy* (2nd ed.). New York: Pergamon.

Worley, N., & Albanesa, N. (1989). Independent living for the chronically mentally ill. *Journal of Psychosocial Nursing and Mental Health Services, 27*(9), 18–23.

Wrisley, Jack L. (1989). Use of milieu as a problem-solving strategy in addiction treatment. *Nursing Clinics of North America, 24,* 69–79.

Wykle, M. (1983). Adaptive behaviors. In W. Phipps, B. Long, & N. Woods (Eds.), *Medical surgical nursing* (2nd ed.). St. Louis, MO: Mosby.

Yegidis, B. (1992). Family violence: Contemporary research findings and practice issues. *Community Mental Health Journal, 28*(6), 519–528.

Zerwekh, J., & Michaels, B. (1989). Codependency assessment and recovery. *Nursing Clinics of North America, 24,* 109–120.

Index